AF670105

# Series in BioEngineering

The Series in Bioengineering serves as an information source for a professional audience in science and technology as well as for advanced students. It covers all applications of the physical sciences and technology to medicine and the life sciences. Its scope ranges from bioengineering, biomedical and clinical engineering to biophysics, biomechanics, biomaterials, and bioinformatics.

Indexed by WTI Frankfurt eG, zbMATH.

Almir Badnjević • Lemana Spahić • Tamer Bego
Sara Deumić

# Biomedical Instrumentation

## Concepts, Technologies, and Future Innovations

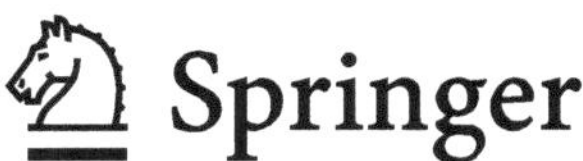

Almir Badnjević
Registers and Data Exchange of B & H
Agency for Identification Documents
Banja Luka, Bosnia and Herzegovina

Tamer Bego
Faculty of Pharmacy
University of Sarajevo
Sarajevo, Bosnia and Herzegovina

Lemana Spahić
Research Institute Verlab
Sarajevo, Bosnia and Herzegovina

Sara Deumić
International Burch University
Ilidža, Bosnia and Herzegovina

ISSN 2196-8861 ISSN 2196-887X (electronic)
Series in BioEngineering
ISBN 978-3-032-10977-4 ISBN 978-3-032-10978-1 (eBook)
https://doi.org/10.1007/978-3-032-10978-1



This Springer imprint is published by the registered company Springer Nature Switzerland AG
The registered company address is: Gewerbestrasse 11, 6330 Cham, Switzerland

# Foreword

Biomedical engineering has emerged as one of the most dynamic and impactful disciplines in modern healthcare, blending principles of engineering, biology, and medicine to develop technologies that improve diagnosis, treatment, and patient outcomes. This book represents a unique contribution to the field, offering a comprehensive and structured exploration of both foundational concepts and cutting-edge applications.

The text begins by establishing the scope and evolution of biomedical engineering, providing readers with a historical perspective that contextualizes current practices. It then systematically addresses core disciplines, including biomechanics, biomaterials, medical imaging, and computational modeling, illustrating how these fields converge to drive innovation in healthcare technology. Subsequent chapters delve into a wide array of medical devices, from electrocardiographs and blood pressure monitors to complex systems such as mechanical ventilators, anesthesia machines, pacemakers, and robotic surgical platforms. Each chapter not only discusses the technical characteristics and types of devices but also examines their clinical applications, regulatory frameworks, and future potential, offering a holistic view of the technologies that define contemporary biomedical practice.

Equally important is the book's attention to ethical, legal, and social considerations, highlighting the responsibilities of biomedical engineers to uphold patient safety, ensure regulatory compliance, and consider societal implications of medical innovations. The inclusion of clinical engineering and healthcare technology management demonstrates the practical realities of deploying, maintaining, and optimizing medical devices in clinical environments. Laboratory instrumentation, such as biochemical analyzers, PCR devices, sequencing machines, and mass spectrometry devices, is also thoroughly addressed, underscoring the critical role of diagnostics in patient care.

Beyond technical mastery, this book emphasizes the interdisciplinary nature of biomedical engineering and the collaborative mindset required to succeed in this field. By integrating historical context, current best practices, and emerging trends, including wearable technologies, smart devices, and the Internet of Medical Things, the text prepares readers to meet both present and future challenges in healthcare innovation.

This book is not only a foundational resource for students seeking a rigorous introduction to biomedical engineering but also an invaluable reference for professionals, clinicians, and researchers aiming to stay at the forefront of medical technology. It reflects the author's deep expertise and thoughtful approach to teaching, making it a landmark contribution to the literature.

In a world where biomedical innovations continue to reshape healthcare, this book stands as a guiding reference, offering clarity, insight, and inspiration to all who seek to contribute meaningfully to the advancement of medical science and technology.

Research Institute Verlab for Biomedical Engineering
Medical Devices and Artificial Intelligence
Ferhadija, Sarajevo, Bosnia and Herzegovina

Lejla Gurbeta Pokvić

# Preface

Biomedical engineering is a rapidly evolving discipline at the intersection of engineering, biology, and medicine, driving innovation across healthcare technologies. The field encompasses a diverse range of areas, from foundational principles and core engineering domains to the design, development, and management of medical devices and laboratory instrumentation. The goal of this book is to provide a comprehensive, structured exploration of biomedical engineering, presenting both theoretical foundations and practical applications, while emphasizing ethical, legal, and societal responsibilities.

The book is organized into five chapters. Chapter 1 introduces the definition, scope, and historical evolution of biomedical engineering, illustrating how the field has developed through scientific discovery, technological innovation, and translational applications in medicine. Chapter 2 focuses on medical devices in healthcare institutions, exploring their components, technical characteristics, clinical applications, regulatory considerations, and emerging trends such as miniaturization, smart devices, and AI integration. Chapter 3 addresses clinical engineering and healthcare technology management, highlighting the competencies required for effective device management, post-market surveillance, quality assurance, compliance, and sustainability. Chapter 4 examines laboratory devices, emphasizing their technical features, clinical relevance, and regulatory frameworks. Finally, Chapter 5 provides a review of key concepts, practice problems for reinforcing knowledge, and a forward-looking perspective on future directions in biomedical instrumentation.

Throughout the book, emphasis is placed on the integration of engineering principles with clinical practice, highlighting how biomedical engineers contribute to patient care, healthcare system efficiency, and innovation. Ethical, legal, and social considerations are interwoven, underscoring the responsibility of engineers to develop technologies that are safe, equitable, and socially responsible. Each chapter is structured to provide a logical progression from foundational concepts to advanced applications, making the book suitable for students, practitioners, and professionals seeking a comprehensive understanding of biomedical engineering.

This book aspires to serve as both a reference and a learning tool, offering theoretical insights, practical examples, and problem-solving exercises to prepare readers for the dynamic and multidisciplinary challenges of biomedical engineering. It is intended to inspire the next generation of engineers, researchers, and healthcare innovators to advance technology responsibly and to improve health outcomes worldwide.

Banja Luka, Bosnia and Herzegovina Almir Badnjević
Sarajevo, Bosnia and Herzegovina Lemana Spahić
Sarajevo, Bosnia and Herzegovina Tamer Bego
Ilidža, Bosnia and Herzegovina Sara Deumić

**Competing Interests** The authors have no competing interests to declare that are relevant to the content of this manuscript.

# Contents

# List of Figures

# List of Tables

# Chapter 1
# Introduction to Biomedical Instrumentation

This section provides a comprehensive introduction to biomedical engineering, tracing its definition, scope, historical evolution, core disciplines, applications, and ethical, legal, and societal considerations. It begins by defining biomedical engineering as an interdisciplinary field that integrates engineering, medical, and biological sciences to develop innovative healthcare solutions, emphasizing problem-solving, system design, and translational applications (Sect. 1.1). The historical development of the field is then explored (Sect. 1.2), highlighting key milestones, hallmarks such as innovation and interdisciplinarity, and the emerging role of artificial intelligence. Core domains, including biomechanics, biomaterials, computational modeling, medical imaging, and medical device design are examined alongside their practical applications in tissue engineering, prosthetics, wearable devices, robotics, minimally invasive surgery, and diagnostic technologies (Sect. 1.3). Finally, the section addresses ethical, legal, and social responsibilities, encompassing patient safety, regulatory compliance, privacy, equity, and sustainability, illustrating the broader societal impact of biomedical engineering (Sect. 1.4).

## 1.1 Definition and Scope of Biomedical Engineering

Biomedical engineering is a dynamic, interdisciplinary field that combines engineering principles, design methods, and advanced technologies to address healthcare challenges and enhance human well-being, thereby uniting biology and medical science. This field plays a significant role in modern medicine, offering innovations that enable better diagnostics, more effective treatments, and enhanced patient care. Biomedical engineering can be described as the bridge between engineering and medicine, providing solutions for health systems, medical technology, and detailed biological systems [1].



A. Badnjević et al., *Biomedical Instrumentation*, Series in BioEngineering,
https://doi.org/10.1007/978-3-032-10978-1_1

Biomedical engineering is an application of engineering principles to perceive and solve problems in biology and medicine. Engineers in this field utilize their knowledge to analyze biological systems, model physiological processes, and design devices and systems that support, restore, or enhance health. It often requires a multi-disciplinary approach to have the precision of engineering matched by the intricacy of medical science. The results of such integration include several state-of-the-art developments, such as imaging systems to visualize body structure, biomaterials that replace tissues damaged by disease or trauma, and rehabilitation devices that restore mobility and independence to patients.

The scope of biomedical engineering is broad, encompassing diverse subfields that address critical healthcare needs. These range from designing and developing medical devices, including pacemakers, prosthetic limbs, and surgical tools, to developing advanced imaging technologies that enable non-invasive diagnostics, biomaterials engineering for implants and drug delivery systems, and bioinformatics for the analysis and interpretation of genetic and clinical data. It also extends into the newest areas of tissue engineering and regenerative medicine, where methods are being developed to replace impaired organs, as well as rehabilitation engineering, which aims to assist individuals with disabilities. The field continues to evolve with advancements in technology and an increasing understanding of human biology.

### *1.1.1 Core Principles of Biomedical Engineering*

Biomedical engineering is an engineering discipline that integrates and applies engineering, biology, and medical sciences to develop innovative and practical solution modalities. First is the principle of systems thinking: biological systems are complicated networks of interconnected components that interact. In this way, a system that is either part of or an interaction within an organ will be modeled to delineate its behavior, such as the cardiovascular or nervous system, and design interventions that can maximize function. The design of an artificial heart would require knowledge of the mechanical properties of heart tissue, fluid dynamics related to blood flow, and the electrical signals that control the heartbeat. These would combine into devices that simulate bodily functions [2].

Another important philosophy is collaboration between disciplines. Biomedical engineering is, by nature, a collaborative effort, bringing together professionals from various backgrounds. It is common for engineers, biologists, physicians, and computer scientists to work together on technically sound and clinically relevant technologies. Examples include developing a robotic surgical system, which will involve mechanical engineers providing input into hardware design, software engineers into the programming of the control systems, and surgeons to guide functionality so that the device's purpose is met clinically. Innovation advances collaboration, and biomedical solutions solve real-world medical challenges [3].

A third guiding principle in biomedical engineering is ensuring that ethical demands for patient safety, efficacy, and accessibility are achieved. In this regard, biomedical engineers should consider the ethical implications of their work, particularly in sensitive areas such as genetic engineering, artificial intelligence in healthcare, and clinical trials [4]. Innovations should be both harmless and effective, and readily available for use, to maintain public confidence and achieve the desired health outcomes. The regulatory framework established by the Food and Drug Administration (FDA) and other governing bodies is designed to provide a basis for biomedical engineers to ensure adherence to ethical and safety standards at all times.

### 1.1.2 Development of Medical Devices

Perhaps the most notable contribution from biomedical engineering is the development of medical devices. These have revolutionized healthcare, allowing doctors to diagnose and monitor diseases, as well as treat them much more effectively than in the past. Diagnostic equipment, such as Magnetic Resonance Imaging (MRI) machines, Computed Tomography (CT) scanners, and ultrasound systems, enables physicians to visualize the body's internal structures in unprecedented detail. These imaging systems enable non-invasive diagnosis and monitoring, thereby facilitating early diagnosis and improved patient outcomes. Similarly, therapeutic devices, including pacemakers, insulin pumps, and ventilators, enable the management of both chronic and acute medical conditions, further enhancing the quality of life for patients [5].

Another significant development within biomedical engineering pertains to surgical tools. Robotic surgical systems are designed for minimally invasive procedures, reducing recovery times and enabling surgeons to achieve greater precision. These include enhanced imaging technologies and real-time monitoring, which are integral to many systems that help guide surgeons to optimal outcomes. Biomedical engineers also design prosthetics and orthotics, developing devices that allow amputees or people with musculoskeletal diseases to regain motor capabilities and function [6]. The use of new materials and biomechanical studies has made modern prosthetics significantly more comfortable, resilient, and capable of mimicking the natural movements of human limbs.

#### Biomechanics

Biomechanics is a specialized area of biomedical engineering that deals with the mechanical properties of biological systems. The interaction between forces and movements, as well as their relationships with the body, will enlighten us concerning the design of devices and systems that enhance human health. The study of mechanics in the joint today can mimic the knee or hip movement, giving some patients with arthritis or injuries a second chance through artificial joints. In this aspect of dynamics, too, muscle action provides designs for exoskeletons and assistive devices that help mobility-impaired people regain some independence.

Biomechanics also has applications in sports, where engineers study the forces acting during an athletic performance to maximize efficiency and minimize the risk of injury. Running shoes, for instance, should have an optimal amount of cushioning and support, requiring a deep understanding of biomechanics related to gait and impact forces. Rehabilitation medicine in biomechanics involves designing therapies and devices to aid in recovery from injury. Robotic systems used in physical therapy guide patients through controlled movements that help rebuild strength and coordination.

### Biomaterials

The study and development of biomaterials is another cornerstone of biomedical engineering. Biomaterials are engineered substances designed to interact with biological systems for medical purposes, such as implants, drug delivery systems, and wound healing products. These materials must meet strict biocompatibility standards, ensuring they do not trigger adverse reactions when introduced into the body. Advances in biomaterials have enabled the creation of implants that mimic the mechanical and biological properties of natural tissues, such as titanium joints for hip replacements and polymer-based stents for cardiovascular treatments.

Biomaterials are also critical in drug delivery systems, where they are used to encapsulate medications and release them in a controlled manner. This approach improves the efficacy of treatments and reduces side effects by targeting drugs to specific sites within the body. Recent developments in nanotechnology have expanded the possibilities for biomaterials, allowing engineers to design nanoparticles that deliver drugs directly to cancer cells or other disease sites, increasing treatment precision. Additionally, integrating biomaterials with tissue engineering has opened new avenues for creating artificial tissues and organs that can replace damaged ones, addressing critical shortages in organ transplantation.

### Biomedical Imaging

Biomedical Imaging is one of the revolutionary areas in biomedical engineering, as it allows healthcare professionals a glimpse into the internal structures of the body and their functioning. It encompasses various significant means for diagnosis and treatment, including X-rays, MRI scans, and ultrasounds, all of which are forms of imaging diagnostics. These systems offer non-invasive means of monitoring the body and aid in diagnosing diseases related to tumors, cardiovascular diseases, and neurological disorders at an early stage. Improvements in imaging have made these techniques not only of higher resolution, but also faster and safer [6, 7].

Biomedical engineers make significant contributions to the creation and advancement of imaging technologies. Innovations to MRI technology, for example, have reduced the time a patient must undergo a scan while improving the resolution of the images captured, thereby improving the procedure's efficacy and comfort. The creation of functional imaging—the ability to visualize the activity of organs or systems within the body in real-time—has allowed researchers to observe brain activity, greatly enhancing our understanding of neurological processes and potentially leading to new treatments. Moreover, imaging is being integrated with surgical systems to an ever-greater degree, thereby enabling real-time visualization in surgery and, consequently, generating better outcomes [8, 9].

### Tissue Engineering and Regenerative Medicine

Tissue engineering and regenerative medicine represent the frontiers of biomedical engineering, integrating biology, materials science, and engineering to repair, regenerate, or replace damaged tissues and organs. This area is inspired by the increasing demand for alternatives to organ transplantation and finding a cure for chronic tissue damage brought about by physical injuries, diseases, or aging. Tissue engineering is the fabrication of scaffolds, which are three-dimensional structures designed to mimic the extracellular matrix of tissues. A scaffold provides an interim structural framework that allows cells to attach, proliferate, and form functional tissue [1].

Engineering tissues requires a combination of several elements, including stem cells, growth factors, and biomaterials, all working together. In a nutshell, the contribution of stem cells to regenerative medicine becomes important because they can differentiate into a wide range of cell types. For example, mesenchymal stem cells from either bone marrow or fat can serve to regenerate cartilage, bone, or even cardiac muscle. Some methodologies in tissue engineering have already begun to include proteins that regulate cell proliferation and differentiation, commonly referred to as growth factors, to enhance the repair process [10]. Most of these factors are delivered in a controlled manner through the use of biodegradable scaffolds, which ensure their sustained release and optimal tissue regeneration. The application and development of tissue engineering relate to various fields. For example, researchers are developing artificial cartilage and bones in orthopedics to treat osteoarthritis and fractures. In dermatology, skin substitutes made by bioengineering are used to treat burn wounds and chronic ulcers. The cardiovascular field has been able to develop heart valves and blood vessels; these are likely to replace damaged structures and restore circulatory function. Benefits accruing from such advances have also allowed the engineering of bioartificial kidneys and livers, among other organs, to alleviate the acute shortage of donor organs for transplantation [11].

Regenerative medicine encompasses gene therapy, which involves replacing defective or missing genes with healthy ones to treat genetic disorders. Conventionally, this is typically achieved by using viral vectors to insert healthy genes into the target cells of the body in question, thereby making them functional. This new combination of tissue engineering with gene therapy has opened up new routes for treating diseases such as cystic fibrosis, muscular dystrophy, and specific types of cancer [12]. As technologies in this area continue to improve, the possibility of cultivating fully functional organs either in the laboratory or naturally regenerating those with the innate capacity of the body instills fresh hope into patients worldwide.

### Bioinformatics

Bioinformatics plays a crucial role in biomedical engineering, as it utilizes bioinformatics tools and techniques to analyze vast amounts of biological data and interpret complex biological information. Due to the advent of big data, the volume of information generated from genomic sequencing, proteomics, and clinical research has increased exponentially. Bioinformatics enables methodologies and platforms for structuring, analyzing, and visualizing data within this framework, facilitating unimaginable discoveries.

One of the significant bioinformatics applications in biomedical engineering involves using genomics, whereby bioinformatics algorithms are applied to sequence and interpret DNA. Thereafter, it has enabled many advances in personalized medicine, whereby treatments can be tailored and allocated based on a subject's genetic profile. In this respect, the analysis of genetic mutations associated with diseases such as cancer enables bioinformatic tools to identify specific drug targets. This approach ensures that therapies are more effective and have fewer side effects, marking a shift from a one-size-fits-all model toward precision healthcare.

Another area to which bioinformatics has made significant contributions is proteomics, the study of proteins and their functions. Proteins perform crucial tasks in cells, and understanding how they interact can help explain the mechanisms of disease. Bioinformatics allows researchers to chart maps of protein networks, predict protein structures, and investigate post-translational modifications. Such insights are invaluable in drug discovery and the development of diagnostic biomarkers that can detect diseases at an early stage [12]. Beyond genomics and proteomics, it plays a vital role in clinical data analysis, from electronic health records to medical imaging. Machine learning algorithms are increasingly being applied to identify patterns in these datasets, enabling predictive modeling for disease progression and treatment outcomes. For example, various research studies on patient data using bioinformatics have helped increase our understanding of complex disorders, such as diabetes, Alzheimer's disease, and cardiovascular disorders, by developing better policies for preventing and managing these life-threatening conditions [13].

Incorporating artificial intelligence and machine learning in bioinformatics has also greatly extended this. Deep learning models are being applied to medical imaging, such as MRI or CT scans, to yield finer and faster processing. Similarly, algorithms in natural language processing are being used to synthesize valuable information from the growing body of medical literature and patient records that inform clinical decision-making. Bioinformatics will remain at the heart of biomedical engineering as computational power and algorithmic sophistication advance, driving improvements in diagnostics, therapeutics, and personalized medicine [7, 14].

### Rehabilitation Engineering

Rehabilitation engineering, a sub-discipline within biomedical engineering, focuses on the design and construction of devices utilizing various technologies to enhance the quality of life for individuals with physical, cognitive, or sensory impairments. This area of study aims to be in line with the disabilities that affect one's life by helping individuals gain independence, mobility, and other functionalities. In general, rehabilitation engineering is a multidisciplinary field that integrates concepts from biomechanics, robotics, and assistive technologies to design equipment and systems that help recover and adapt human organisms [15].

One of the most valuable contributions of rehabilitation engineering is in the design of prosthetics and orthotics. Contemporary prosthetic limbs are fabricated with state-of-the-art sensors and actuators that can truly emulate natural limbs. These devices often interface with the nervous system, allowing users to control them through neural signals. For instance, myoelectric prosthetics rely on electrical impulses generated by muscle contractions to actuate the movement of the prosthetic limb, thereby providing a high degree of functionality and dexterity. Orthotic devices, braces, and supports are meant to correct musculoskeletal disorders and improve mobility [6, 16]. Rehabilitation engineering has also further developed exoskeletons, wearable robotic systems that assist individuals with spinal cord injuries or neurological disorders in walking. These devices, which utilize a combination of motors and sensors, replicate patterns of natural ambulation, enabling users to stand, walk, and even climb stairs. In addition to improving mobility, using exoskeletons is also beneficial for therapeutic purposes, as it encourages muscle activity and circulation that help reduce complications from prolonged periods of immobilization.

Other focuses of rehabilitation engineering are communication and sensory assistive technologies. Communication devices and sensory technology include those used by individuals with speech or hearing disabilities, such as augmentative and alternative communication systems and cochlear implants. Examples of Augmentative and Alternative Communication (AAC) devices include speech-generating systems for individuals with non-verbal communication needs, while cochlear implants restore auditory input by direct stimulation of the auditory nerve. Developments in haptic feedback and virtual reality are also being explored in the development of sensory substitution devices, which aim to provide alternative means of perceiving the environment [1].

The other side of rehabilitation engineering deals with software and applications that support the rehabilitation process. For example, it finds its place in virtual reality-based therapies, which have created an immersive environment for patients to practice their motor skills and cognitive tasks in a highly controlled environment [6]. A few of the promising treatments for conditions like stroke, traumatic brain injury, and Post-Traumatic Stress Disorder (PTSD) have been developed using these therapies. Indeed, rehabilitation engineering utilizes technology and knowledge of human physiology and psychology to continually enhance the lives of individuals with disabilities.

### 1.1.3 Interdisciplinary Nature of Biomedical Engineering

Biomedical engineering is an interdisciplinary field, and it uniquely prepares a new generation of researchers and practitioners to tackle the most complex medical challenges. The field's knowledge base includes mechanical engineering, electrical engineering, computer science, biology, and medicine. Innovation arises from their interaction, enabling biomedical solutions to be both technically robust and clinically relevant.

Knowledge in physics, specifically regarding the principles of radiation and magnetism, as well as computer science, particularly in the processing and analysis of images, and clinical expertise in defining applications, are all required to develop state-of-the-art medical imaging [17]. The design of a drug delivery system similarly requires expertise in chemical engineering to create biocompatible materials, pharmacological knowledge regarding the action of drugs, and biomedical engineering expertise to ensure that the system is safe, functional, and effective [18]. There is also a need for collaboration between academia, research, industry, and healthcare providers. Many biomedical engineers collaborate with clinicians, beginning with an unmet clinical need and progressing to a practical solution. In designing a wearable health monitor, physicians may suggest which physiological parameters to measure, engineers may develop the hardware, and software specialists may design the user interface. This collaborative approach ensures that the final product best meets the needs of both patients and healthcare providers.

The academic and learning elements of biomedical engineering are also at the heart of any interdisciplinary study. Programs in biomedical engineering encompass a wide range of subjects, including anatomy and physiology, as well as electronics and materials science. This broad-based education enables students to function effectively in multidisciplinary teams and equips them with a wide range of problem-solving skills. As biomedical engineering continues to change, its dependency on interdisciplinary collaboration will drive its success.

### 1.1.4 Ethical and Regulatory Considerations

Ethics and regulation play a crucial role in biomedical engineering, ensuring that innovations in this field prioritize patient safety, efficacy, and accessibility. Biomedical engineers must balance a delicate landscape of ethical debates and regulatory requirements, especially when constantly developing technologies create new questions about privacy, consent, and equity.

From the perspective of biomedical engineering, the safety and reliability of medical devices and technology are among the most critical ethical concerns. The engineers must ensure that their design meets critical safety standards and poses no risks to patients. Such a responsibility is significant in various devices, including implantable defibrillators or robotic surgical systems, since failures of those devices may be life-threatening. These guidelines and testing protocols are mandated by regulatory agencies, such as the FDA in the United States and the EMA in Europe, to ensure that medical devices are deemed safe and effective before they are approved for clinical use [19].

Other important ethical issues involve privacy and data security, especially in the modern era of digital health and wearable technologies. Biomedical engineers developing devices to collect and transmit patient data should ensure that these systems are secure and comply with all relevant regulations, such as the Health Insurance Portability and Accountability Act (HIPAA). Ethical issues also encompass Artificial Intelligence (AI) in healthcare, where biased algorithms may lead to unequal treatments or misdiagnoses. It is expected that engineers will be able to overcome all these challenges by developing systems that are transparent, fair, and accountable [20, 21]. Other ethical considerations include access and equity. Biomedical engineers must utilize their skills and ingenuity to make technologies accessible and reasonably affordable for people from diverse backgrounds. This would ensure health improvements accrue to everyone, not just those who can afford them. Attention should be paid to the healthcare gap, and consideration should be given to the needs of underserved communities when designing new technologies [15].

Ethical and regulatory dimensions in biomedical engineering are crucial for sustaining the public's trust and ensuring that the application and development of this technology continue to evolve in an accountable manner. Indeed, by adhering to such tenets, biomedical engineers strike a balance between innovation and the ethical obligation to prioritize patient welfare and benefit society [22].

## 1.2 History and Evolution of Biomedical Engineering

Biomedical Engineering (BME) is a dynamic and rapidly evolving field that integrates engineering principles with biological and medical sciences to develop technologies that improve healthcare [23]. It is an interdisciplinary domain that spans multiple specializations, including medical device design, tissue engineering, bioinformatics, medical imaging, rehabilitation engineering, and neural engineering [7]. The progress of biomedical engineering is intrinsically linked to humanity's longstanding pursuit of understanding, diagnosing, and treating disease. Its history reflects the coalescence of scientific knowledge and technological innovation over millennia.

The development of biomedical engineering is deeply rooted in human civilization, dating back to ancient times when early medical practitioners devised tools and techniques to mend injuries and alleviate suffering. Archaeological evidence suggests that early humans used rudimentary prosthetics, splints, and surgical instruments, demonstrating an innate drive to manipulate materials for medical purposes [24]. These early innovations, though primitive, laid the groundwork for more sophisticated developments in later centuries. The field continued to evolve as civilizations such as the Egyptians, Greeks, Romans, and Chinese advanced their medical knowledge and engineering capabilities, creating surgical tools, prosthetic limbs, and even early forms of bioelectrical therapy.

During the Renaissance period, the study of human anatomy flourished, primarily driven by the works of scholars such as Leonardo da Vinci and Andreas Vesalius. Anatomical illustrations, precise dissections, and the application of mechanical principles to understand human movement set the stage for future biomedical innovations [25]. However, it was not until the Industrial Revolution that biomedical engineering became a formalized field of study. This era witnessed the emergence of mechanical devices, steam-powered machinery, and electrical discoveries, which were soon applied to medical instrumentation. The nineteenth and early twentieth centuries brought groundbreaking developments in diagnostic and therapeutic technologies, including the invention of the stethoscope, electrocardiogram (ECG), and X-ray imaging.

The mid-twentieth century marked the formal recognition of biomedical engineering as an academic and professional field. World War II and the subsequent technological boom led to significant advancements in prosthetics, medical imaging, and biomaterials [26]. Establishing biomedical engineering departments in universities and increasing funding for medical research fostered a new generation of engineers and scientists dedicated to healthcare innovation. The rise of computer technology in the latter half of the twentieth century further transformed the field, enabling the development of sophisticated diagnostic tools, medical simulations, and computational modeling techniques that continue to shape modern medicine [27].

Today, biomedical engineering stands at the forefront of medical innovation, encompassing cutting-edge fields such as artificial intelligence in medicine, bioinformatics, nanotechnology, and regenerative medicine [19]. Advances in 3D printing have revolutionized prosthetics and organ transplantation, while breakthroughs in genetic engineering and personalized medicine are paving the way for highly targeted therapies. Integrating engineering and biology has enhanced diagnostic and therapeutic capabilities, significantly improving patient outcomes and quality of life.

As this chapter unfolds, we will examine the historical trajectory of biomedical engineering, exploring key milestones, technological breakthroughs, and transformative discoveries that have shaped the field. The first section will provide an in-depth history of BME, tracing its origins from ancient medical practices to the sophisticated biomedical technologies of today. The second section will highlight the hallmarks of BME, outlining fundamental contributions, defining characteristics, and landmark innovations that have established BME as a cornerstone of modern healthcare. Lastly, we will examine BME now, exploring contemporary trends, emerging research areas, and the future direction of biomedical engineering.

Biomedical engineering continues to redefine the boundaries of human health, bridging the gap between engineering ingenuity and medical necessity. As discoveries unfold, the field remains committed to solving some of the most pressing challenges in healthcare, from improving early disease detection to developing life-saving medical devices and pioneering regenerative therapies. The journey of biomedical engineering is one of relentless progress, driven by the pursuit of knowledge, technological advancement, and the fundamental goal of improving human health and well-being.

## *1.2.1 History of Biomedical Engineering*

### Early Civilizations and the Dawn of Medical Technology

The origins of biomedical engineering can be traced back to the earliest civilizations, where humans sought ways to treat injuries, alleviate pain, and improve bodily function using rudimentary tools. Ancient societies, including those of the Egyptians, Greeks, Romans, Chinese, and Indians, developed foundational medical practices that incorporated engineering principles and empirical observations [28].

#### Ancient Egyptian Medical Practices

Ancient Egypt (c. 3000 BCE) is one of the earliest known civilizations to have made significant contributions to medicine and biomedical engineering. Egyptian physicians utilized various bronze and copper tools, including forceps, scalpels, and surgical needles [29]. The famous Ebers Papyrus (c. 1550 BCE) details medical treatments for various conditions, including wound care, prosthetic use, and splinting techniques.

Additionally, archaeological discoveries suggest that the Egyptians used prosthetic devices, such as artificial toes and fingers made from wood and leather, demonstrating an early understanding of biomechanics. These prosthetics were designed for cosmetic reasons and to aid mobility (Fig. 1.1).

#### Ancient Greek and Roman Contributions

The ancient Greeks and Romans expanded upon Egyptian medical knowledge and introduced more systematic medical practices. Hippocrates (c. 460–370 BCE), often called the "Father of Medicine," emphasized clinical observation and ethical medical practice, laying the foundation for evidence-based medicine [30]. Greek physicians also developed sophisticated surgical tools, including bone drills, scalpels, and forceps [29].

The Romans further advanced biomedical engineering through public health innovations, including aqueducts, sewage systems, and hospitals. Their engineering expertise in water supply and sanitation significantly reduced the spread of disease and improved population health [28]. Galen of Pergamon (c. 129–216 CE), a Roman physician, made significant contributions to human anatomy through dissections of

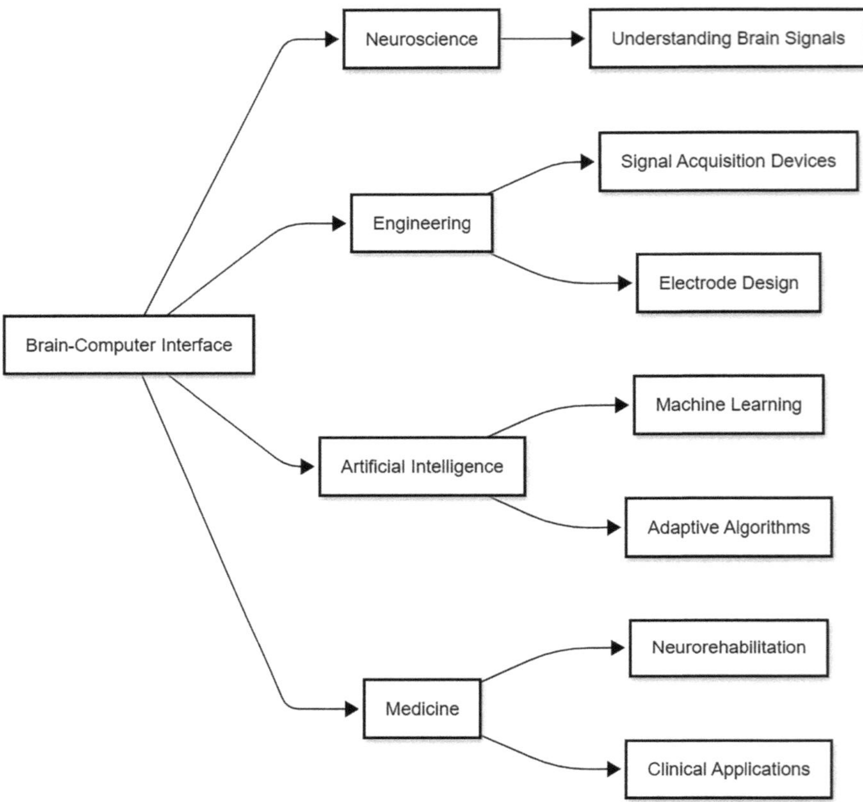


**Fig. 1.1** An ancient Egyptian wooden prosthetic toe, one of the earliest known examples of a prosthetic device (https://commons.wikimedia.org/wiki/File:Prosthetic_toe.jpg)

animals, providing insights that influenced medical practice for over a millennium (Fig. 1.2).

### Traditional Chinese and Indian Medicine

Parallel to the advancements of the Greco-Roman civilization, ancient Chinese and Indian civilizations developed unique biomedical methodologies. Traditional Chinese Medicine (TCM) introduced acupuncture, herbal medicine, and pulse diagnosis, emphasizing the balance of vital energy (Qi) for health [31]. Early Chinese engineers also developed mechanical models of the human body, which contributed to the understanding of biomechanics.

In India, an ancient surgeon, Sushruta (c. 600 BCE), documented detailed surgical procedures, including early reconstructive surgery and prosthetic development.

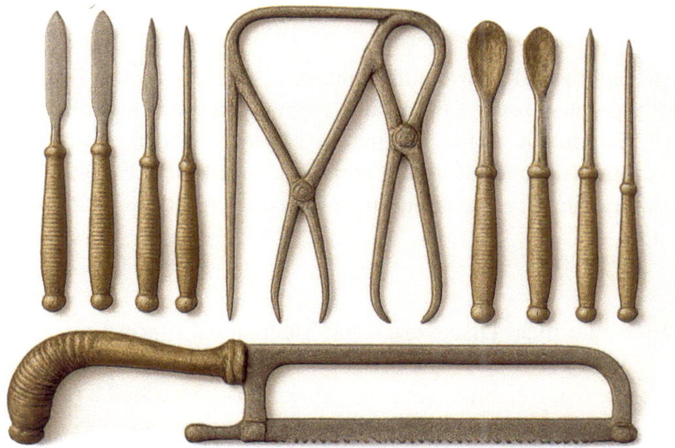

**Fig. 1.2** A reconstruction of a Roman surgical toolkit, including scalpels, forceps, and bone saws

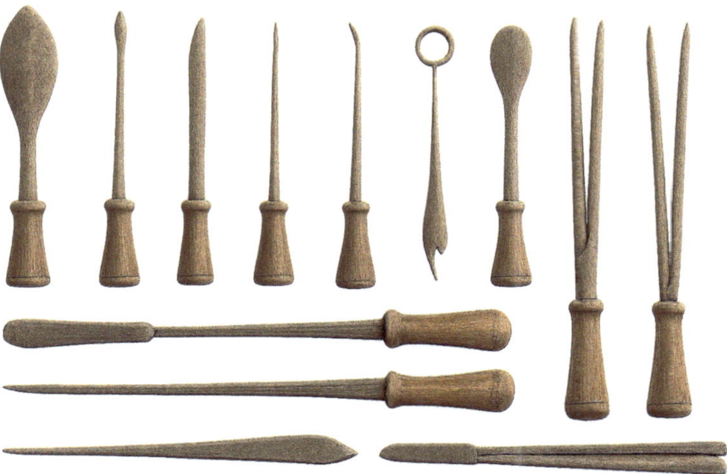

**Fig. 1.3** An ancient Indian surgical instrument set based on the descriptions in the Sushruta Samhita

His work, the Sushruta Samhita, describes over 120 surgical instruments and numerous procedures for wound healing, bone-setting, and plastic surgery (Fig. 1.3).

### The Middle Ages and Renaissance: The Growth of Medical Engineering

Following the fall of the Roman Empire, medical advancements in Europe slowed, but progress continued in the Islamic world and later revived during the European Renaissance.

### Islamic Golden Age Contributions

Between the eighth and fourteenth centuries, scholars in the Islamic world preserved and expanded upon Greek and Roman medical knowledge. Al-Zahrawi (936–1013 CE), known as the "Father of Modern Surgery," developed over 200 surgical instruments, many of which are still in use today. He also pioneered early forms of orthopedic surgery, including methods for setting fractures and dislocations (Fig. 1.4).

### Renaissance: Anatomical Discoveries and Mechanical Innovation

The Renaissance (fourteenth to seventeenth centuries) marked a revival of scientific inquiry and the application of engineering in medicine. Leonardo da Vinci (1452–1519) conducted detailed anatomical studies, producing highly accurate sketches of the human body that enhanced the understanding of musculoskeletal mechanics [32].

The sixteenth century saw the rise of Andreas Vesalius (1514–1564), whose book "De Humani Corporis Fabrica" revolutionized anatomical knowledge by correcting many of Galen's errors. These anatomical insights laid the foundation for prosthetics, biomechanics, and surgical innovations.

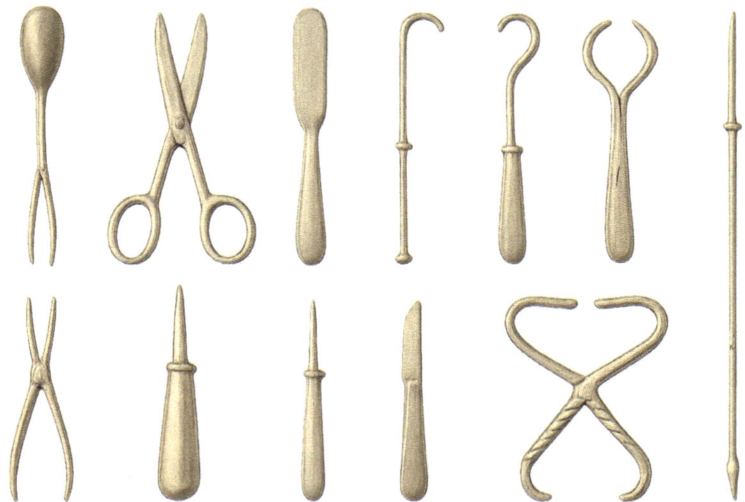

**Fig. 1.4** Illustrations from Al-Zahrawi's medical texts showing early surgical instruments

### The Industrial Revolution and the Birth of Biomedical Engineering

Mechanization and Medical Instrumentation

The Industrial Revolution (eighteenth to nineteenth centuries) introduced new materials, precision manufacturing techniques, and mechanical innovations that greatly influenced biomedical engineering.

One of the most significant medical advancements of this era was the invention of the stethoscope by René Laennec (1816), which improved the ability to diagnose respiratory and cardiovascular conditions. Around the same time, electrical discoveries led to the development of electrophysiology, with Luigi Galvani demonstrating bioelectricity in frog muscles, laying the groundwork for modern neural engineering (Fig. 1.5).

X-Rays and Early Medical Imaging

The discovery of X-rays by Wilhelm Röntgen in 1895 revolutionized medical diagnostics, allowing for non-invasive visualization of internal structures. This breakthrough spurred the development of medical imaging, one of the most significant domains within biomedical engineering [33].

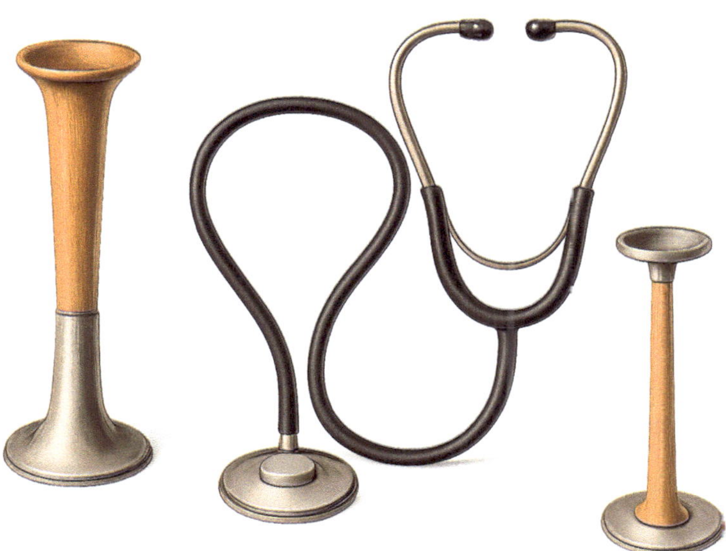

**Fig. 1.5** Early designs of the stethoscope

### The Twentieth Century: The Formalization of Biomedical Engineering

The twentieth century saw the formal establishment of biomedical engineering as a distinct discipline, driven by technological advancements and increased collaboration between engineers and medical professionals [34].

#### Development of Medical Devices

Rapid advancements in prosthetics, surgical techniques, and medical instrumentation occurred during the two World Wars. Willem Einthoven's development of the electrocardiogram (ECG) in 1903 allowed for real-time cardiac monitoring, while the invention of the artificial pacemaker in the 1950s revolutionized the treatment of heart conditions [19] (Fig. 1.6).

#### The Rise of Medical Imaging and Computational Biology

The mid-to-late twentieth century witnessed an explosion in biomedical imaging technologies, including computed tomography (CT) in the 1970s and magnetic resonance imaging (MRI) in the 1980s. These imaging techniques vastly improved diagnostic accuracy [35].

In parallel, the advent of computers enabled bioinformatics and computational modeling, leading to personalized medicine and improved disease prediction [34] (Fig. 1.7).

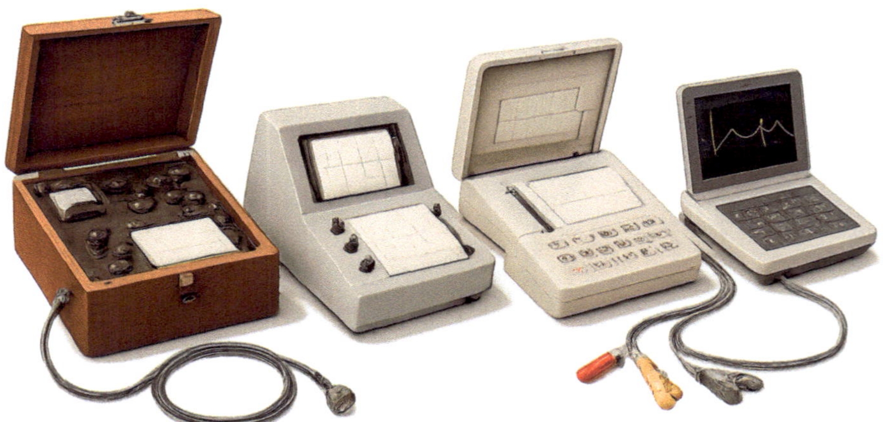

**Fig. 1.6** Evolution of ECG machines from early designs to modern digital systems

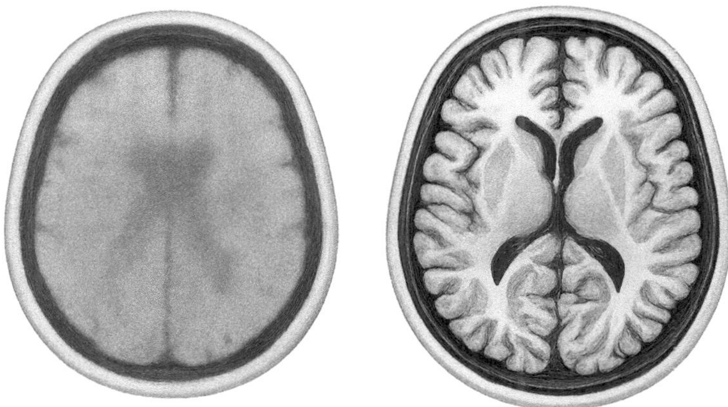

**Fig. 1.7** Comparison of early and modern high-resolution MRI images

**The Twenty-First Century: Biomedical Engineering Today and Future Directions**

AI, Robotics, and Regenerative Medicine

The twenty-first century has witnessed groundbreaking advancements in artificial intelligence (AI) for diagnostics, robotic surgery, and regenerative medicine, utilizing systems like the da Vinci Surgical System, as well as the use of stem cells and 3D-printed organs [36] (Fig. 1.8).

The Future of Biomedical Engineering

With the rise of nanotechnology, wearable health monitors, and brain-computer interfaces, biomedical engineering is poised to revolutionize healthcare further [27]. Future trends include fully personalized medicine, enhanced neural prosthetics, and further integration of AI into medical decision-making [37, 38].

### *1.2.2 Hallmarks of Biomedical Engineering*

Biomedical engineering (BME) is defined by the technologies it produces and the principles and approaches that drive its evolution. It is a field that merges medicine, engineering, and biology, always striving to enhance human health and well-being [13]. Historically, BME has been shaped by a few key characteristics—hallmarks that define its impact and set it apart from other disciplines. These include relentless technological innovation, an inherently interdisciplinary nature, a deep

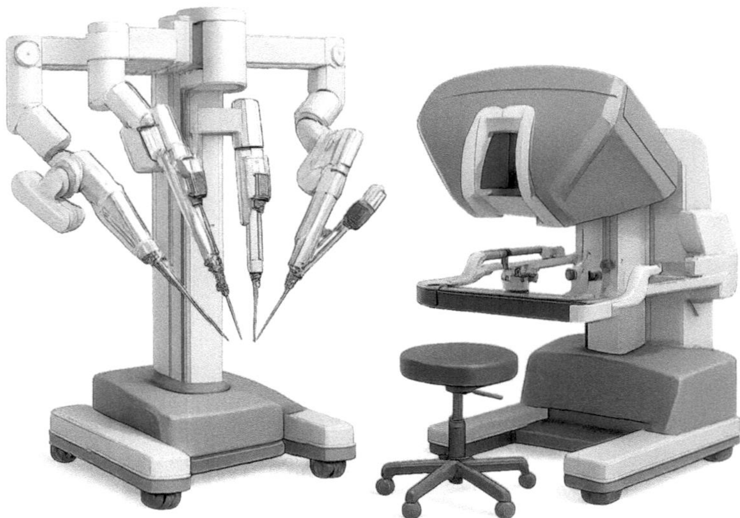

**Fig. 1.8** A robotic surgery system and a 3D-printed organ model

commitment to patient-centered solutions, strict ethical considerations, and a strong focus on translational research. Each of these elements has played a crucial role in shaping modern healthcare, ensuring that biomedical engineering continues to push the boundaries of what is possible.

### Innovation as the Driving Force

Innovation is at the heart of biomedical engineering. The field thrives on discovering new ways to diagnose, treat, and prevent disease [27]. From early mechanical medical devices to today's AI-assisted diagnostics and robotic surgeries, the evolution of BME has been defined by a continuous stream of breakthroughs [39].

One of the most significant innovations in biomedical engineering has been the development of medical imaging technologies. The ability to visualize the inside of the human body without invasive procedures has revolutionized medicine. The journey began with the discovery of X-rays in 1895, which allowed doctors to see bones and internal structures for the first time. This was followed by ultrasound technology in the 1950s, CT scans in the 1970s, and MRI soon after. These advancements provided greater clarity and detail, enabling more accurate diagnoses and better patient outcomes [34].

The field of prosthetics and artificial organs has also seen remarkable progress. What once were simple mechanical replacements for lost limbs have evolved into highly sophisticated devices. Today's prosthetic limbs incorporate neural interfaces, allowing users to control them using their thoughts, bringing movement and dexterity closer to that of natural limbs. Similarly, artificial organs such as pacemakers, ventricular assist devices, and bioengineered kidneys have provided life-saving alternatives for patients with failing organs [40].

Biomedical engineers do not just improve existing medical tools but also develop new ways of approaching medical challenges. 3D bioprinting, for example, is pushing the boundaries of regenerative medicine by allowing scientists to print human tissues and, in the future, potentially entire organs. Such innovations do not exist in a vacuum; they arise from the collaborative and interdisciplinary nature of BME.

### The Interdisciplinary Nature of BME

Biomedical engineering is inherently multidisciplinary, combining principles from mechanical engineering, electrical engineering, materials science, biology, and medicine [10]. This fusion is essential because the problems biomedical engineers seek to solve are too complex to be addressed by a single discipline alone.

Consider the development of brain-computer interfaces (BCIs)—devices that enable direct communication between the brain and external systems. These interfaces are being developed to restore movement in paralyzed individuals, allowing users to control prosthetic limbs through thought alone [19]. To create such a system, expertise from multiple fields is required (Fig. 1.9):

- Neuroscientists study brain activity and identify relevant neural signals.
- Electrical engineers design the electrodes that can safely and effectively interface with neurons.
- Computer scientists develop the algorithms to decode brain signals and translate them into commands.
- Medical doctors ensure the devices are safe and clinically viable for patient use.

Without this interdisciplinary approach, BCIs would remain theoretical rather than functional. Another prime example of interdisciplinary collaboration is wearable medical technology. Devices such as smartwatches that monitor heart rate and oxygen levels, as well as detect arrhythmias, rely on contributions from bioengineers, software developers, and medical professionals [41]. These technologies have enabled individuals to track their health in real-time, shifting healthcare from a reactive to a proactive approach [42].

### Patient-Centered Design in Biomedical Engineering

A defining aspect of biomedical engineering is that every technology and innovation is ultimately developed with the patient in mind. Unlike other engineering fields that might focus on efficiency or cost reduction, BME places the highest priority on improving quality of life.

A key example is assistive technology—devices designed to help individuals with disabilities regain independence. Cochlear implants, for instance, have restored hearing to individuals with profound deafness, completely transforming

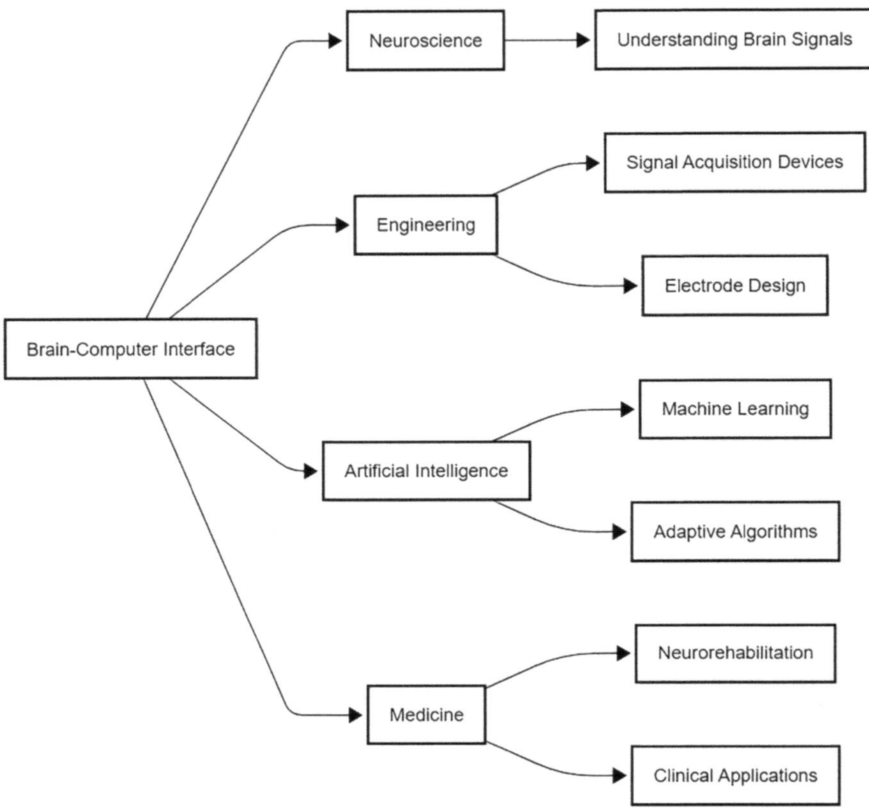


**Fig. 1.9** The interdisciplinary nature of a brain-computer interface

their ability to interact with the world [43]. Exoskeletons, once a concept seen only in science fiction, are now used to help individuals with paralysis walk again. Each of these technologies was developed with a deep understanding of human needs, ensuring that they integrate seamlessly into a patient's daily life rather than disrupt it. Personalized medicine is another area where patient-centered design is at the forefront. Traditional treatments often employ a one-size-fits-all approach, but biomedical engineering has enabled customized therapies tailored to a person's unique genetics, physiology, and lifestyle. Targeted drug delivery systems, for example, enable medications to reach only the affected area, reducing side effects and increasing effectiveness. Similarly, 3D-printed implants can be custom-designed for a perfect anatomical fit, improving surgical outcomes (Fig. 1.10).

### Ethical Considerations in Biomedical Engineering

As biomedical engineering advances, it introduces profound ethical challenges. While promising, new technologies must be implemented responsibly to ensure they are safe, accessible, and equitable.

One primary concern is the accessibility of medical technology. While groundbreaking devices and treatments are being developed at an incredible pace, they are often prohibitively expensive. Should life-saving technologies be available only to those who can afford them, or should they be considered a universal right? Biomedical engineers must collaborate with policymakers and healthcare professionals to ensure that innovations do not exacerbate inequalities in healthcare access [44].

Another pressing ethical issue is data privacy in AI-driven medicine. The increasing reliance on machine learning models for diagnosing diseases and predicting patient outcomes means that vast amounts of patient data. This raises concerns about how data is stored, who has access to it, and how it is used. If AI algorithms are trained on biased datasets, they can unintentionally reinforce disparities in

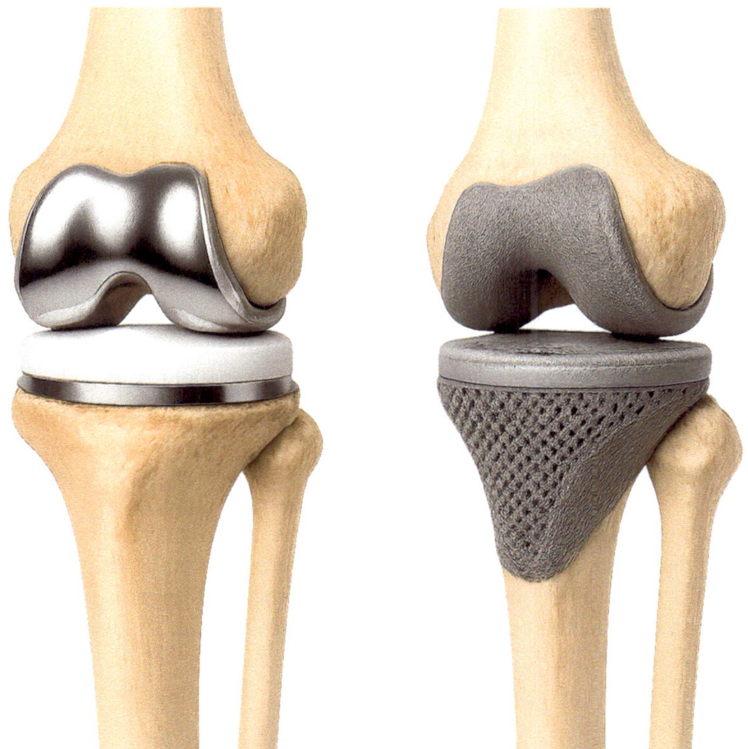

**Fig. 1.10** A comparison of a traditional knee implant vs. a custom 3D-printed knee implant

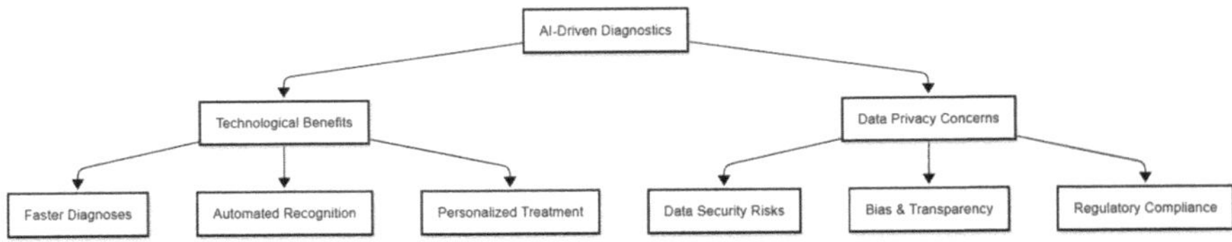


**Fig. 1.11** AI-driven diagnostics, illustrating the balance between technological benefits and data privacy concerns

healthcare. Engineers and healthcare professionals must work together to establish guidelines that ensure fairness, transparency, and patient consent [44, 45] (Fig. 1.11).

A final ethical dilemma involves the line between treatment and human enhancement. Technologies such as gene editing (CRISPR) and brain augmentation pose significant questions about how far biomedical engineering should go. While they have the potential to cure genetic disorders and restore lost functions, they also introduce the possibility of human enhancement beyond natural abilities [46]. Where should society draw the line between medical necessity and elective enhancement?

## Translational Research: From Lab to Clinic

One of the most defining aspects of biomedical engineering is its focus on translational research, which ensures that scientific discoveries lead to real-world medical applications. Unlike theoretical disciplines, BME thrives on bringing research from the laboratory to the patient's bedside [47].

Take the development of artificial heart valves as an example. Early concepts required years of refinement, testing, and clinical trials before they were safe for human implantation. Minimally invasive transcatheter aortic valve replacement (TAVR) allows surgeons to replace faulty heart valves without open-heart surgery, drastically reducing recovery time and improving patient survival rates [48] (Fig. 1.12).

The journey from research to implementation is long and complex, requiring collaboration between engineers, researchers, regulatory agencies, and medical practitioners. However, this dedication to turning ideas into real-world solutions transforms biomedical engineering [49]. Biomedical engineering is defined by its innovation, interdisciplinarity, patient-centered approach, ethical responsibility, and translational impact. These hallmarks ensure that the field remains at the forefront of medical advancements, continuously improving lives and shaping the future of healthcare [4].

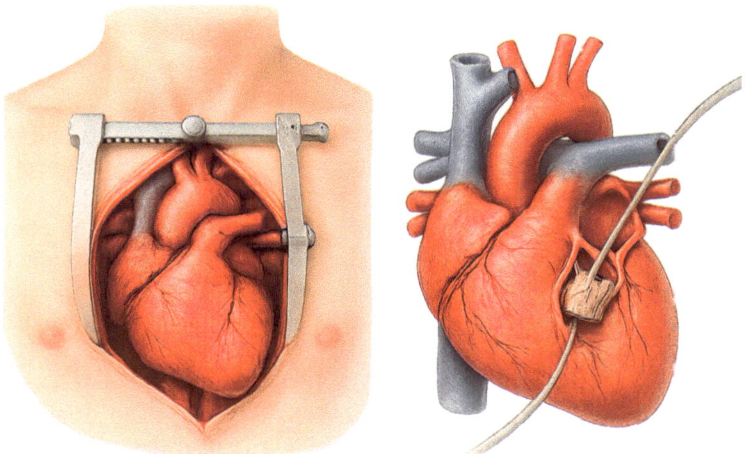

**Fig. 1.12** A comparison of traditional open-heart surgery vs. TAVR

### *1.2.3 BME Now: The Current Landscape of Biomedical Engineering*

Biomedical engineering has never been more influential in shaping the future of medicine. In the modern era, the field is characterized by rapid technological advancements, increasing reliance on AI, the miniaturization of medical devices, and the rise of personalized medicine [34]. Integrating cutting-edge computational tools, advanced materials, and robotics has transformed how we diagnose diseases, monitor patients, and develop treatments [27].

The role of biomedical engineers has evolved to address some of the most pressing healthcare challenges, including the management of chronic diseases, the need for early disease detection, and the push for minimally invasive therapies. As healthcare systems worldwide strive to become more efficient, biomedical innovations are shifting towards automation, precision medicine, and remote patient monitoring [50]. This chapter examines the state of biomedical engineering, focusing on three key areas: medical devices, artificial intelligence in healthcare, and computational modeling and simulation.

#### Medical Devices: The Backbone of Modern Medicine

Medical devices are the most tangible products of biomedical engineering, and their impact on healthcare is immeasurable. They range from simple diagnostic tools, such as electronic thermometers, to complex implantable systems, including pacemakers and neurostimulators. In recent years, significant trends in medical device innovation have focused on miniaturization, wireless connectivity, and enhanced automation [51, 52].

### Wearable and Portable Health Monitoring Devices

Advancements in sensor technology and microelectronics have led to a surge in wearable medical devices, enabling patients to monitor their health in real-time. Devices such as smartwatches, continuous glucose monitors (CGMs), and wearable electrocardiograms (ECGs) have transformed chronic disease management by providing continuous feedback to patients and healthcare providers [53].

For example, CGMs have revolutionized diabetes management by eliminating the need for frequent finger-prick blood tests. Instead, a small sensor under the skin continuously monitors blood glucose levels, sending data to a smartphone app or an insulin pump. This enables real-time adjustments in treatment, reducing the risk of complications [34] (Fig. 1.13).

Wearables are also being increasingly used in cardiac monitoring. Devices like the Apple Watch and Fitbit can detect irregular heart rhythms and atrial fibrillation and even measure blood oxygen levels, providing critical data for early disease detection. These consumer-friendly devices blur the lines between personal health technology and medical-grade diagnostics [54].

### Implantable and Bioelectronic Medical Devices

In addition to external devices, biomedical engineers have made remarkable progress in implantable medical technology, particularly cardiovascular, neural, and orthopedic applications. Pacemakers and implantable cardioverter defibrillators (ICDs) have long been the standard for managing heart rhythm disorders. However,

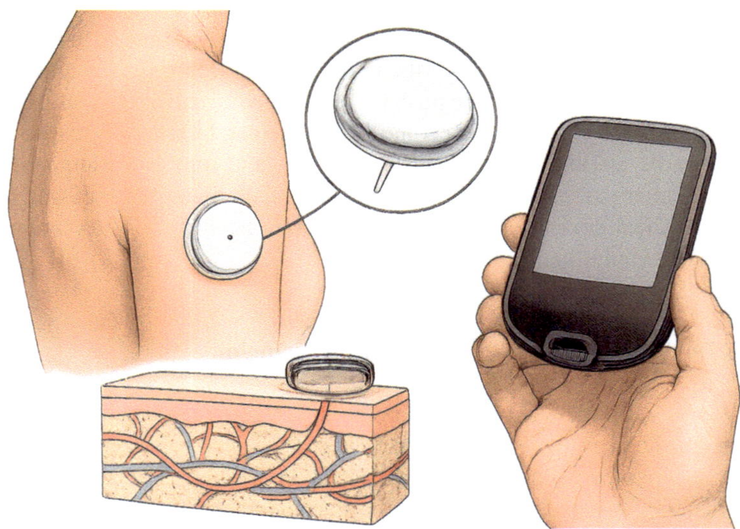

**Fig. 1.13** A continuous glucose monitor

newer developments include leadless pacemakers, which are smaller, longer-lasting, and easier to implant [55].

A fascinating frontier is bioelectronic medicine, where devices like spinal cord stimulators and vagus nerve stimulators are being used to treat chronic pain, epilepsy, and even depression. These devices modulate electrical signals in the nervous system to restore normal function, providing an alternative to pharmaceuticals [56] (Fig. 1.14).

### Minimally Invasive and Robotic-Assisted Surgical Systems

Minimally invasive surgery has significantly benefited from robotic assistance and precision imaging. The da Vinci Surgical System has been widely adopted for urology, gynecology, and cardiothoracic surgery, allowing for greater precision, reduced recovery times, and minimal scarring.

More recently, companies are developing AI-assisted robotic surgery systems that integrate machine learning algorithms to enhance surgeon decision-making, reduce fatigue, and improve patient outcomes. This convergence of robotics, imaging, and AI is paving the way for fully autonomous surgical procedures [57].

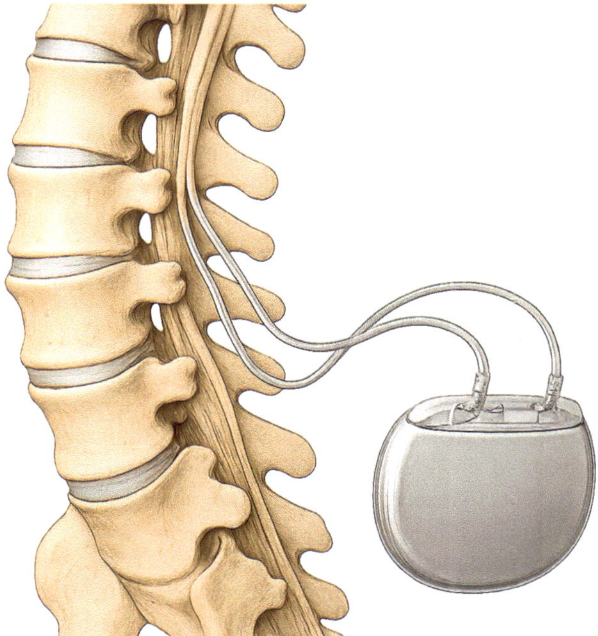

**Fig. 1.14** A spinal cord stimulator

### 1.2.4 *Artificial Intelligence in Biomedical Engineering*

AI has become one of the most disruptive forces in healthcare, accelerating diagnostics, drug discovery, and patient management. By leveraging vast amounts of medical data, AI-powered tools enhance decision-making, reduce diagnostic errors, and personalize treatment plans [58, 59].

#### AI in Medical Imaging and Diagnostics

Medical imaging is one of the most significant areas where AI has made a major impact. Traditional imaging techniques such as MRI, CT scans, and X-rays rely on human interpretation, which is time-consuming and subject to errors. AI algorithms, particularly those based on deep learning, can analyze medical images faster and more accurately [60, 61].

For example, AI-powered radiology assistants can identify abnormalities in lung scans, flag potential tumors, and even predict disease progression based on historical data. AI-based image segmentation also improves early detection of cancers, strokes, and neurodegenerative diseases [9, 62].

#### AI-Driven Personalized Medicine and Drug Discovery

AI is transforming drug discovery by significantly reducing the time and cost required to develop new treatments. Traditionally, developing a new drug takes 10–15 years and billions of dollars, but AI shortens this cycle by predicting how different compounds will interact with the human body.

AI also makes personalized medicine a reality by analyzing genetic and molecular data. AI algorithms can tailor drug prescriptions based on an individual's genetic makeup, metabolism, and disease characteristics, improving efficacy and reducing adverse effects [58].

#### AI in Remote Patient Monitoring and Telemedicine

The COVID-19 pandemic accelerated the adoption of telemedicine and remote monitoring systems, and AI is now playing a crucial role in making these systems more effective [63]. AI-powered chatbots, symptom checkers, and virtual health assistants allow patients to receive preliminary diagnoses and guidance without visiting a hospital [64] (Fig. 1.15).

Moreover, AI-powered predictive analytics in remote patient monitoring devices can detect early signs of deterioration in conditions such as heart failure, sepsis, and respiratory diseases, allowing for timely interventions and reduced hospitalizations [65] (Fig. 1.16).

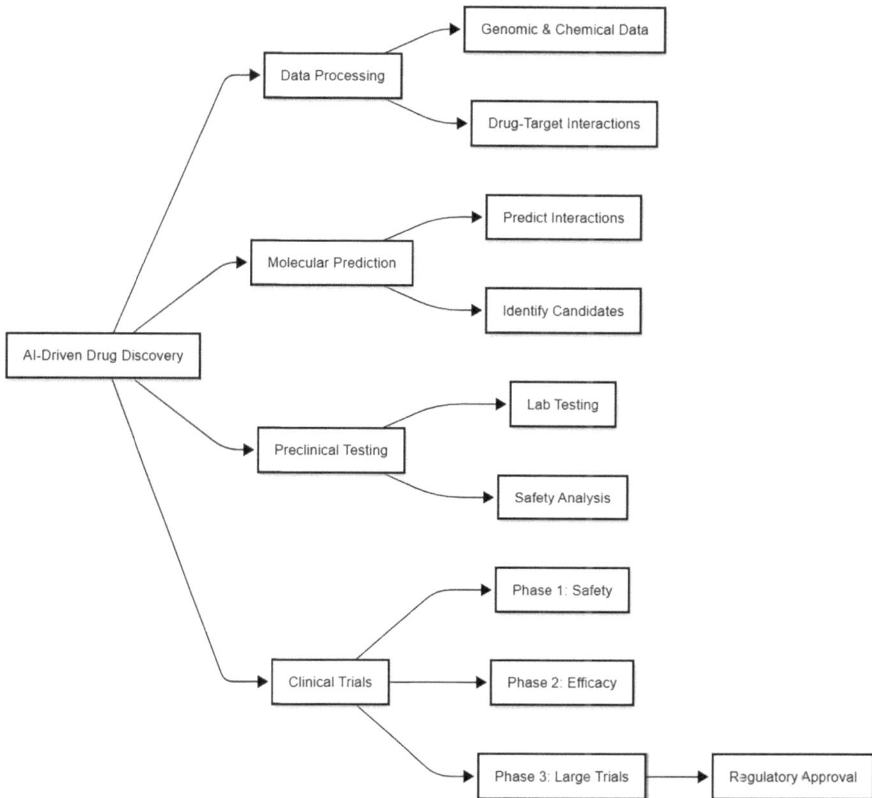


**Fig. 1.15** A flowchart of AI-driven drug discovery

## Computational Modeling and Simulations in Biomedical Engineering

With the increasing computational power available today, simulation-based medicine is emerging as a critical component of biomedical engineering. Instead of relying solely on clinical trials and traditional experimentation, scientists use biomechanical modeling and computational simulations to predict how medical treatments interact with the human body [66].

## Patient-Specific Modeling for Surgery and Treatment Planning

One of the most exciting applications is patient-specific modeling, where virtual simulations of an individual's heart, brain, or musculoskeletal system are created to predict their response to surgery or treatment. These models allow surgeons to

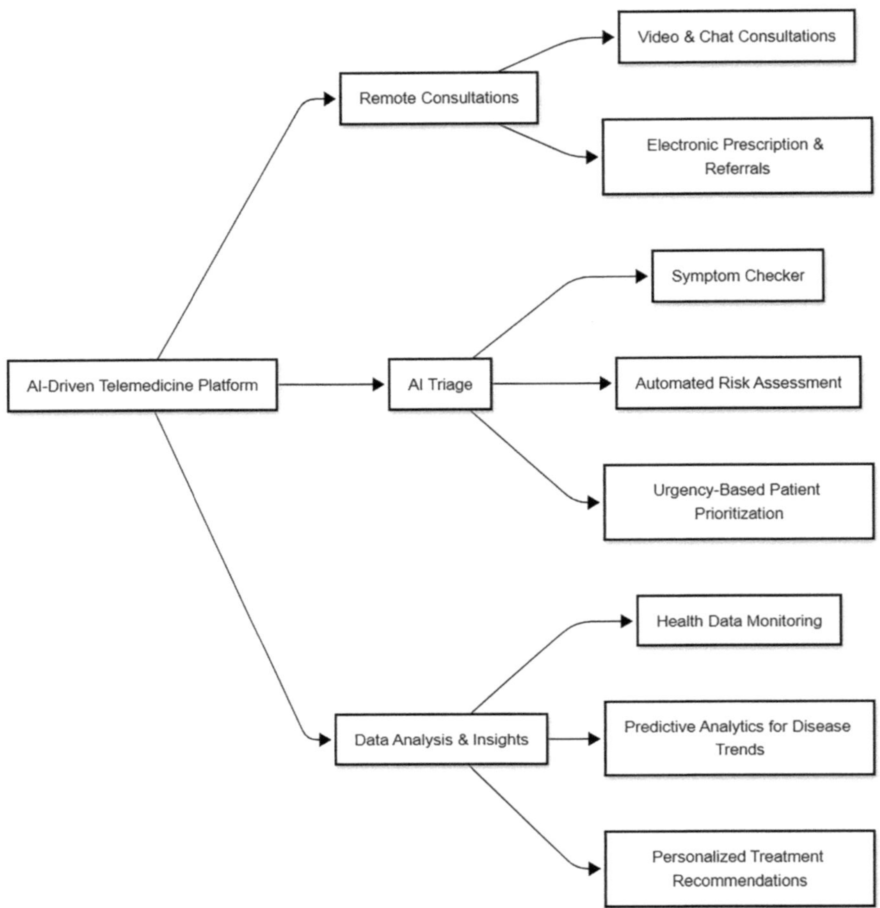


**Fig. 1.16** A diagram illustrating an AI-driven telemedicine platform, showing remote consultations, AI triage, and data analysis

rehearse complex procedures before operating, reducing complications and improving outcomes.

For example, computational fluid dynamics (CFD) models in cardiovascular surgery can simulate blood flow through arteries, helping surgeons determine the best placement of stents and grafts [67].

**AI and Simulations in Drug Testing**

Computational models are also being used to test new drugs and therapies without the need for extensive animal testing or early-stage human trials. These models can simulate how drugs interact at a molecular level, predicting their effectiveness and potential side effects.

Biomedical engineering today stands at the forefront of medical innovation. The field accelerates the transition towards personalized, predictive, and preventive medicine with innovative medical devices, AI-driven healthcare, and advanced computational modeling. As we move forward, biomedical engineers will continue to play a pivotal role in shaping the future of healthcare, ensuring that medicine becomes more efficient, accessible, and patient-centered than ever before.

## 1.3 Key Disciplines and Applications

Biomedical Engineering (BME) is an interdisciplinary field at the intersection of engineering, biology, and medicine. It is a dynamic and evolving discipline that harnesses the principles of various engineering fields to address complex biological and medical problems. By combining cutting-edge technology with a deep understanding of human biology, biomedical engineers develop innovative solutions that advance healthcare outcomes, improve patient quality of life, and enable more effective medical treatments.

Integrating engineering principles into medicine has led to numerous groundbreaking advancements, including improvements in diagnostic tools, medical devices, therapeutic techniques, and rehabilitation methods. As BME continues to expand and evolve, it gives rise to increasingly specialized domains, each dedicated to addressing specific healthcare challenges using tailored approaches and technologies [68]. This chapter explores the fundamental disciplines that form the foundation of BME, providing insight into the core areas that have shaped the field as we know it today.

The interdisciplinary nature of BME allows it to draw from a wide range of scientific and engineering domains. Determining the field's boundaries can be challenging. However, several core disciplines can be identified that encompass the key areas where engineering solutions are applied to biological and medical systems. These disciplines are critical in advancing the fundamental understanding of biological processes and developing new technologies that improve medical care [19].

Biomechanics is one of the most established and fundamental disciplines in biomedical engineering. It involves the study of the mechanical properties and behavior of biological systems, particularly focusing on the forces exerted by muscles and bones during movement. By understanding how forces interact within the body, biomedical engineers can design better medical devices, improve rehabilitation strategies, and optimize surgical procedures [69, 70].

Biomechanics has significant applications in designing prosthetic limbs, orthopedic implants, and assistive devices that help individuals recover from injuries or disabilities. Understanding the human body's response to physical forces also aids in improving the ergonomics of tools and work environments, preventing injury, and optimizing performance in various physical activities [71].

Biomaterials, either natural or synthetic, are another critical component of BME. They are materials designed to interact with biological systems for medical purposes. Biomaterials are pivotal in developing medical implants, prosthetics, and drug delivery systems, offering solutions to repair or replace damaged tissues and organs [72] (Fig. 1.17).

For instance, biomaterials are used to construct artificial joints, dental implants, and vascular stents. They must be biocompatible to avoid rejection by the immune system while also being durable enough to withstand the mechanical forces placed on them. The development of advanced biomaterials is a rapidly evolving field, with innovations such as biodegradable scaffolds used in tissue engineering and regenerative medicine.

Medical imaging technologies enable healthcare professionals to visualize the internal structures of the body without the need for invasive procedures. This area of Biomedical Engineering encompasses technologies such as X-rays, magnetic resonance imaging (MRI), ultrasound, and computed tomography (CT) scans, all of which have revolutionized how physicians diagnose and treat various medical conditions [61] (Table 1.1).

Medical imaging engineers work on improving the resolution, speed, and safety of these devices. One goal is to minimize patients' exposure to harmful radiation while obtaining high-quality diagnostic images [73]. Moreover, ongoing research is being conducted on the use of artificial intelligence (AI) in image interpretation, enabling radiologists to detect abnormalities more quickly and accurately.

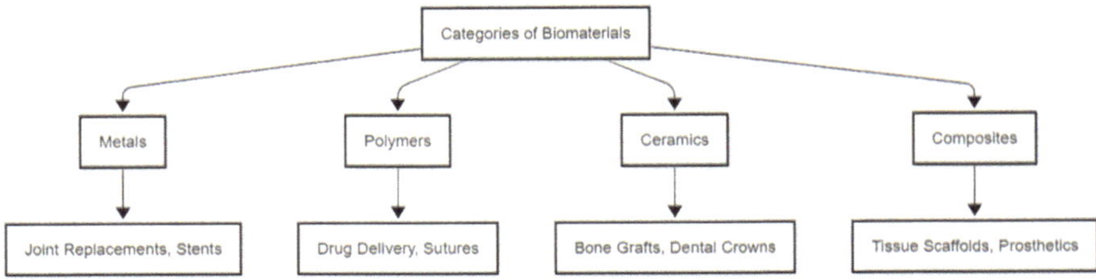


**Fig. 1.17** A flowchart showing the different categories of biomaterials

**Table 1.1** Medical imaging modalities

| CT | MRI | PET | SPECT | Ultrasound |
|---|---|---|---|---|
| | | | | |

Bioinformatics and systems biology use computational and statistical techniques to analyze biological data. Bioinformatics focuses on storing, retrieving, and analyzing data such as genetic sequences, while systems biology takes a broader approach, modeling the interactions within complex biological systems [74].

These fields are integral to personalized medicine, where treatments are tailored to the individual based on their genetic makeup, lifestyle, and environment. Integrating bioinformatics and systems biology into clinical settings enables more accurate predictions of disease risk and more effective treatment strategies tailored to a patient's unique biological profile.

This chapter will explore these disciplines in greater detail, examining how they interact and contribute to the development of advanced medical technologies. These disciplines serve as the foundation for numerous BME applications that directly impact the healthcare sector, and understanding them is crucial for appreciating the transformative power of BME in the modern medical landscape.

As we continue, the subsequent sections will delve deeper into the applications of BME across various medical fields, exploring the real-world challenges these disciplines address and the cutting-edge solutions being developed to improve patient care.

### *1.3.1 Disciplines of Biomedical Engineering*

**Biomechanics**

Biomechanics is one of the core disciplines within biomedical engineering, emphasizing the application of mechanical principles to biological systems. It involves understanding the forces exerted by muscles, the mechanical properties of tissues such as bones and cartilage, and the effects of movement on the body. Biomechanics aims to decipher how the body functions as a mechanical system and how it can be supported or enhanced through engineered solutions [69].

One of the foundational areas of biomechanics is the study of kinematics and kinetics. Kinematics focuses on describing motion without considering the forces that cause it, analyzing parameters such as velocity and acceleration. On the other hand, Kinetics explores the forces themselves, examining how they impact tissues and the body [75]. Understanding these forces allows biomedical engineers to design devices and systems for movement, rehabilitation, and injury prevention.

Biomechanics is pivotal in designing and developing medical devices, particularly those used for prosthetics and orthotics. Prosthetics aim to replace lost limbs, while orthotics are designed to support and correct body parts that are impaired or injured. Engineers use their knowledge of biomechanics to ensure that prosthetic limbs mimic natural human movement as closely as possible, creating devices that restore function and provide comfort and durability [76]. Joint implants such as those used in hip and knee replacements depend heavily on biomechanics. These implants must be designed to bear loads and endure stresses similar to natural bones, requiring careful analysis of the mechanical properties of the materials and the human tissues they interact with [77].

Additionally, biomechanics is crucial in developing rehabilitation engineering technologies, including devices like robotic exoskeletons. These systems assist patients with spinal cord injuries or other mobility impairments by augmenting their ability to walk or move. As technology advances, biomechanics is playing an increasing role in designing systems that help patients regain mobility, often through complex, computer-controlled devices that provide real-time feedback and assistance [78] (Fig. 1.18).

### Biomaterials

Biomaterials, natural or synthetic, form the foundation of many medical devices, implants, and therapeutic interventions in biomedical engineering. They are specifically designed to interact with the human body without causing harm. The key to

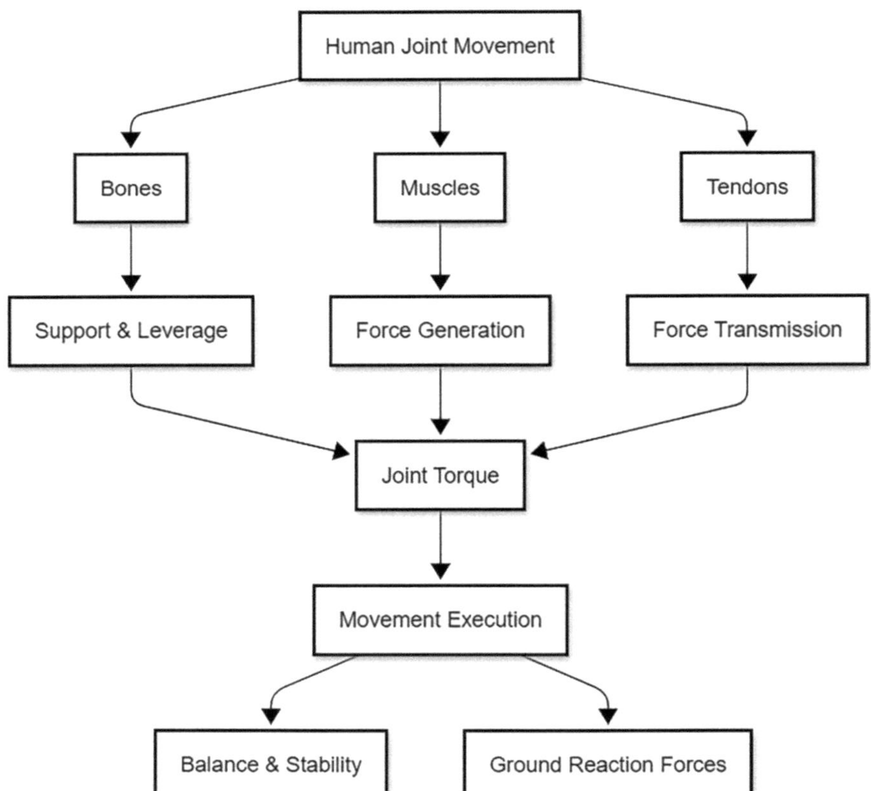


**Fig. 1.18** The interaction between bones, muscles, and tendons in human joint movement

their success lies in their biocompatibility, ensuring they do not elicit an adverse response from the immune system or cause toxicity or inflammation [79].

Biomaterials development often requires engineers to balance several important characteristics: mechanical properties, biodegradability, and tissue integration. For instance, in the design of orthopedic implants such as joint replacements, materials like titanium or cobalt-chromium alloys are often chosen for their strength and durability. These materials must endure the mechanical stresses of walking, running, and other daily activities. However, strength alone is not enough. The material must also integrate with the surrounding biological tissues to avoid complications such as implant failure or rejection [80]. Engineers must, therefore, consider factors such as the material's surface properties, which might be engineered to encourage tissue growth around it.

Biodegradability is crucial in specific biomaterial applications, such as drug delivery systems. Some medical devices are designed to slowly degrade over time, releasing drugs or healing agents at specific rates. Materials such as biodegradable polymers or hydrogels are often used in these applications because they can break down safely within the body without requiring surgical removal [81]. In the case of tissue engineering, biomaterials are used as scaffolds to support the growth of new tissues. These scaffolds can provide a framework for cells to grow and develop into functional tissues, a process vital for developing regenerative therapies or creating lab-grown organs [82].

Tissue engineering is one of the most exciting areas in which biomaterials are applied. Biomaterial-based tissue scaffolds serve as the foundation for the growth of new tissues, helping to regenerate damaged organs or even creating entirely new ones. This research has the potential to revolutionize medicine, offering solutions to organ shortages and improving the outcomes for patients with severe tissue damage [83].

### Computational Modeling and Simulation

Computational modeling and simulations are powerful tools that allow biomedical engineers to analyze complex biological systems and predict patient-specific outcomes. By simulating biological processes, such as blood flow, tissue growth, or drug delivery, engineers can make informed decisions about treatments, device designs, and surgical procedures. Computational models are increasingly used to predict the progression of diseases such as atherosclerosis or cancer, enabling healthcare providers to tailor interventions to individual patients [84].

Finite Element Analysis (FEA) and Computational Fluid Dynamics (CFD) are commonly used to model mechanical systems in the body, such as bone structures, joints, or blood vessels. These models help optimize the design of medical devices, like prosthetic limbs, implantable devices, and vascular stents, ensuring that they function as intended under real-world conditions [85] (Fig. 1.19).

Simulations are also used to enhance the development of drug delivery systems. Engineers can optimize drug formulations and improve their efficacy by modeling how drugs interact with tissues or travel through the body. This area of computational modeling helps in personalized medicine, where drug regimens can be adjusted based on individual patient profiles.

## Medical Imaging

Medical imaging is perhaps one of the most revolutionary advancements in modern medicine, allowing clinicians to peer inside the body without making a single incision. This discipline employs various technologies to visualize internal structures, diagnose diseases, monitor treatment progress, and guide interventions. The significance of medical imaging in healthcare cannot be overstated, as it enhances the accuracy of diagnoses and provides valuable insights that help shape patient care.

The most common imaging technologies include X-ray, CT, MRI, positron emission tomography (PET), and ultrasound. Each technology has strengths and limitations, making it suitable for different examinations. For instance, X-rays and CT scans are excellent for imaging bones and detecting fractures or tumors, while MRI provides detailed images of soft tissues, including the brain, spinal cord, and muscles. PET and other nuclear imaging techniques are used to evaluate metabolic activity, often in the context of cancer detection and monitoring. Ultrasound, a non-invasive and safe imaging modality, is widely used in obstetrics and cardiology [86].

A critical aspect of medical imaging is the resolution of the images produced. High-resolution imaging detects minute abnormalities, such as small tumors or subtle fractures, and is key to early disease detection. Advances in contrast agents have also improved the effectiveness of medical imaging. These agents enhance the visibility of specific tissues, making it easier to distinguish between healthy and abnormal areas. For instance, in MRI, contrast agents can highlight blood vessels or detect inflammation (Fig. 1.20).

Many medical imaging modalities rely on ionizing radiation, which can be harmful if used excessively. As a result, there is a growing focus on developing imaging technologies that either reduce radiation exposure or eliminate it, such as ultrasound or MRI. Additionally, engineers and medical professionals continuously work on improving imaging software, employing advanced image processing algorithms to

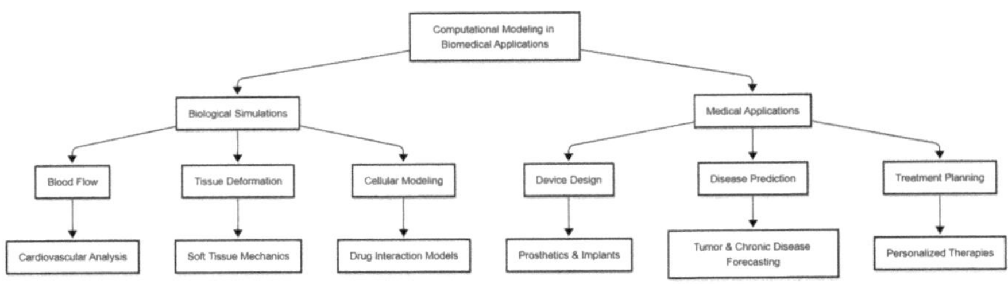


**Fig. 1.19** The computational modeling process to simulate biological systems and its applications in device design and disease progression prediction

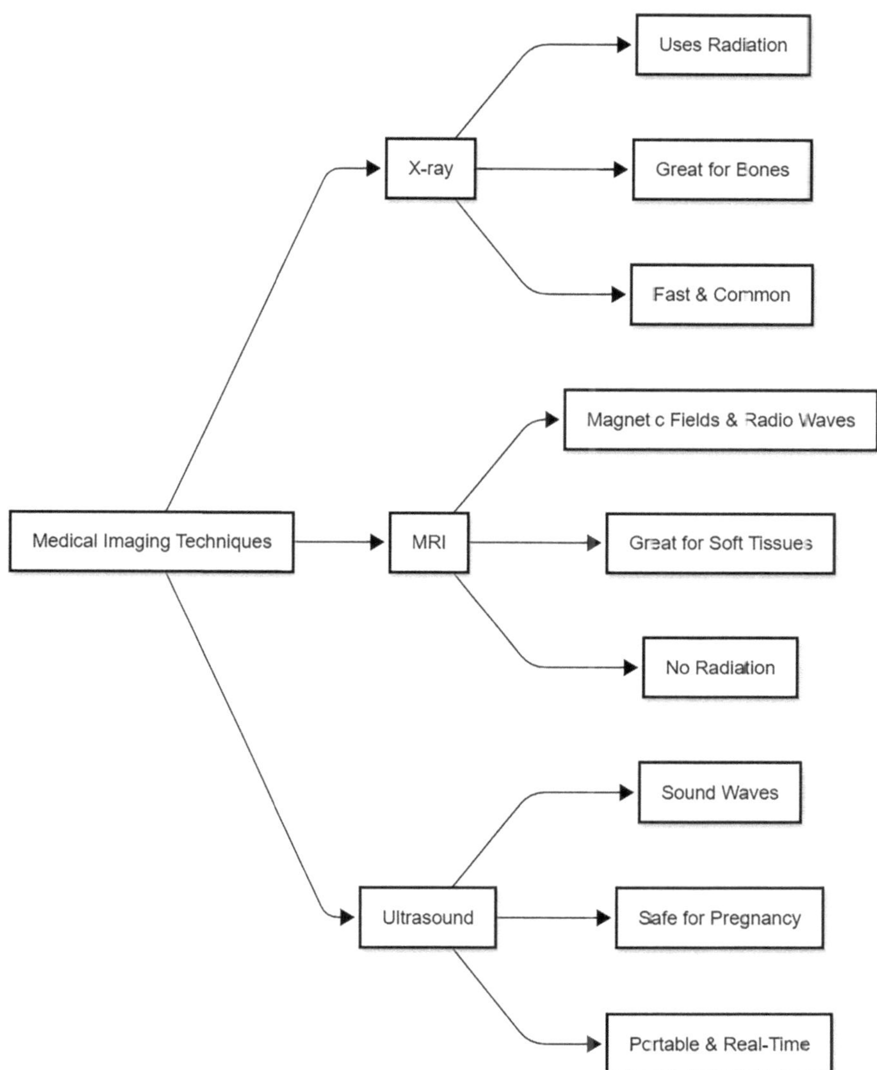


**Fig. 1.20** The principles of various medical imaging techniques

enhance image quality, reduce noise, and provide more accurate interpretations of the data [87].

Medical imaging is vital in interventional procedures, such as robot-assisted surgeries. In these surgeries, imaging systems are often used in real-time to guide the surgical tools, ensuring greater precision and minimizing the risk of complications. The integration of imaging with robotic systems is rapidly advancing, leading to the development of more sophisticated surgical techniques that are minimally invasive and highly effective [88].

## Medical Device Design

Medical device design is another essential discipline within biomedical engineering, concerned with creating tools, instruments, and devices for diagnosing, monitoring, and treating medical conditions. These devices range from simple tools like stethoscopes and thermometers to sophisticated instruments such as pacemakers, insulin pumps, and robotic surgery systems. The design process involves a thorough understanding of both engineering principles and biological systems to ensure that the devices are safe, effective, and capable of meeting the specific needs of patients and healthcare providers [12, 89]. One of the foundational aspects of medical device design is human factors engineering or ergonomics.

This principle focuses on designing user-friendly devices, particularly when healthcare professionals must operate them in high-stress environments. For instance, surgical instruments must be carefully crafted to allow precise manipulation, minimizing the risk of human error. Similarly, the design of patient-monitoring devices requires simplicity and intuitiveness so that clinicians can interpret results quickly and act accordingly. A practical design must balance technological complexity with ease of use, as even the most advanced device is ineffective if it cannot be operated or interpreted correctly [90].

Another significant aspect of medical device design is biocompatibility. Medical devices often come into direct contact with the body, so materials used in their construction must not cause an adverse biological reaction. This is crucial for implantable devices like pacemakers, stents, and joint replacements. Biocompatible materials, such as titanium, silicone, and specific polymers, are selected to ensure the device will function effectively without provoking immune system responses, infections, or other complications. The design of these devices often involves extensive testing to evaluate how the material will interact with body tissues over time [45, 91]. For instance, a stent inserted into an artery must be durable enough to withstand the mechanical forces exerted by blood flow while being gentle on the inner vessel walls to avoid irritation.

Sterility is another critical consideration in medical device design. Any device used in invasive procedures must be designed to maintain sterility through disposable components or by incorporating sterilization procedures into the device's design and manufacturing process [92]. The sterilization process—whether autoclaving, irradiation, or chemical sterilization—must be compatible with the materials used in the device to ensure that it remains functional and safe for use.

Medical device design also includes regulatory compliance. Regulatory bodies such as the U.S. Food and Drug Administration (FDA) and the European Medicines Agency (EMA) have stringent standards for medical devices before marketing. These regulations ensure that the devices are safe for patient use and perform as intended [93]. Engineers must collaborate with medical professionals to ensure that devices meet these standards, often conducting clinical trials and pre-market evaluations to demonstrate their efficacy and safety. The design process must account for these regulations at every step, from the initial concept to the final product, and include detailed documentation and testing to support regulatory submissions [94] (Fig. 1.21).

Prototyping and testing are fundamental stages of the design process. A prototype allows engineers to evaluate a device's functionality, usability, and safety before it goes into mass production. Testing may include mechanical tests, clinical trials, and simulations to assess the device's performance in real-world settings [95]. For example, a new type of catheter may undergo stress tests to ensure it does not break or cause harm when inserted into the body. If a device is implantable, it may undergo biocompatibility tests to ensure it does not cause an inflammatory response in the body [96].

In some cases, devices must be designed to operate in specialized environments, such as the intensive care unit (ICU) or operating room (OR). Devices used in these settings, like ventilators, infusion pumps, or surgical robots, must be robust, highly reliable, and able to function in high-pressure, critical conditions. The design of these devices often incorporates advanced technologies like wireless communication, allowing for remote monitoring and management of patients [97].

## *1.3.2 Applications of Biomedical Engineering*

### Tissue Engineering and Regenerative Medicine

Tissue engineering and regenerative medicine represent some of the most innovative areas of biomedical engineering, offering the potential to repair or replace damaged tissues and organs. Engineers can create scaffolds that promote tissue regeneration by combining biomaterials, cells, and growth factors. For example, engineered skin grafts and bone scaffolds are already being used to treat burn victims and fractures, and research is ongoing to develop more complex organs, such as livers and kidneys, to reduce the need for organ transplants [12, 98].

An up-and-coming area within regenerative medicine is stem cell therapy, which aims to harness stem cells' regenerative potential to treat various diseases. Researchers are exploring using stem cells to repair damaged cardiac tissue in heart disease, regenerate neurons in neurodegenerative disorders, and repair joints in osteoarthritis. This application holds immense promise for revolutionizing treatments in various medical fields [99] (Fig. 1.22).

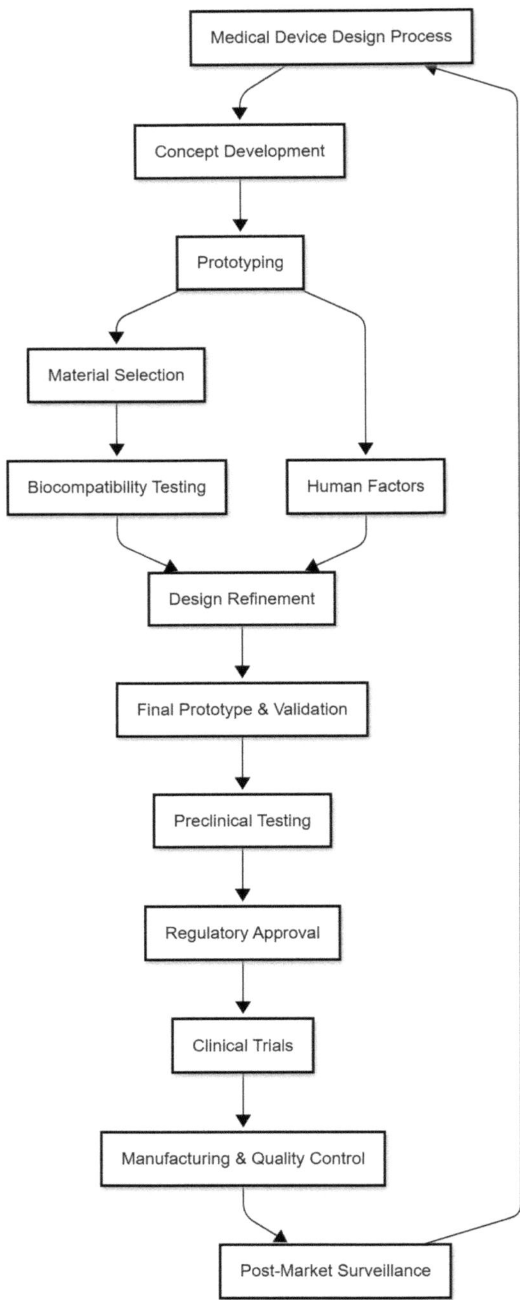


**Fig. 1.21** A flowchart illustrating the stages of medical device design, from concept and prototyping to regulatory approval and testing

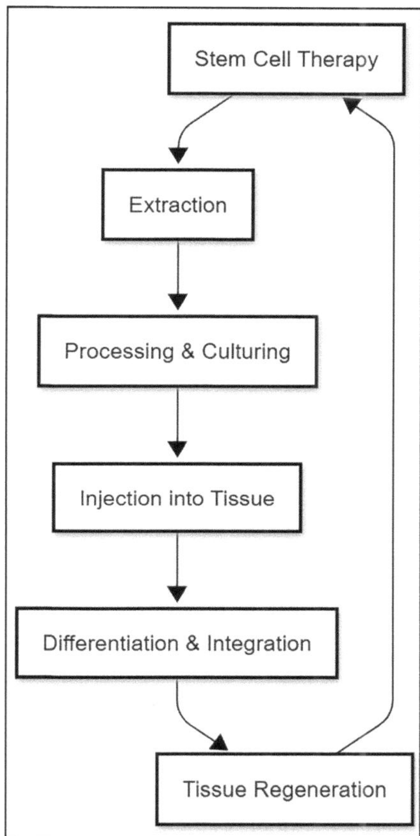


**Fig. 1.22** A diagram illustrating the use of stem cells to repair tissue

## Prosthetics and Assistive Technologies

The development of prosthetics and assistive technologies has dramatically improved the lives of individuals with disabilities. Advances in bionic limbs, robotic prosthetics, and neuroprosthetics have enabled patients to regain mobility and function. Modern prosthetics, which are often controlled by brain signals or muscle movements, offer a more natural range of motion and better integration with the user's body [100].

For example, neuroprosthetics use electrodes to detect electrical signals from the brain or muscles, which can then control the movements of prosthetic limbs. These devices enable users to perform complex tasks such as grasping, walking, or even fine motor movements, giving them greater autonomy. AI-powered prosthetics take this further, learning the user's preferences and adapting to their movements [101] (Fig. 1.23).

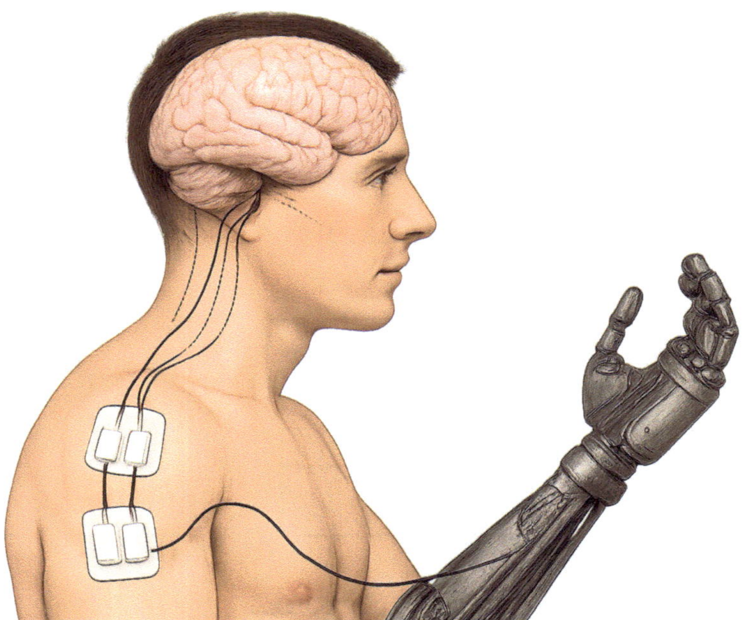

**Fig. 1.23** The connection between a neuroprosthetic limb and the brain through EMG signals, allowing for advanced movement control

Assistive technologies extend beyond prosthetics, including devices that help individuals with hearing or visual impairments. Hearing aids amplify sound and filter background noise, giving patients better access to speech and communication. Smart wheelchairs equipped with sensors can assist with navigation and movement, allowing greater independence for users with limited mobility [102].

## Biomedical Sensors and Wearable Health Technologies

Wearable health technologies and biomedical sensors have emerged as powerful tools in monitoring and managing health. These devices continuously collect physiological data, enabling real-time health assessments and early detection of abnormalities. For example, wearable fitness trackers monitor heart rate, step count, and even sleep patterns, providing valuable insights into an individual's health. More advanced devices, such as continuous glucose monitors (CGMs), offer diabetic patients continuous feedback on their blood sugar levels, enabling proactive management of the condition.

In clinical settings, biomedical sensors track various patient metrics, such as oxygen saturation, blood pressure, and heart rate. These sensors are increasingly integrated into telemedicine platforms, allowing healthcare providers to monitor

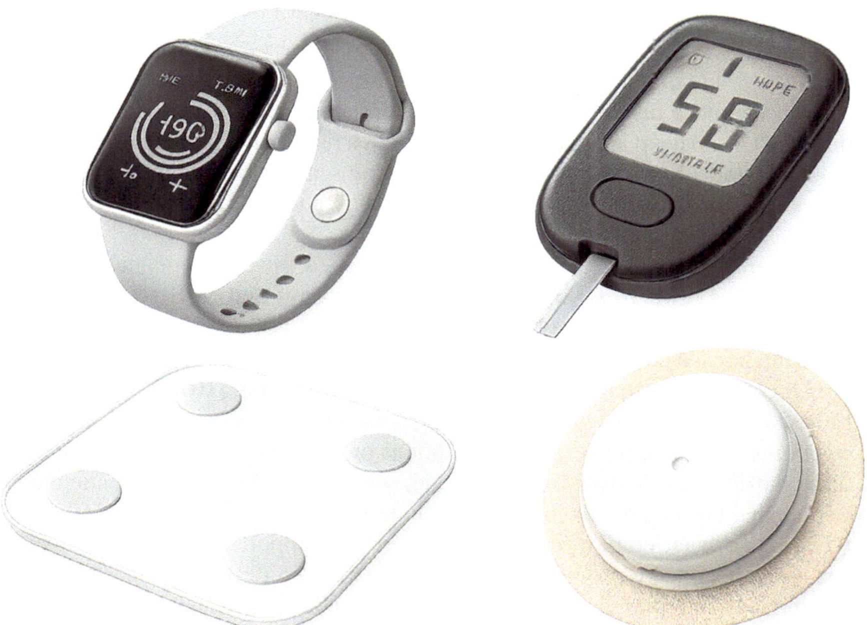

**Fig. 1.24** Various wearable health devices

patients remotely. This integration is particularly beneficial for patients in rural or underserved areas, as it improves access to healthcare and reduces the need for frequent in-person visits [55, 65] (Fig. 1.24).

### Robotics and Minimally Invasive Surgery

Medical robotics and minimally invasive surgery are revolutionizing the field of surgery. Robotic systems, such as the da Vinci Surgical System, allow surgeons to perform procedures with greater precision and control. These systems improve the accuracy of surgical procedures, particularly in delicate areas like the prostate, heart, and brain, reducing the risk of complications and speeding up recovery times [103, 104].

Robotic surgery also allows for minimally invasive procedures, which reduce the size of incisions and the associated risks of infection and scarring. Surgeons can operate through small incisions with the help of robotic arms, video cameras, and other advanced technologies. This approach has applications in various types of surgery, including urological, cardiovascular, and gynecological procedures [105].

**Artificial Intelligence in Diagnostics**

Integrating AI into diagnostic systems has revolutionized how healthcare providers detect and diagnose diseases. AI algorithms, particularly those based on machine learning (ML) and deep learning (DL), have shown remarkable potential in processing vast amounts of medical data, such as imaging scans, electronic health records, and genomic data, to provide accurate diagnoses and predict patient outcomes [59, 106].

AI-driven systems have already been implemented in various diagnostic areas, such as radiology, where algorithms can analyze X-rays and MRI scans to detect anomalies like tumors, fractures, or lesions. AI models trained on large datasets of medical images have achieved diagnostic accuracy comparable to human experts, making them valuable tools for early detection and screening [107, 108].

Moreover, AI plays a key role in genomics, where machine learning models analyze genomic data to identify genetic mutations or predict the likelihood of disease. AI also contributes to personalized medicine, where algorithms process patient data to recommend tailored treatment plans, optimizing therapeutic outcomes [109].

AI has also been employed in clinical decision support systems, where algorithms assist healthcare providers in making data-driven decisions. These systems help clinicians interpret lab results, identify potential risks, and select the most appropriate treatment for patients, improving the overall efficiency and quality of care [9, 11, 110] (Fig. 1.25).

## 1.4 Ethical, Legal, and Social Considerations

Biomedical engineering (BME) is one of the most dynamic and transformative fields in modern science and healthcare. As it continues to evolve, it presents an ever-expanding range of innovative solutions that promise to revolutionize the treatment of diseases, the management of health conditions, and the overall functioning of healthcare systems. With such rapid advancements, however, comes a range of significant challenges that require careful consideration. As biomedical engineers develop groundbreaking technologies, they must do so within a framework that considers the ethical, legal, and social implications of their work [111]. Ethical, legal, and social domains guide biomedical engineers to create solutions that advance medicine, ensure patient safety, promote fairness, and protect human rights.

The ethical questions surrounding biomedical engineering innovations often delve into fundamental issues of human dignity, autonomy, and justice. Biomedical engineers must consider how their inventions will affect individuals and society, asking whether the benefits of a new technology outweigh the risks, and whether the technology respects patients' rights and promotes overall well-being. Ethical considerations are particularly pressing in fields like genetic engineering, artificial intelligence (AI) for diagnostics, and robotic surgery, where new technologies may blur the lines between what is considered safe and what could potentially introduce

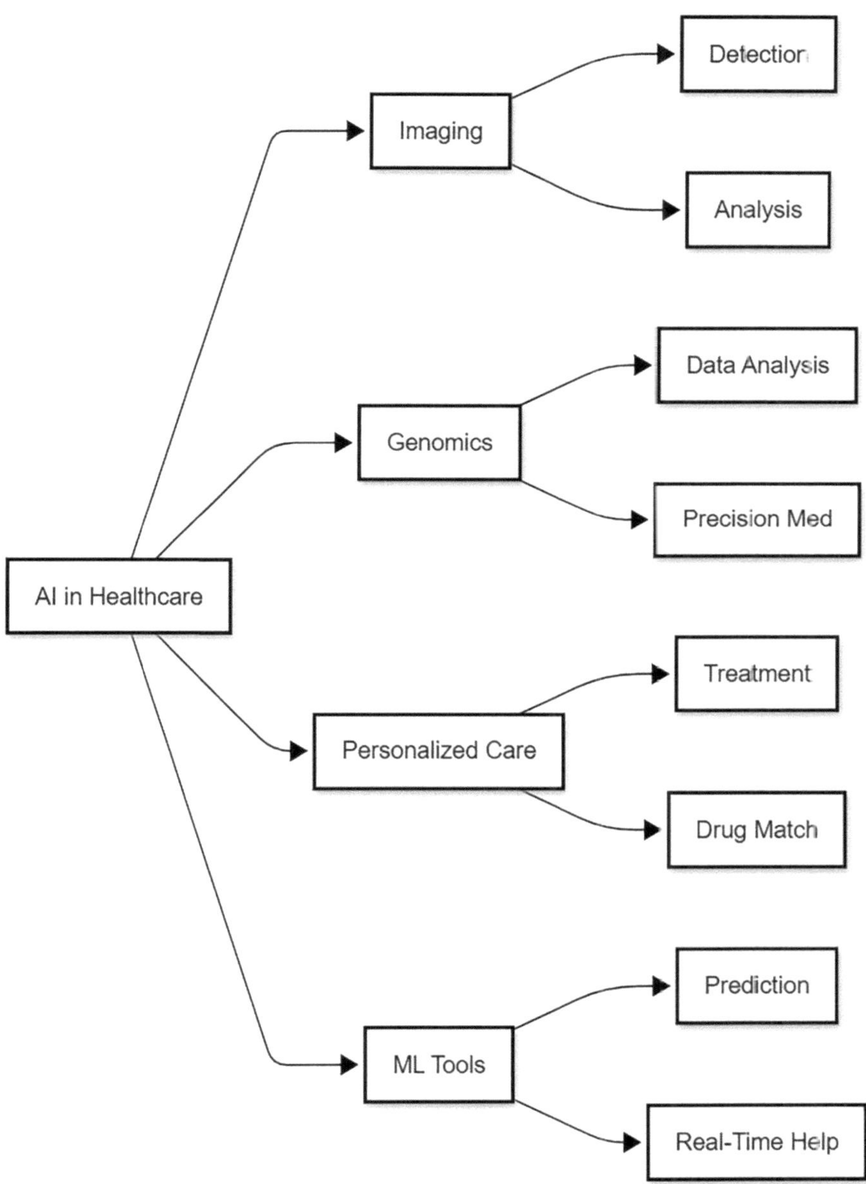


**Fig. 1.25** AI applications in diagnostic imaging, genomics, and personalized medicine

harm or exploitation [112]. The principle of "do no harm" is particularly pertinent in this context, where the potential for error or unintended consequences may have far-reaching impacts.

Legal considerations serve as the guardrails for biomedical engineering, ensuring that inventions meet specific safety and regulatory standards and are used appropriately. Legal frameworks help ensure biomedical engineers follow established protocols for designing, testing, and deploying medical devices, treatments, and technologies. These legal frameworks aim to protect the patients who will ultimately use these technologies and the professionals who may use them in clinical settings regulations, and the ethics of human subject research. For example, how do we regulate emerging technologies such as AI in medical imaging or predictive diagnostics to ensure they comply with accuracy, fairness, and transparency standards? These questions are vital in protecting the rights of individuals and ensuring that medical advancements are both practical and accessible.

The social considerations of biomedical engineering explore the broader implications of technological advances on society. While the primary aim of biomedical engineering is to improve healthcare, its impact extends beyond individual patients to entire populations and communities. New biomedical technologies may improve access to healthcare, save lives, and enhance quality of life, but they also have the potential to create or exacerbate social inequalities [113, 114]. For example, introducing sophisticated medical devices or cutting-edge genetic treatments may be inaccessible to underserved communities due to their high costs. Furthermore, cultural, regional, and societal differences may exist in how new technologies are perceived or accepted. These differences must be carefully considered when developing and deploying biomedical innovations. The goal is to ensure that new technologies do not disproportionately benefit one group at the expense of another and that healthcare solutions are equitable and inclusive. This chapter explores the growing recognition that biomedical engineers must take social responsibility seriously, ensuring that the innovations they develop serve the broader needs of society.

The interrelationship between ethics, law, and society is integral to biomedical engineering. These domains are not standalone but are interconnected and profoundly influence each other. Biomedical engineers must balance their technical expertise with a deep understanding of the ethical, legal, and social issues that accompany their work. By incorporating these considerations into their practice, biomedical engineers can help ensure that the technologies they develop are innovative, effective, but also responsible, ethical, and fair [111].

This chapter aims to provide a comprehensive overview of these three critical domains—ethics, law, and social responsibility—and explore how they intersect and guide the work of biomedical engineers. As students, professionals, and practitioners in biomedical engineering, we must deeply understand the ethical, legal, and social implications of the technologies we create, the policies we advocate for, and the innovations we bring into the world. These considerations are not merely regulatory or theoretical concerns but fundamental to the sustainable and responsible development of biomedical engineering solutions.

In this chapter, we will first introduce the ethical considerations that govern biomedical engineering. From patient rights and informed consent to the ethical challenges of new technologies such as gene editing and Artificial Intelligence (AI), we will discuss how biomedical engineers must navigate complex moral landscapes when designing and implementing new tools and systems. The legal considerations section will examine the regulatory environment that influences the biomedical field, with a focus on the significance of safety standards, patent laws, and the evolving role of international law in regulating biomedical technologies. Finally, we will examine the social considerations of biomedical engineering, addressing how societal factors such as healthcare access, socioeconomic disparities, and cultural values influence the development and adoption of biomedical innovations.

### *1.4.1 Ethical Principles in Biomedical Engineering*

At the heart of ethical considerations in biomedical engineering lies the understanding of the core principles of bioethics, which include autonomy, beneficence, nonmaleficence, and justice. These principles are foundational guidelines that help biomedical engineers navigate the complex decision-making landscape when creating and deploying medical technologies [115].

Autonomy refers to a patient's right to make their own decisions regarding their healthcare, informed by all relevant information. Autonomy is a guiding principle in biomedical engineering when engineers design technologies that require patient interaction, such as wearable devices or diagnostic tools. Respecting patient autonomy means providing individuals with all necessary information to make informed decisions about their treatment and allowing them to retain control over their health data [116] (Fig. 1.26).

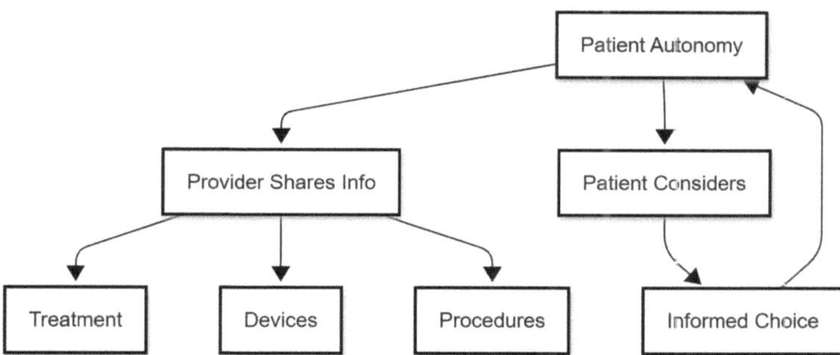


**Fig. 1.26** A concept of patient autonomy in decision-making, where the patient is informed about treatment options, medical devices, and procedures, with a balance of information presented by the healthcare provider

Beneficence refers to the obligation of doing good and promoting the well-being of patients. Biomedical engineers must design technologies and systems that contribute to individuals' health and quality of life, ensuring that their work positively impacts the patients it is intended to serve. In practice, this means that engineers must evaluate the potential benefits of a new medical device or system and ensure that it improves patient outcomes, whether it is through greater accuracy in diagnosis or enhanced efficiency in treatments [117].

Non-maleficence is the principle of "do no harm," a fundamental ethical guideline for all biomedical engineering practices. Biomedical engineers must ensure that the technologies they develop do not harm patients, directly through malfunctioning devices or indirectly through unforeseen consequences. This principle applies to everything from medical equipment safety to the potential for over-treatment or unnecessary risk in clinical settings [118].

Justice refers to fairness in the distribution of healthcare benefits and the prevention of discrimination. Biomedical engineers must ensure that their innovations are accessible and equitable, with particular attention given to underserved populations who may not have access to the latest technologies. The ethical principle of justice in BME also encompasses issues like affordability, cultural considerations, and the prioritization of healthcare resources.

### Ethical Issues in Biomedical Engineering Technologies

Biomedical engineers must deal with various ethical issues throughout medical technologies' design, development, and deployment [119]. These issues include:

#### Informed Consent and Patient Privacy

Informed consent is a critical ethical issue in BME, especially when new technologies are introduced into clinical settings. Patients must be provided with clear and comprehensive information about medical procedures, devices, or technologies being used. This ensures they fully understand potential risks, benefits, and alternatives. Informed consent also extends to the use of medical data, where the privacy and confidentiality of patient information must be maintained [120] (Fig. 1.27).

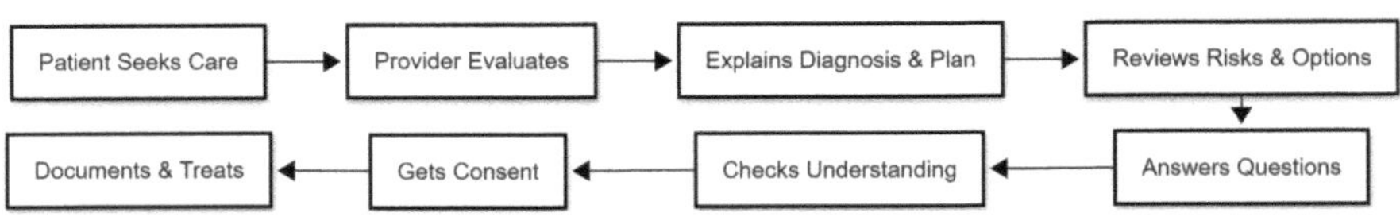


**Fig. 1.27** The steps in the informed consent process for patients when using new medical devices or undergoing procedures

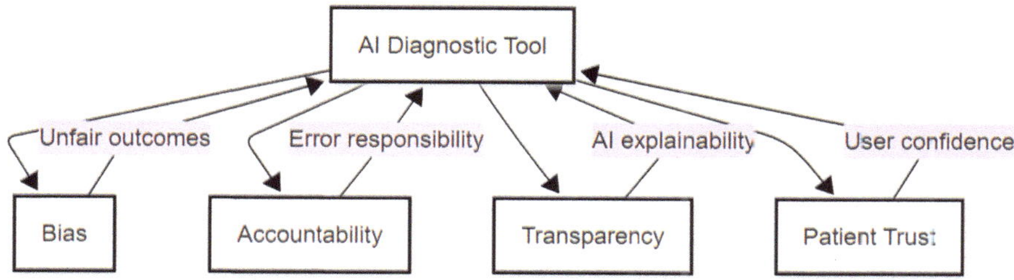


**Fig. 1.28** The ethical considerations in AI-based diagnostic tools

### The Use of Artificial Intelligence in Healthcare

AI and machine learning technologies are transforming medicine by enabling more accurate diagnostics, personalized treatments, and predictive analytics. However, these advancements raise several ethical concerns, including the reliability of AI in decision-making, algorithmic bias, and the issue of accountability. To prevent inequalities in healthcare delivery, it is essential to ensure that AI systems are transparent, explainable, and free from bias [61, 121] (Fig. 1.28).

### Genetic Engineering and CRISPR Technology

Clustered Regularly Interspaced Short Palindromic Repeats (CRISPR) technology has opened up new possibilities for genetic engineering, enabling gene editing and the treatment of genetic disorders. However, genetic modifications also raise significant ethical questions, including concerns about the unintended consequences of altering the human genome, the potential for "designer babies," and the implications of gene editing for future generations [122].

### Robotics and Human Enhancement

Robotics plays a growing role in surgery, prosthetics, and rehabilitation. The ethical issues associated with robotic systems include patient safety, the dehumanization of care, and the balance between technological advancement and human touch (Almand, 2023). Additionally, robotics may raise questions about the potential for human enhancement, such as using robotic systems to augment human physical capabilities beyond natural limits [6, 123] (Figs. 1.29 and 1.30).

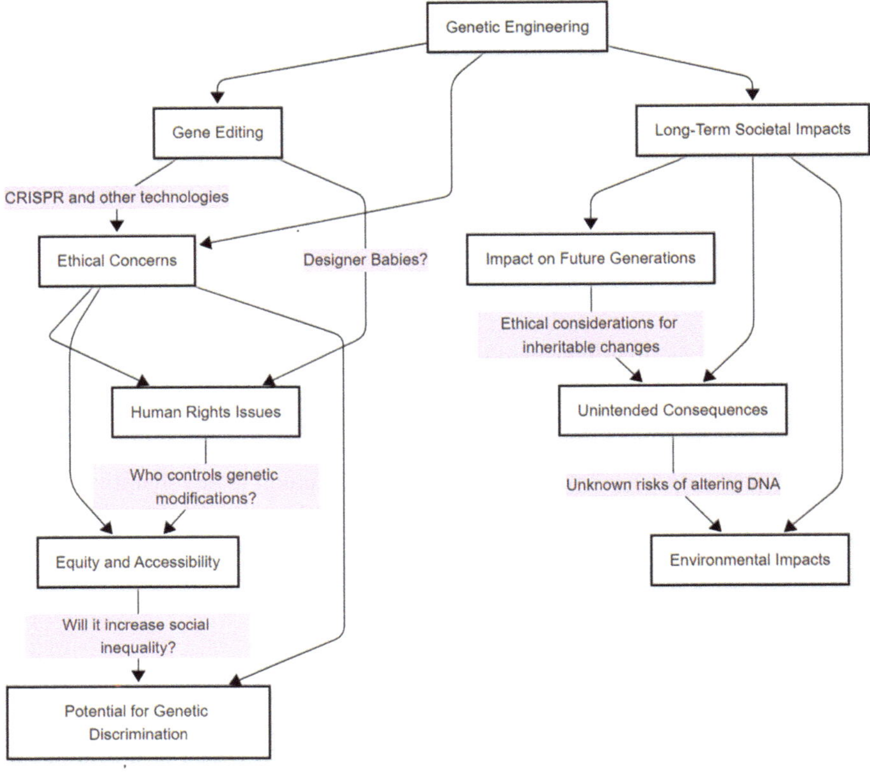


**Fig. 1.29** The ethical concerns and considerations in genetic engineering

## Ethical Issues in Clinical and Research Settings

Biomedical engineers work in both clinical and research settings, and in both environments, they must address several ethical challenges. Clinical trials are essential for testing new medical technologies, treatments, and devices. However, conducting research involving human subjects requires strict adherence to ethical guidelines, including ensuring informed consent, minimizing risks to participants, and maintaining the integrity of the research process [124]. Ethical concerns also arise when research involves vulnerable populations, such as children, the elderly, or individuals with disabilities [125] (Fig. 1.31).

Biomedical engineers often collaborate with pharmaceutical companies, medical device manufacturers, and other stakeholders. However, these relationships can create potential conflicts of interest. Engineers must ensure that their decisions are guided by the best interests of patients and the integrity of their work, rather

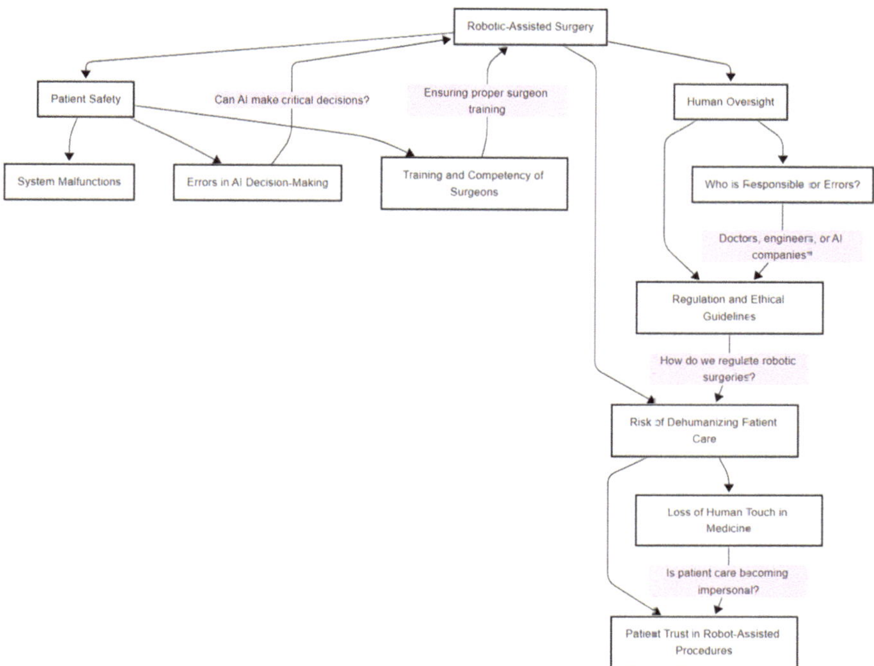


**Fig. 1.30** The ethical challenges in robotic-assisted surgery

than by financial incentives or external pressures [126]. Biomedical engineers play a vital role in addressing these ethical challenges through careful design, thoughtful implementation, and a commitment to patient safety and well-being. As the field of biomedical engineering continues to advance, engineers must develop a strong understanding of ethical principles and work closely with medical professionals, patients, regulatory bodies, and policymakers to ensure that the technologies they develop are not only practical but also ethical and socially responsible [127].

The field of biomedical engineering is rapidly advancing, and with these advancements come complex ethical, legal, and social challenges. The role of ethical considerations in BME cannot be overstated, as engineers must ensure that their innovations contribute to the greater good of society while minimizing harm. From the ethical principles of autonomy, beneficence, non-maleficence, and justice, to the practical concerns surrounding informed consent, patient privacy, and the responsible use of emerging technologies, biomedical engineers must work diligently to address these issues [128]. As biomedical engineers continue to shape the future of medicine, they must remain steadfast in their commitment to ethical practices, ensuring that the technologies they create are not only revolutionary but also grounded in a strong ethical framework that respects patient rights, promotes justice, and ensures the equitable distribution of healthcare

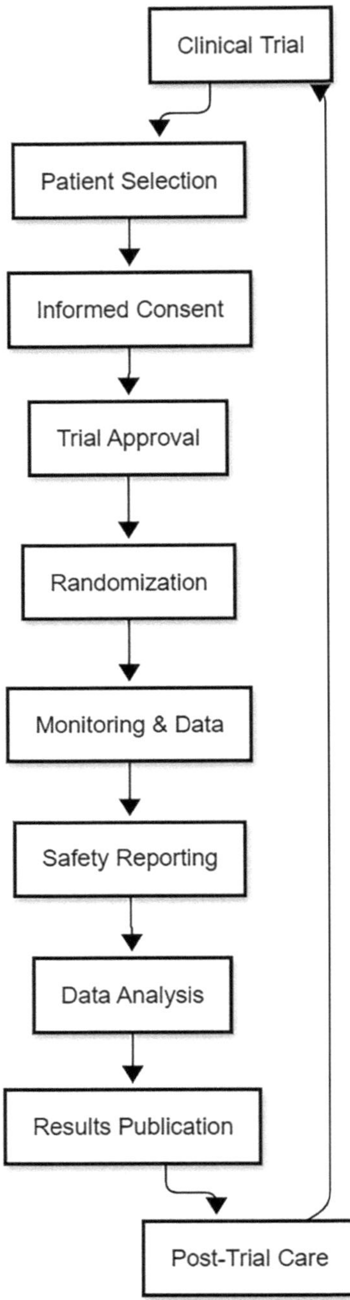


**Fig. 1.31** The process of conducting ethically sound clinical trials, from patient selection to post-trial care and reporting

resources [71]. Through careful consideration of ethical issues and a deep commitment to responsible innovation, biomedical engineers can continue to drive progress in the healthcare sector while preserving the trust and well-being of patients worldwide [129].

### 1.4.2 Legal Implications of Biomedical Engineering

The legal implications of BME encompass various issues that biomedical engineers, healthcare professionals, and organizations must navigate to ensure that innovations are practical and ethical and comply with applicable laws and regulations. Understanding these legal aspects is essential for maintaining public safety, patient rights, and the responsible development of medical technologies. Biomedical engineering has far-reaching implications across various facets of law, including intellectual property, regulatory compliance, product liability, privacy laws, and medical malpractice. This chapter will explore the key legal issues in biomedical engineering and examine the frameworks and regulations that govern the' design, development, and deployment of medical technologies.

#### Regulatory Framework for Biomedical Engineering

One of the most critical legal considerations in biomedical engineering is ensuring that medical devices, technologies, and procedures comply with the regulatory requirements established by governmental bodies. These regulations are in place to protect patients and ensure that medical products are safe, effective, and properly labeled [130].

In most countries, regulatory agencies oversee the approval and monitoring of medical devices and technologies. In the United States, the Food and Drug Administration (FDA) is central in regulating medical devices, including those developed by biomedical engineers. The FDA classifies medical devices into three categories—Class I, Class II, and Class III—based on the level of risk they pose to patients. The regulatory requirements vary depending on the class of the device, with Class III devices (such as pacemakers or artificial heart valves) undergoing more rigorous testing and approval processes than lower-risk devices [131]. In Europe, the European Medicines Agency (EMA), along with national regulatory authorities, oversees medical devices under the European Union's Medical Device Regulation (MDR) and In Vitro Diagnostic Regulation (IVDR). These regulations ensure that medical devices are subjected to strict pre-market and post-market surveillance processes, including clinical evaluations, risk assessments, and compliance with essential safety and performance requirements [22, 132].

For a medical device to be legally sold or distributed, it must often bear certification marks, such as the CE mark in the European Union, indicating that the device complies with relevant health, safety, and environmental protection standards [133].

The FDA approval or clearance is another necessary certification for devices in the U.S. Biomedical engineers must understand these certifications and the associated processes to navigate the legal landscape effectively [134] (Fig. 1.32).

### Intellectual Property in Biomedical Engineering

Biomedical engineering is strongly driven by creativity and technological progress, leading to continuous development of new concepts, designs, innovations, and inventions. Biomedical engineers often work with groundbreaking technologies that may have the potential for significant commercial success. Understanding IP laws is essential for safeguarding these innovations and ensuring their creators and developers benefit from their work [135].

One of the primary tools for protecting biomedical inventions is the patent system. A patent grants the inventor exclusive rights to their invention for a specified period (typically 20 years). This protection is crucial in the biomedical field, where novel devices, technologies, and methods must be protected from unauthorized use or reproduction [136]. The patent application process requires a detailed description of the invention, including its novel features, technical specifications, and potential applications. Biomedical engineers often patent their innovations in medical devices, diagnostic tools, and therapeutic technologies [137]. However, the patent process is complex, as patents must meet specific criteria, including novelty, non-obviousness, and utility. In addition to the patent, engineers must consider potential licensing agreements and disputes with other patent holders or companies [138].

In some cases, biomedical engineers may choose to protect their innovations through trade secrets rather than patents. Trade secrets involve keeping valuable information confidential and protecting it from unauthorized disclosure. This can include proprietary algorithms, design specifications, or manufacturing processes crucial to a medical device's success [139]. Unlike patents, trade secrets do not require public disclosure, which can offer a competitive advantage in rapidly evolving markets. However, trade secrets must be carefully safeguarded, as their legal protection relies on maintaining confidentiality [140] (Figs. 1.33 and 1.34).

### Product Liability and Biomedical Engineering

Product liability is a key area of law that addresses the responsibility of manufacturers and designers when their products cause harm or injury to users. Biomedical engineers must be acutely aware of the potential risks associated with their designs and innovations to avoid legal consequences of defective products [141].

In the context of biomedical engineering, product liability concerns may arise from defective medical devices that cause harm to patients. These can be categorized

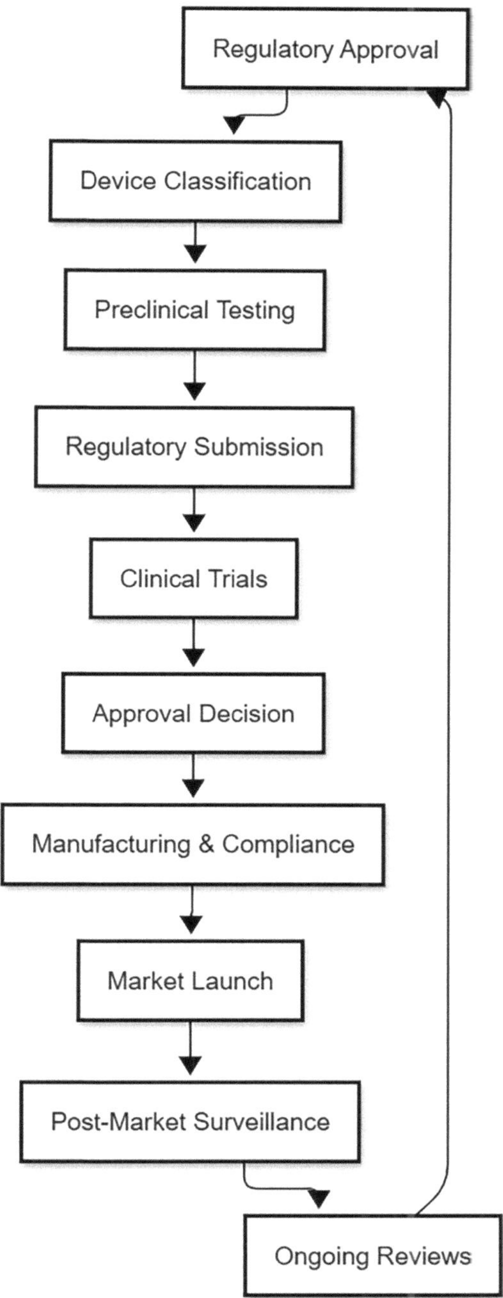


**Fig. 1.32** The regulatory approval process for medical devices

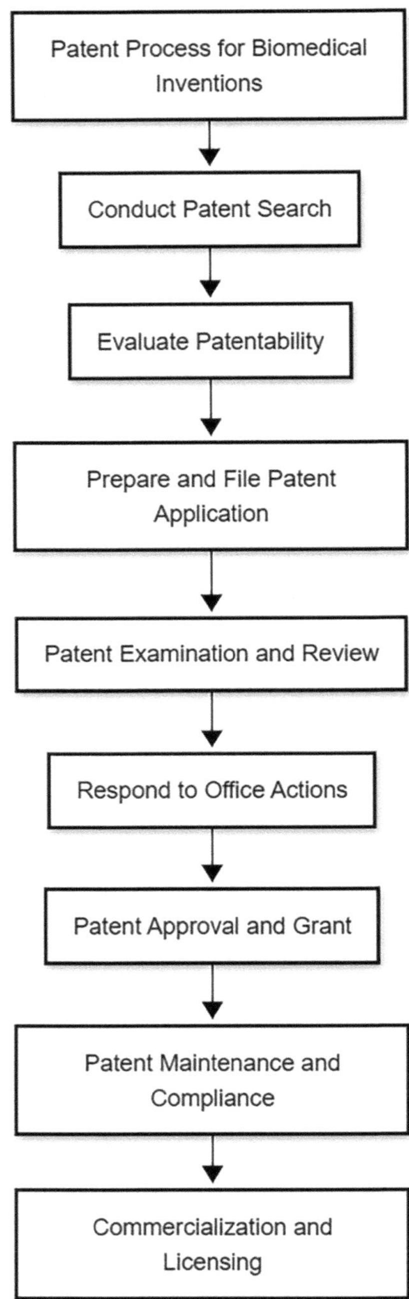


**Fig. 1.33** The steps involved in the patent process for biomedical inventions

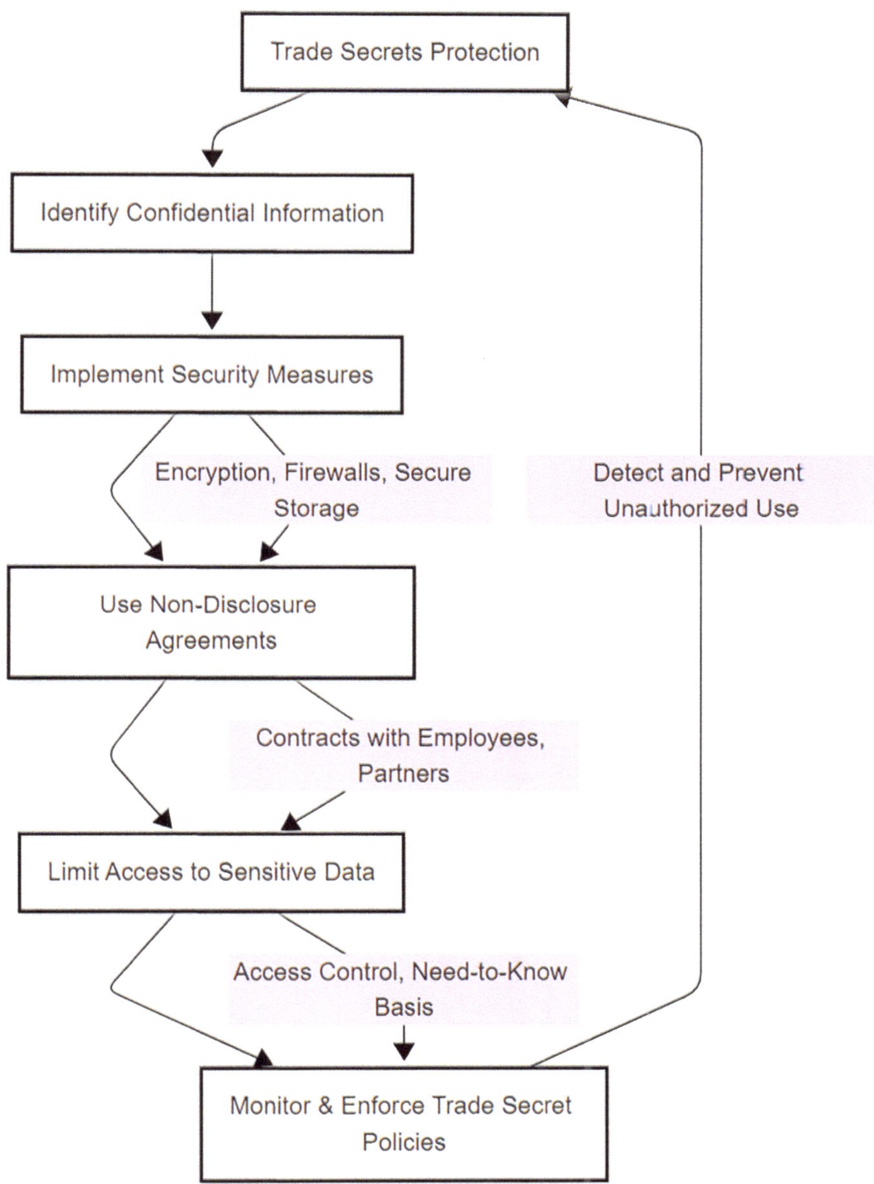


**Fig. 1.34** The concept of trade secrets, including non-disclosure agreements and secure data management

as manufacturing, design, or marketing (e.g., failure to provide adequate warnings or instructions). If a medical device malfunctions or causes injury due to a defect, the manufacturer, designer, and even the biomedical engineer may be liable for damages [4]. Manufacturers must ensure that their devices are safe, and engineers must follow stringent testing and quality control processes to minimize the risk of defects. Patients who suffer harm from defective products can take legal action, and in some cases, class-action lawsuits may be filed if many individuals are affected [132] (Fig. 1.35).

In the development and commercialization of biomedical devices, companies must follow structured procedures and clearly defined phases to mitigate the legal risks associated with product liability. This includes conducting rigorous testing, including preclinical and clinical trials, and ensuring compliance with regulatory standards and safety protocols [142]. Regular post-market surveillance is also essential to identify any emerging issues with medical devices once they are in widespread use [143].

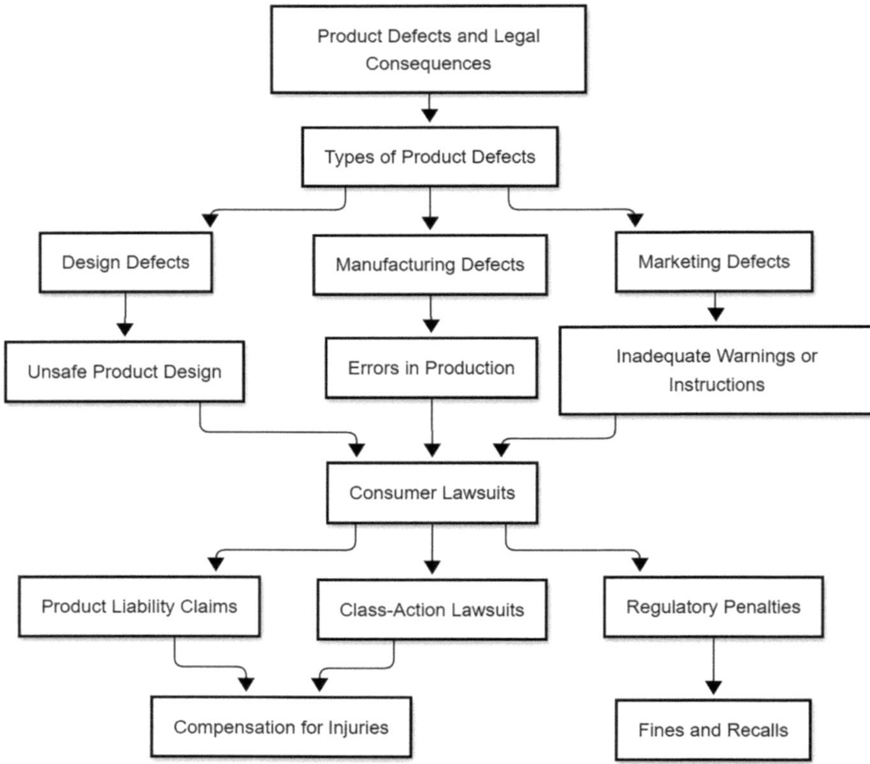


**Fig. 1.35** A flowchart illustrating the different types of product defects and their potential legal consequences, including lawsuits and regulatory penalties

### Privacy Laws and Data Protection

Patient data collection, storage, and use are critical legal considerations in biomedical engineering. Ensuring patient privacy and data protection is paramount with the increasing use of digital health technologies, wearables, and AI-driven diagnostics. Violations of privacy laws can lead to legal actions, fines, and reputational damage to organizations [144].

In many countries, privacy laws regulate the use and sharing of health information. In the United States, the Health Insurance Portability and Accountability Act (HIPAA) sets strict guidelines for the confidentiality and security of health data. Biomedical engineers must design technologies that comply with these privacy regulations, ensuring patient information is protected from unauthorized access or breaches [145].

With the rise of big data and AI in healthcare, data ownership and access issues have become increasingly important. Critical legal questions are who owns patient data and has the right to access it. Biomedical engineers must design systems that allow patients to control their health data while ensuring it is accessible to authorized healthcare providers and researchers [146].

### Medical Malpractice and Liability

Medical malpractice involves the failure of healthcare providers to meet accepted standards of care, leading to patient harm.

In biomedical engineering, medical malpractice may occur if a medical device fails to function as intended, resulting in injury or death. Engineers, manufacturers, and healthcare providers may face liability for medical malpractice if they are found to have contributed to the harm caused by a defective device (Figs. 1.36, 1.37 and 1.38).

The legal landscape surrounding biomedical engineering is complex and multifaceted. To ensure their innovations are legally compliant and ethically sound, biomedical engineers must be well-versed in medical device regulatory requirements, intellectual property laws, product liability, privacy regulations, and medical malpractice [147]. By understanding these legal implications and taking proactive steps to address them, biomedical engineers can minimize legal risks and contribute to the responsible development and deployment of medical technologies that improve patient care and outcomes. In this rapidly evolving field, staying informed about the latest legal trends and developments is crucial for biomedical engineers. Legal frameworks will continue to evolve alongside technological advancements, and engineers must be adaptable, proactive, and ethical in their design, development, and deployment [148]. By working with regulatory bodies, legal professionals, and healthcare providers, biomedical engineers can help ensure that their innovations are groundbreaking, legally sound, and beneficial to society [149].

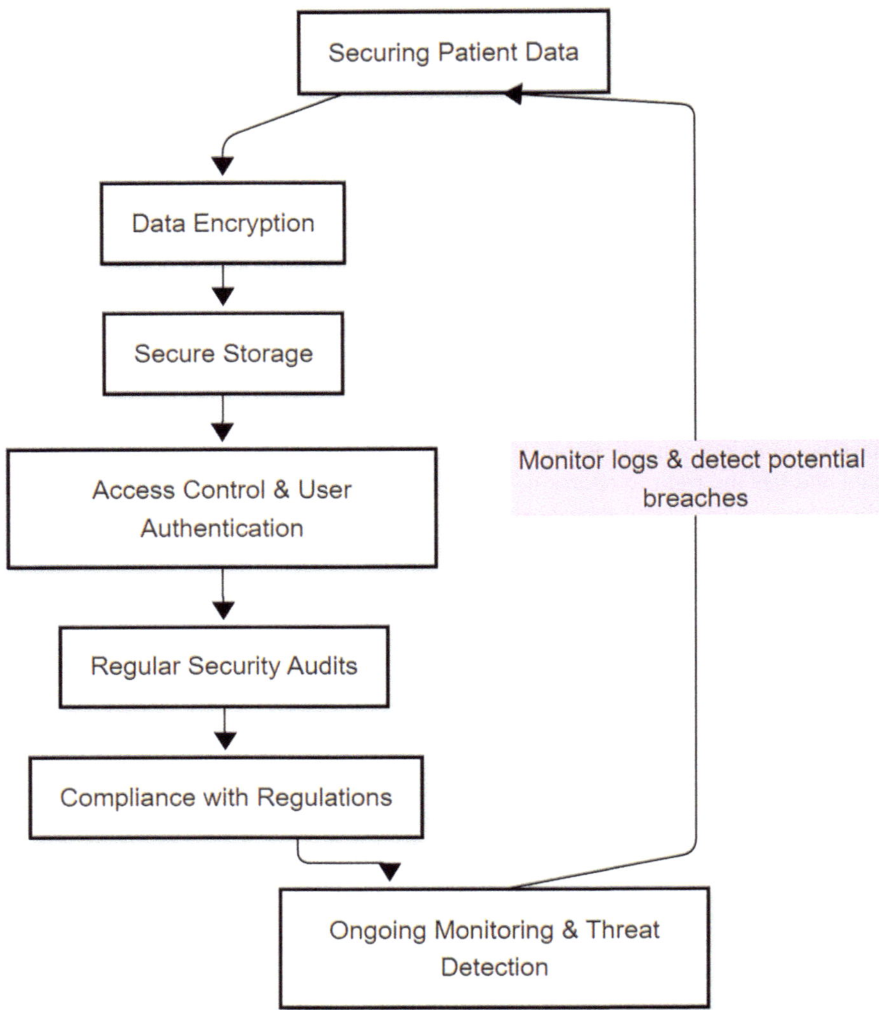


**Fig. 1.36** The steps involved in securing patient data

### *1.4.3 Societal Implications of Biomedical Engineering*

Biomedical engineering has made remarkable strides in recent decades, revolutionizing the healthcare landscape with innovations from life-saving medical devices to personalized diagnostic tools. However, with these advancements come important societal implications that must be addressed to ensure that the benefits of BME are distributed equitably, ethically, and sustainably. As biomedical technologies

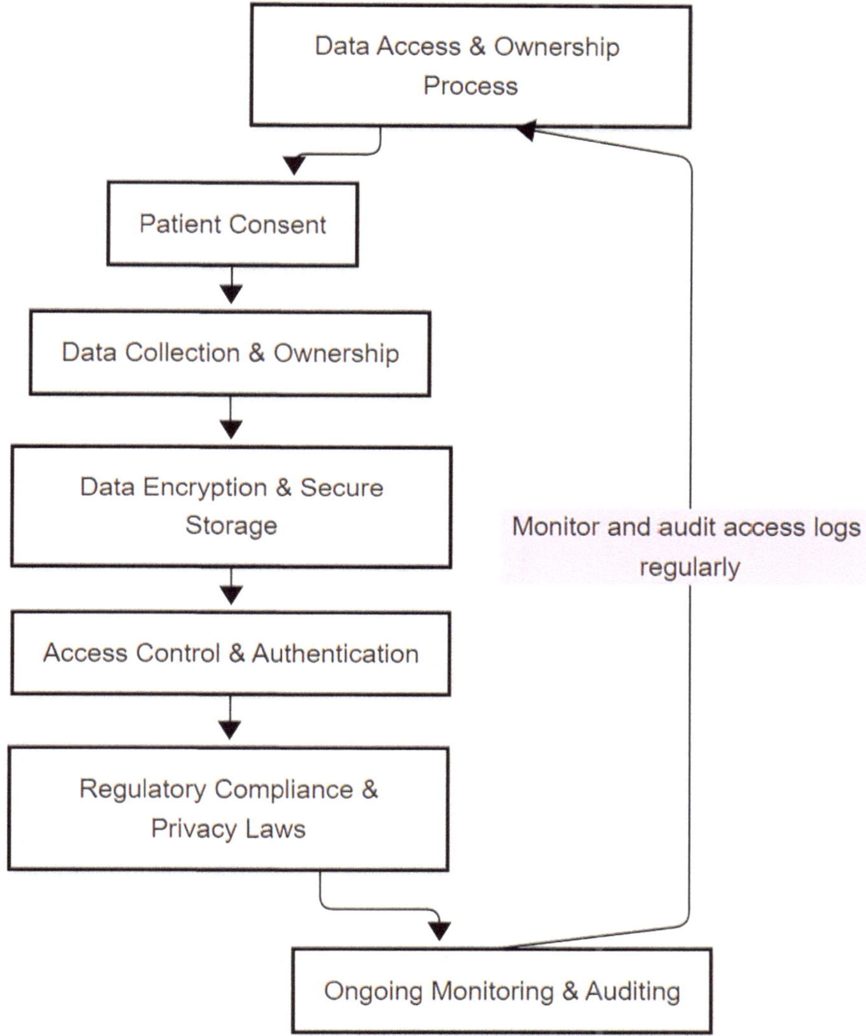


**Fig. 1.37** The process of data access and ownership

increasingly influence public health, patient care, and even individual lifestyles, it becomes vital to consider the broader impact on society, culture, and the environment. The societal implications of BME can be viewed through various lenses, including access to healthcare, the potential for social inequality, the impact of new technologies on human behavior, and the environmental footprint of biomedical innovations. This chapter delves into these dimensions, examining the impact of BME on society and the necessity for responsible innovation.

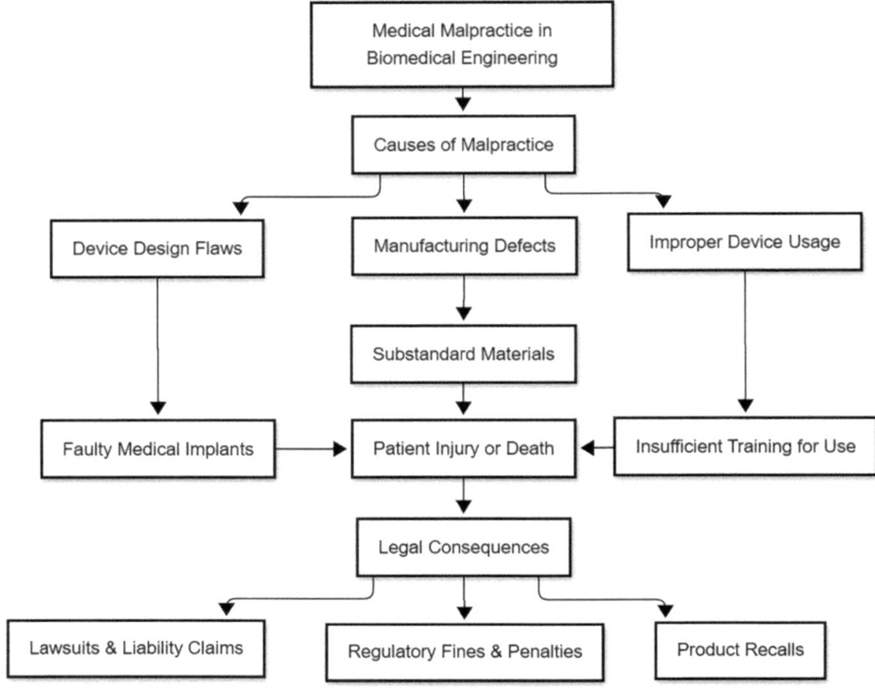


**Fig. 1.38** The concept of medical malpractice in the context of biomedical engineering

## Access to Healthcare

One of the most profound societal impacts of BME is its potential to improve or limit access to healthcare. Biomedical engineering innovations, such as medical devices, diagnostic tools, and assistive technologies, can transform healthcare delivery, particularly in under-resourced areas. Devices such as portable ultrasound machines, low-cost prosthetics, and diagnostic kits are already making healthcare more accessible in developing countries. However, there are significant challenges in ensuring these innovations reach everyone who needs them [52, 150]. The cost of cutting-edge medical devices and technologies can be prohibitive, particularly in low-income communities. Biomedical engineers must consider these economic constraints during the design and development phases to create affordable solutions that can be scaled globally.

While innovations in BME promise to alleviate many global health challenges, disparities in healthcare access remain a significant issue. Many of the most advanced biomedical technologies are developed and marketed in high-income countries, with substantial demand and purchasing power. Meanwhile, low-income countries may lack the infrastructure, resources, or regulatory frameworks to adopt these technologies [151]. Biomedical engineers can play a role in bridging this gap

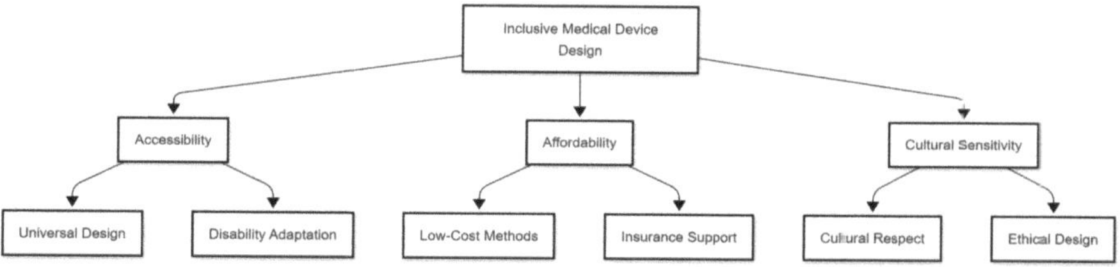


**Fig. 1.39** Inclusive medical device design

by focusing on developing affordable, portable, and culturally appropriate medical devices tailored to the needs of these populations.

The design of medical technologies must also account for health equity and inclusion. This includes ensuring that devices and diagnostic tools are accessible to all population groups, including vulnerable populations such as the elderly, people with disabilities, and marginalized communities [152]. Incorporating inclusive design principles in BME is essential to ensure that new technologies do not inadvertently exacerbate existing inequalities. Moreover, integrating technology into healthcare delivery systems must ensure that it complements traditional care practices and addresses the unique needs of diverse populations [153] (Fig. 1.39).

## Social Inequality and Technological Divide

While biomedical engineering can potentially enhance the quality of life for many, it also raises concerns regarding social inequality. The rapid pace of technological innovation, particularly in fields like personalized medicine, genetic engineering, and AI-powered diagnostics, may widen the gap between the "haves" and the "have-nots" [150]. As the healthcare industry increasingly adopts digital health technologies, such as telemedicine, wearable health monitors, and AI-driven diagnostic tools, there is a risk that those without access to technology may be left behind [154]. The digital divide could disproportionately affect low-income communities, rural areas, and the elderly, who may lack access to the internet, smartphones, or the technical literacy necessary to benefit from digital health innovations [155]. The development of user-friendly technologies that are both affordable and accessible is critical to addressing this divide. For instance, while smartphones are becoming increasingly ubiquitous, some people in underserved regions may still lack reliable internet access, rendering telemedicine or remote monitoring solutions less viable [17, 156]. Addressing these disparities requires a concerted effort to design and implement solutions that consider socioeconomic factors and ensure broader access to the benefits of BME.

The potential for biomedical technologies to exacerbate social inequalities is not limited to access. There are also concerns about the social implications of genetic engineering, gene editing, and other cutting-edge biotechnologies [157]. Technologies such as CRISPR and gene therapies hold tremendous promise in treating genetic diseases. However, they also raise ethical questions about the potential for genetic modification to enhance 0 traits in ways that could perpetuate social

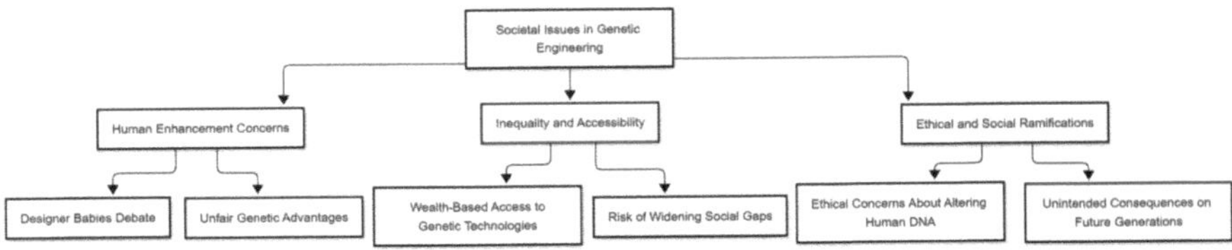


**Fig. 1.40** A potential societal issue related to genetic engineering

inequality (Schultz-Bergin, 2018). This could lead to new forms of discrimination, where individuals with access to genetic enhancements are viewed as superior, while those without are marginalized [158] (Fig. 1.40).

## Impact on Human Behavior

Biomedical engineering technologies have the power to influence patient care and human behavior. The ability to monitor, analyze, and even alter biological processes through medical technologies can raise fundamental questions about autonomy, privacy, and the role of technology in human life [119].

Medical technologies, particularly those involving monitoring or intervention, can affect an individual's autonomy. For example, wearable devices that track a person's health data may empower individuals to take charge of their health. However, they also raise concerns about privacy and personal data control [159]. Invasive medical devices or interventions, such as deep brain stimulators or genetic therapies, challenge the boundaries of personal autonomy by altering the biological functions of the human body [160].

Ethical debates also emerge when considering the balance between the potential benefits of these technologies (such as improving quality of life or extending life expectancy) and the loss of personal control. Striking this balance requires careful consideration of biomedical interventions' moral and philosophical implications [161].

Advances in biomedical engineering can also have unintended consequences on human behavior. For example, technologies that enable constant monitoring of an individual's health or genetic predispositions could lead to a "surveillance society," where individuals feel pressured to conform to specific health standards or lifestyle choices [162]. Employers may increasingly require employees to wear health-monitoring devices to track their physical activity or stress levels in the workplace, raising concerns about privacy and the potential for discrimination based on health data [163].

## Environmental Impact

Another critical societal implication of biomedical engineering is its environmental impact. The production, use, and disposal of biomedical devices and materials can have significant environmental consequences [164]. Biomedical engineering has the potential to reduce the environmental footprint of healthcare by developing sustainable medical technologies that are both effective and environmentally friendly [165].

The biomedical industry is a significant producer of medical waste, including single-use devices, packaging materials, and biohazardous materials [166]. Proper disposal and recycling of medical waste are essential to prevent environmental damage and reduce pollution [167]. Biomedical engineers are increasingly tasked with designing medical devices that are more sustainable, using biodegradable or recyclable materials and reducing the need for single-use items [45]. New manufacturing processes that minimize waste and reduce energy consumption are also emerging to mitigate the environmental impact of the healthcare sector [168] (Fig. 1.41).

Green innovation refers to the development of environmentally sustainable technologies that minimize environmental harm while still meeting the needs of healthcare providers and patients [169]. For example, biodegradable medical implants, eco-friendly diagnostic devices, and energy-efficient medical equipment can all contribute to a more sustainable healthcare system [170]. Biomedical engineers can drive these innovations by integrating sustainability into the design and development processes [171] (Fig. 1.42).

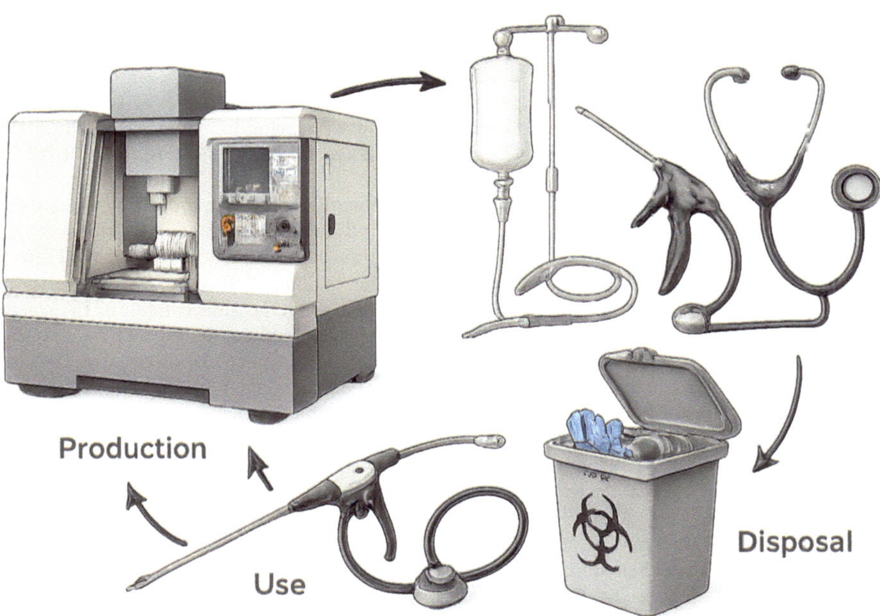


**Fig. 1.41** The lifecycle of medical devices from production to disposal

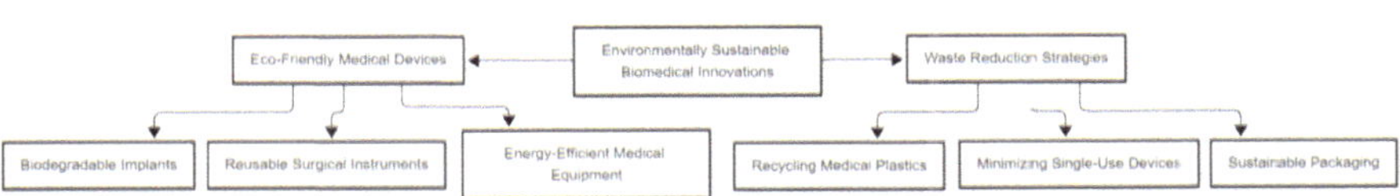


**Fig. 1.42** Examples of environmentally sustainable biomedical innovations

## References


1. Vashishth TK, Sharma V, Sharma KK, Chaudhary S, Kumar B, Kumar P. Future trends and emerging technologies in biomedical engineering. In: Innovations in biomedical engineering. Academic Press; 2025. p. 519–50.
2. Quon S, Low S. Bridging the gap in biomedical engineering education by integrating local context. Res Dev Med Educ. 2024;13(1):18.
3. Javaid M, Haleem A, Singh R, Suman R. Sustaining the healthcare systems through biomedical engineering. Biomed Technol. 2023;1:39.
4. Badnjević A, Pokvić LG, Hasičić M, Bandić L, Mašetić Z, Kovačević Ž. Evidence-based clinical engineering: machine learning algorithms for prediction of defibrillator performance. Biomed Signal Process Control. 2019;54:101629.
5. Badnjević A, Gurbeta L, Jimenez ER, Iadanza E. Testing of mechanical ventilators and infant incubators in healthcare institutions. Technol Health Care. 2017;25(2):237–50.
6. Badnjević A, Gurbeta Pokvić L, Spahić L, Kovačević Ž. Prediction of medical device performance using machine learning techniques: infant incubator case study. Health Technol. 2020;10(1):151–5.
7. Shalkharov S, Shalkharova Z, Shalkharova Z, Rysbekov K, Shalkharova S, Paromova Y, Petrova Y. Biomedical engineering as a modern component of science in biology and medicine. J Biomim Biomater Biomed Eng. 2021;53:67–75.
8. Enderle J, Bronzino J, editors. Introduction to biomedical engineering. London: Academic Press; 2012.
9. Hafizović L, Čaušević A, Deumić A, Bećirović LS, Pokvić LG, Badnjević A. The use of artificial intelligence in diagnostic medical imaging: systematic literature review. In: 2021 IEEE 21st international conference on bioinformatics and bioengineering (BIBE). IEEE; 2021. p. 1–6.
10. Hayaliev R, Nurkhodjaev S, Nazarova N, et al. Interdisciplinary approach of biomedical engineering in medical devices. J Biomim Biomater Biomed Eng. 2021;53:85–92.
11. Qamar SUR, Spahić L, Benolić L, Živanović M, Filipović N. Treatment of peripheral artery disease using injectable biomaterials and drug-coated balloons: safety and efficacy perspective. Pharmaceutics. 2023;15(7):1813. https://doi.org/10.3390/pharmaceutics15071813.
12. Spahić L, Mašetić Z, Badnjević A, Kurjak A, Pokvić LG. Artificial intelligence-based ultrasound imaging classification for infant neurological impairment disorders: a review. In: Mediterranean conference on medical and biological engineering and computing; 2023.
13. Mann M, Qavi I, Zhang N, Tan G. Engineers in medicine: bridging disciplines. Crit Rev Biomed Eng. 2023;51(2):19–32.
14. Merdović N, Spahić L, Hundur M, Pokvić LG, Badnjević A. Advancement of post-market surveillance of medical devices leveraging artificial intelligence: infusion pumps case study. Technol Health Care. 2024;33(2):915–21.
15. Nam S, Kim D, Jung W, Zhu Y. Understanding the research landscape of deep learning in biomedical science: Scientometric analysis. J Med Internet Res. 2022;24(4):e28114.
16. Šećkanović A, Šehovac M, Spahić L, Ramić I, Mamatnazarova N. Review of artificial intelligence application in cardiology. In: 2020 9th Mediterranean conference on embedded computing (MECO). IEEE; 2020. p. 1–5. https://doi.org/10.1109/MECO49872.2020.9134339.
17. Spahić L, Jeremić L, Lalatović I, Muratović T, Džuho A, Gurbeta Pokvić L, Badnjević A. Machine learning for improved medical device management: a focus on defibrillator performance. Technol Health Care. 2024;33:737–43.
18. Hashimoto S. How do students learn artificial intelligence in interdisciplinary field of biomedical engineering? J Syst Cybern Inform. 2023;21(4):87–91.
19. Gupta A, Kumar S. A study on biomedical engineering in healthcare. IJMLNCE. 2020;3:229–38.
20. Sitti M. Introducing progress in biomedical engineering. Prog Biomed Eng. 2020;2(2):020201.
21. Vuković D, Šumar S, Dupovac S, Badnjević A. Cost effectiveness analysis of medical devices in legal metrology system. In: Badnjević A, Cifrek M, Magjarević R, Džemić Z, editors. Inspection of medical devices, Biomedical engineering. Cham: Springer; 2024.

22. Badnjević A, Pokvić LG, Deumić A, Bećirović LS. Post-market surveillance of medical devices: a review. Technol Health Care. 2022;30(6):1315–29.
23. Penhaker M. Biomedical engineering in the 21st century and in the future. In: 2022 IEEE 20th jubilee world symposium on applied machine intelligence and informatics (SAMI). IEEE; 2022. p. 11–2.
24. Khan MY, Chen M-H. A review on role of biomaterials in biomedical field. Int J Biomed Res. 2019;8(9):2788–93.
25. Paul S, Riffat M, Yasir A, Mahim MN, Sharnali BY, Naheen IT, et al. Industry 4.0 applications for medical/healthcare services. J Sens Actuator Netw. 2021;10(3):43.
26. Kennedy SM, Vasanthanathan A, Jeen Robert RB, Vignesh Moorthi Pandian A. Impact of mechanical engineering innovations in biomedical advancements. In Vitro Models. 2024;3(1):5–18.
27. Sindhwani S, Chan WC. Nanotechnology for modern medicine: next step towards clinical translation. J Intern Med. 2021;290(3):486–98.
28. Taher M, Alam MK, Khan MM, Mannan M, Hossain MA. A brief analysis of the ancient Roman medical system. Int J Unani Integr Med. 2019;3:37.
29. Güemes LEA, Cusumano AM. Education and medical practice in ancient Greece, the Alexandrian period and the Western Roman empire: advantages and disadvantages from a contemporary perspective. Asian J Educ Soc Stud. 2022;35(2):54–63.
30. Supady J. Ancient Greek medicine during Hellenistic age and the Roman empire. Med Rev J. 2020;11:28–34.
31. Panegyres K. The Greco-Roman contribution to lifestyle medicine. Lifestyle Med. 2024;5(3):e111.
32. Schuez I, Alt KW. Leonardo da Vinci and dental anatomy. J Anat. 2022;240(2):183–96.
33. Standring S. A brief history of topographical anatomy. J Anat. 2016;229:1–5.
34. Akhtar ZB. Exploring biomedical engineering (BME): advances within accelerated computing and regenerative medicine for a computational and medical science perspective exploration analysis. J Emerg Med OA. 2024;2:1–23.
35. Mohsen M, Hussain M, Mustafa K, Mostafa M. Advancements in optical technologies for medical imaging and diagnosis. Int J Sci Res. 2023;2:92–117.
36. Gharibshahian M, Torkashvand M, Bavisi M, Aldaghi N, Alizadeh A. Recent advances in artificial intelligent strategies for tissue engineering and regenerative medicine. Skin Res Technol. 2024;30(9):e70016.
37. Cannard C, Wahbeh H, Delorme A. Electroencephalography correlates of well-being using a low-cost wearable system. Front Hum Neurosci. 2021;15:745135.
38. Spahić L, Sredović U, Kurpejović Z, Mrdanović E, Pokvić G, Badnjević A. Machine learning for improved medical device management: a focus on infant incubators. Technol Health Care. 2025;33:2034.
39. Pokvić LG, Deumić A, Softić A, Badnjević A. Application of artificial intelligence for management of maintenance and prediction of performances. In: Badnjević A, Cifrek M, Magjarević R, Džemić Z, editors. Inspection of medical devices, Biomedical engineering. Cham: Springer; 2024.
40. Neumann T, Brück R, Gaus O. Business plan ready—an interdisciplinary approach in teaching and learning how to start-up in biomedical engineering. In: 2023 IEEE global engineering education conference (EDUCON). IEEE; 2023. p. 1–6.
41. Jones S. An engineering design-oriented first year biomedical engineering curriculum. 2021.
42. Cadwalladera J, Mellemab S, Lightnera NJ. Using simulation to provide insights into the concept development of patient-centered care services. Adv Hum Asp Healthc Med. 2021;248:1–6.
43. Flood M, Ennis M, Ludlow A, Sweeney FF, Holton A, Morgan S, et al. Research methods from human-centered design: potential applications in pharmacy and health services research. Res Social Adm Pharm. 2021;17(12):2036–43.
44. Rothstein M. Translational bioethics and health privacy. Ethics Hum Res. 2023;45(3):40–4.

45. Badnjevic A, Deumic A, Biskovic D, Pokvic LG. A novel method for conformity assessment testing of dialysis machines for post-market surveillance purposes. Technol Health Care. 2023;31(1):357–65.
46. Khokhlov AL, Belousov DY, Kagramanyan IN, Mokhov AA, Tsyzman LG, Samarina EI. Bioethical aspects of translational medicine. Kutafin Law Rev. 2022;9(1):175–90.
47. Hostiuc S, Moldoveanu A, Dascalu M, Unnthorsson R, Jóhannesson ÓI, Marcus I. Translational research—the need of a new bioethics approach. J Transl Med. 2016;14:1–7.
48. Sunderland M, Nayak R. Reengineering biomedical translational research with engineering ethics. Sci Eng Ethics. 2015;21:1019–31.
49. Tornini VA, Peregalli Politi S, Bruce L, Latham SR. Maximizing biomedical research impacts through bioethical considerations. Dis Model Mech. 2023;16(4):dmm050046.
50. Charfare RH, Desai AU, Keni NN, Nambiar AS, Cherian MM. IoT-AI in healthcare: a comprehensive survey of current applications and innovations. Int J Robot Control Syst. 2024;4(3):1–25.
51. Yang J. Flexible biosensors and intelligent medical devices in health and disease. Front Bioeng Biotechnol. 2022;10:849617.
52. Kovačević Ž, Gurbeta Pokvić L, Spahić L, Badnjević A. Prediction of medical device performance using machine learning techniques: infant incubator case study. Health Technol. 2020;10(1):151–5. https://doi.org/10.1007/s12553-019-00386-5.
53. Zhang S. Current development on wearable biosensors towards biomedical applications. Front Bioeng Biotechnol. 2023;11:1264337.
54. He T, Lee C. Evolving flexible sensors, wearable and implantable technologies towards BodyNET for advanced healthcare and reinforced life quality. IEEE Open J Circuits Syst. 2021;2:702–20.
55. Deumić S, Crnčević N, Ajayi DM, Zubčević T, Kolić H. Implantable and ingestible biosensors. In: MEDICON'23 and CMBEBIH'23. Cham: Springer; 2023. p. 1–7.
56. Paternò L, Lorenzon L. Soft robotics in wearable and implantable medical applications: translational challenges and future outlooks. Front Robot AI. 2023;10:1075634.
57. Wang Y, Xie Z, Huang H, Liang X. Pioneering healthcare with soft robotic devices: a review. Smart Med. 2024;3(1):e20230045.
58. Gangwal A, Lavecchia A. Artificial intelligence in natural product drug discovery: current applications and future perspectives. J Med Chem. 2025;68:3948–69.
59. Badnjević A, Gurbeta L, Custovic E. An expert diagnostic system to automatically identify asthma and chronic obstructive pulmonary disease in clinical settings. Sci Rep. 2018;8(1):11645.
60. Song Y. Artificial intelligence algorithms in biomedical application. In: 2023 International conference on Intelligent Supercomputing and BioPharma (ISBP). IEEE; 2023. p. 42–7.
61. Badnjević A, Avdihodžić H, Gurbeta Pokvić L. Artificial intelligence in medical devices: past, present and future. Psychiatr Danub. 2021;33(Suppl 3):101–6.
62. Qi C, Lei Y. Artificial intelligence applications in medical sciences: illustrations in pharmaceutical and medical imaging areas. In: Third international conference on computer science and communication technology (ICCSCT 2022). SPIE; 2022. p. 846–51.
63. Kurpad NB, Dhanyashree S, Shivank V, Shobith TS, Jinny SV. AI-infused telemedicine for rural wellness: a comprehensive approach. In: 2024 5th International conference on innovative trends in information technology (ICITIIT). IEEE; 2024. p. 1–6.
64. Abbasi N. Artificial intelligence in remote monitoring and telemedicine. J Artif Intell Gen Sci. 2024;1(1):258–72.
65. Talati D. Telemedicine and AI in remote patient monitoring. J Knowl Learn Sci Technol. 2023;2(3):254–5.
66. Hrvat F, Spahić L, Pokvić LG, Badnjević A. Artificial neural networks for prediction of medical device performance based on conformity assessment data: infusion and perfusor pumps case study. In: 2020 9th Mediterranean conference on embedded computing (MECO). IEEE; 2020. p. 1–4.

67. Shorna SA, Sultana R, Hasan MAR. Big data applications in remote patient monitoring and telemedicine services: a review of techniques and tools. SSRN Electron J. 2024; https://doi.org/10.2139/ssrn.5026572.
68. Miller M, Brightman A. BME 2.0: engineering the future of medicine. BME Front. 2022;4:0001.
69. Kiwerski JE. The application of biomechanics on orthopaedic rehabilitation. Orthop Surg Sports Med. 2019; https://doi.org/10.31579/2641-0427/015.
70. Kovačević Ž, Gurbeta Pokvić L, Spahić L, Badnjević A. Prediction of medical device performance using machine learning techniques: infant incubator case study. Health Technol. 2019;10(1):151–5.
71. Atheena MPS, Rashika M, Sudherson M, Mohammed SS. The influence of biomedical engineering in India. I-Manager's J Future Eng Technol. 2024;19:23.
72. Huang H, Feng W, Chen Y. Two-dimensional biomaterials: material science, biological effect and biomedical engineering applications. Chem Soc Rev. 2021;50(20):11381–405.
73. Tavares J, Fernandes P. Special issue: CMBBE2018—15th international symposium on computer methods in biomechanics and biomedical engineering and 3rd conference on imaging and visualization, vol. 8; 2020. p. 231.
74. Unal E, Bozdoganoglu M. Medical engineering applications in modern medicine. Med Eng Adv. 2018; https://doi.org/10.31031/RMES.2018.04.000598.
75. Zhao F. The application of sports biomechanics in sports injury prevention and rehabilitation. Front Sports Res. 2024;6(3):142–7.
76. Kim D-H, Yu MNSC, Arel EJM, Lim MJU, Velasquez AT, Lavadia W, Vicerra RRP. Understanding of the biomechanics of tendons and ligaments and its application in designing prosthetics. In: 2022 IEEE 14th international conference on humanoid, nanotechnology, information technology, communication and control, environment, and management (HNICEM). IEEE; 2022.
77. Li Q, Zhang X, Wang Y, Chen L, Liu H. Computational optimization for biomechanics and biomedical engineering. J Mech Behav Biomed Mater. 2017;20:387–97.
78. Erdmann W. Engineering support of orthopedics and rehabilitation. Signif Bioeng Biosci. 2021; https://doi.org/10.31031/SBB.2021.04.000593.
79. Manoukian OS, Sardashti N, Stedman T, Gailiunas K, Ojha A, Penalosa A, et al. Biomaterials for tissue engineering and regenerative medicine. In: Encyclopedia of biomedical engineering. Elsevier; 2019.
80. Singh AK, Sundram S, Malviya R. Human-derived biomaterials for biomedical and tissue engineering applications. Curr Pharm Des. 2023;29(8):584–603.
81. Li J, Zreiqat H. Tissue response to biomaterials. In: Encyclopedia of biomedical engineering. Elsevier; 2019.
82. Antmen E, Vrana NE, Hasirci V. The role of biomaterials and scaffolds in immune responses in regenerative medicine: macrophage phenotype modulation by biomaterial properties and scaffold architectures. Biomater Sci. 2021;9(24):8090–110.
83. Christman KL. Biomaterials for tissue repair. Science. 2019;363(6425):340–1.
84. Li S, Liu Y, Du J, Zeybek B, Zani L, Lewis M, et al. Computational modelling of mechanical behavior of biological tissues for biomedical applications. Loughborough Univ Biomed Eng J. 2016;1:1940–1949.
85. Lacroix D. The future of tissue engineering design for bioreactor stimulation. Multiscale Mechanobiology in Tissue Engineering. Springer Singapore. 2018;195–199.
86. Reid L. An introduction to biomedical computational fluid dynamics. Adv Exp Med Biol. 2021;1334:205.
87. Danan E, Shabairou N, Danan Y, Zalevsky Z. Signal-to-noise ratio improvement for multiple-pinhole imaging using supervised encoder–decoder convolutional neural network architecture. Photonics. 2022;9(2):69.

88. Miller DL, Kakar S, Jiang L, Spelic D, Burk L. The U.S. Food and Drug Administration's role in improving radiation dose management for medical X-ray imaging devices. Br J Radiol. 2021;94:20210373.
89. Singh J, Patel P. Methods for medical device design, regulatory compliance and risk management. J Eng Res Rep. 2024;26:373–89.
90. Gangadhar RS, Rajeshwari BV. Biocompatibility of medical devices: a review. J Evol Med Dent Sci. 2021;10(36):3152–9.
91. Bernard M, Jubeli E, Pungente M, Yagoubi N. Biocompatibility of polymer-based biomaterials and medical devices: regulations, in vitro screening, and risk management. Biomater Sci. 2018;6(8):2025–53.
92. Reifschneider A. The new U.S. FDA regulations on biocompatibility and reprocessing for medical devices. Master's thesis. 2017.
93. Umapathi UT, Vijayakumar V, Muthusamy S, Ramamurthy VA, Natarajan D. Regulatory requirement for medical devices. Int J Drug Regul Aff. 2024;12:9.
94. Manita A, Deep V, Rana A, Sharma PC. Regulation and clinical investigation of medical device in the European Union. Appl Clin Res Clin Trials Regul Aff. 2019;6:163.
95. Niimi S. Practice of regulatory science (development of medical devices). Yakugaku Zasshi. 2017;137(4):431–7.
96. Peters K, Unger R, Kirkpatrick C. Biocompatibility testing. Biomed Mater. 2020.
97. Goodarzy F, Skafidas ES, Gambini S. Feasibility of energy-autonomous wireless microsensors for biomedical applications: powering and communication. IEEE Rev Biomed Eng. 2015;8:17–29.
98. Simeoni R, Francisco JC, Cunha R, Cardoso MA, Carvalho KAT, Souza LCG. Co-cultivated cells integration into bacterial cellulose scaffold as a new device for tissue regeneration. Front Nanosci Nanotechnology. 2016;2:1–2.
99. Hueck IS, Frimodig J, Itkin-Ansari P, Gough DA. Encapsulation of stem cells in research and therapy. Springer; 2018.
100. Pulicharla MR, Premani V. AI-powered neuroprosthetics for brain-computer interfaces (BCIs). World J Adv Eng Technol Sci. 2024;12:109.
101. Montgomery RM. Enhancing neuroprosthetic control through AI-powered adaptive learning: a simulation study. Wired Neurosci. 2024; https://doi.org/10.62162/1000000.
102. Kale NA. Research and development in biomedical prosthetics. Int J Sci Res Eng Manag. 2024;8:1–5.
103. Haidegger T, Speidel S, Stoyanov D, Satava R. Robot-assisted minimally invasive surgery—surgical robotics in the data age. Proc IEEE. 2022;110:835–46.
104. Merdović N, Spahić L, Hundur M, Pokvić LG, Badnjević A. Advancement of post-market surveillance of medical devices leveraging artificial intelligence: infusion pumps case study. Technol Health Care. 2025;33(2):915–21.
105. Zhou XY, Guo Y, Shen M, Yang GZ. Artificial intelligence in surgery. https://doi.org/10.48550/arXiv.2001.00627.
106. Zeb S, Nizamullah FNU, Abbasi N, Fahad M. AI in healthcare: revolutionizing diagnosis and therapy. Int J Multidiscip Sci Arts. 2024;3(3):118–28.
107. Egert M, Steward JE, Sundaram CP. Machine learning and artificial intelligence in surgical fields. Indian J Surg Oncol. 2020;11(4):573–7.
108. Mujkić A, Baralić E, Ombašić A, Bećirović LS, Pokvić LG, Badnjević A. Machine intelligence in biomedical data modeling, processing, and analysis. In: 2022 11th Mediterranean conference on embedded computing (MECO). IEEE; 2022. p. 1–10.
109. Fatunmbi TO. Leveraging robotics, artificial intelligence, and machine learning for enhanced disease diagnosis and treatment: advanced integrative approaches for precision medicine. World J Adv Eng Technol Sci. 2022;6(2):121–35.
110. Elhaddad M, Hamam S. AI-driven clinical decision support systems: an ongoing pursuit of potential. Cureus. 2024;16(4):e1–7.

111. Guerrini CJ, McGuire A, Lázaro-Muñoz G. Ethical, legal, and social implications. In: Handbook of clinical adult genetics and genomics. Academic Press; 2020.
112. Komesaroff P, Felman ER. How to make sense of the ethical issues raised by artificial intelligence in medicine. Intern Med J. 2023;53:1–7.
113. Brown JEH, Koenig B. Ethical, legal, and social implications of fetal gene therapy. Clin Obstet Gynecol. 2021;64:933–40.
114. Magjarević R, Badnjević A. Inspection and testing of electrocardiographs (ECG) devices. In: Inspection of medical devices: for regulatory purposes. Cham: Springer; 2023. p. 139–71.
115. Ginghină S. Principles of biomedical ethics. Logos Univ Ment Educ Novelty Soc Sci. 2023;12:110–22.
116. Ismayilova P. Key characteristics of autonomy, confidentiality, beneficence, non-maleficence, justice, and privacy principles in medical law within the context of human rights. Anal Comp Jurisprud. 2024; https://doi.org/10.24144/2788-6018.2024.03.112.
117. Teays W. Applied ethics: principles and perspectives. In: Doctors and torture. Springer; 2019.
118. Morgan MB, Mates J. Ethics of artificial intelligence in breast imaging. J Breast Imaging. 2023;5:195–200.
119. Moffatt S. Ethics of biomedical engineering: the unanswered questions. Sci Biomed Eng. 2017;1(1):1–10.
120. Kaplan B, Liaw T, Subbian V, Courtney K, Hochheiser H, Goodman K. Promoting ethical and professional responsibility in biomedical informatics education. SSRN. 2017;ID:3099251.
121. Saheb T, Saheb T, Carpenter D. Mapping research strands of ethics of artificial intelligence in healthcare: a bibliometric and content analysis. Comput Biol Med. 2021;135:104660.
122. Cahn N. CRISPR parents and informed consent. SMU Sci. & Tech. L. Rev. 2021;23:3.
123. Chang V, Kamanooru MR, Darko GT. Ethical discussions for autonomous robotic surgeries. Second International Conference on Industrial IoT, Big Data, and Supply Chain. SPIE. 2021;12128:188–199.
124. Kimbrough CW, Pawlik TM. Ethics in academic surgery. Surgical Ethics: Principles and Practices. 2019;85–96.
125. Jafar U, Usama M, Hase NE, Yaseen H, Nayyar A, Rabinowitz JB, Aziz H. Analysis of conflicts of interest in studies related to robotics in gastrointestinal and abdominal wall surgery. J Am Coll Surg. 2023;238:54–60.
126. Fink N. Conflicts of interest and an approach to managing them. EJIFCC. 2020;31:292–301.
127. Grundy Q, Mayes C, Holloway K, Mazzarello S, Thombs B, Bero L. Conflict of interest as ethical shorthand: understanding the range and nature of non-financial conflict of interest in biomedicine. J Clin Epidemiol. 2019;120:1.
128. Celis MA, Halabe J, Arrieta O, Burgos R, Campillo C, Llata MD, Domínguez J, Islas S, Jasso L, Lifshitz A, Moreno M, Plancarte R, Reyes-Sánchez A, Ruiz-Argüelles G, Soda A, Verástegui E, Sotelo J. Conflicts of interest in medicine: CETREMI recommendations. Gac Med Mex. 2020;155(5):519–20.
129. Rajendran N, Thomas D, Madhavan SS, Herman RA. Ethics in clinical research. Clinical Pharmacy Education, Practice and Research. Elsevier. 2019;345–364.
130. Williams MR, Solomon D, Drummond CK. Moot court cases: bringing standards to life. In: ASEE proceedings of the north central section meeting; 2022.
131. Sharkey CM. A products liability framework for AI. Columbia Sci Technol Law Rev. 2024;25(2).
132. Leeuwen BV, Verbruggen P. Resuscitating EU product liability law? Contemplating the effects of Boston Scientific Medizintechnik GmbH v. AOK Sachsen-Anhalt and Betriebskrankenkasse RWE. Eur Rev Priv Law. 2015;23:899–915.
133. Nori L, Teja P, Sai Jeevan T, Varma T, Raju KV. CE marking—an insignia for medical devices in European Union. Curr Trends Pharm Pharm Chem. 2023;5(1):4–9.
134. Priyadharshini S, Sivaranjani PS, Nagalakshmi S. The registration of medical device in FDA, EU and CDSCO: overview. J Adv Med Pharm Sci. 2024; https://doi.org/10.9734/jamps/2024/v26i8709.

135. Ramli TS, Putri SA, Ramli AM. Legal review of patent rights with the license agreement on civil law. In: International conference on law reform proceedings; 2018. p. 30–3.
136. Netkovska KA, Ribarska JT, Grozdanova A, Sterjev Z. Patents and licensing in pharmaceutical industry. Maced Pharm Bull. 2015;61(1):51–9.
137. Poddar A, Rao S, Hulsen T, Lee R. Evolving intellectual property landscape for AI-driven innovations in the biomedical sector: opportunities in stable IP regime for shared success. Front Artif Intell. 2024;7:1372161.
138. Thomas K, Cabell A, Hu SS. Relationship between industry royalty and licensing payments and patent authorship among orthopaedic spine surgeons. Spine J. 2020;21:541.
139. Courage N, Calzavara J. Protecting trade secrets in Canada. Cold Spring Harb Perspect Med. 2015;5(9):a024489.
140. Kumar A, Mishra A. Protecting trade secrets in India. J World Intell Prop. 2015;18:335–46.
141. Smith DJ. Product liability and safety legislation. In: Reliability and maintainability in perspective; 2022.
142. Sharma A, Luthra G. A comprehensive review of risk management in the medical device industry. J Pharm Res Int. 2023;35:14–23.
143. Stern G, Baird P, Bills EL, Busdicker M, Grob A, Krenc T, Whanger K, Wu F. Roundtable discussion: in medical device risk management, patients take on increased importance. Biomed Instrum Technol. 2020;54(4):283–90.
144. Sadri M. HIPAA: a demand to modernize health legislation. Undergrad Law Rev UC San Diego. 2024; https://doi.org/10.5070/LR3.21252.
145. Shah WF. Preserving privacy and security: a comparative study of health data regulations—GDPR vs. HIPAA. Int J Res Appl Sci Eng Technol. 2023;11:2189–99.
146. Jadon A, Kumar S. Leveraging generative AI models for synthetic data generation in healthcare: balancing research and privacy. In: International conference on smart applications, communications and networking; 2023.
147. Cindik S. Malpractice in health care services: a study in terms of criminal law (Bachelor's thesis). 2017. Available from: https://revis.openscience.si/IzpisGradiva.php?id=4887&lang=eng&prip=dkum:10976728:d5
148. Aagaard L. Artificial intelligence decision support systems and liability for medical injuries. J Res Pharm Pract. 2020;9:125–7.
149. Pelled O. Aggregating liability for medical malpractice. SSRN Electron J. 2024; https://doi.org/10.2139/ssrn.4746392.
150. Lanier OL, Green MD, Barabino GA, Cosgriff-Hernandez E. Ten simple rules in biomedical engineering to improve healthcare equity. PLoS Comput Biol. 2022;18:e1010525.
151. Gurbeta L, Badnjević A, Maksimovic M, Omanović-Mikličanin E, Sejdić E. A telehealth system for automated diagnosis of asthma and chronic obstructive pulmonary disease. J Am Med Inform Assoc. 2018;25(9):1213–7.
152. Rodriguez NM, Burleson G, Linnes J, Sienko K. Thinking beyond the device: an overview of human- and equity-centered approaches for health technology design. Annu Rev Biomed Eng. 2023;25:257–80.
153. Tandon I. The "I" in inclusion. In: ASEE midwest section conference proceedings; 2021.
154. Saeed S, Masters RM. Disparities in health care and the digital divide. Curr Psychiatry Rep. 2021;23:61.
155. Choy M, O'Brien K, Barnes K, Sturgiss E, Rieger E, Douglas K. Evaluating the digital health experience for patients in primary care: mixed methods study. J Med Internet Res. 2024;26:e50410.
156. Bhoyar A, Vagha S, Mishra V, Agrawal MS, Kambala SR. Addressing the digital divide in health education: a systematic review. Cureus. 2024;16:e70048.
157. Bergel S. The ethical impact of new genetic editing technologies. Rev Bioethics. 2017;25(3):454–61.
158. Subica A. CRISPR in public health: the health equity implications and role of community in gene-editing research and applications. Am J Public Health. 2023;113:e1–9.

159. Sanders EA, Hess J, Miller S, Higbee S. Ethical considerations in biomedical engineering: qualitative student perspectives from a large Midwestern university. In: IEEE frontiers in education conference (FIE); 2022.
160. Murray T. Novel "impacts of biomedical innovations" course integrates ethics. In: Southern biomedical engineering conference proceedings; 2016.
161. Hrvat F, Spahić L, Aleta A. Heart disease prediction using logistic regression machine learning model. In: Mediterranean conference on medical and biological engineering and computing; 2023.
162. Hundur M, Spahić L, Bećirović F, Gurbeta Pokvić L, Badnjević A. Advancement of post-market surveillance of medical devices leveraging artificial intelligence: ECG devices case study. Technol Health Care. 2025; https://doi.org/10.1177/09287329241303727.
163. Catalano G. Integrating compassion into an engineering ethics course. In: ASEE annual conference and exposition; 2016.
164. Manzoor J, Sharma M. Impact of biomedical waste on environment and human health. Environ Claims J. 2019;31(3):311–34.
165. Solorzano ADB, Wu MMH. Environmental impact of medical waste treatment. In: Proceedings of the international conference on industrial engineering and operations management; 2023.
166. Omo QG, Hassan NE. Biomedical waste management and their effects on the environment: a review. World J Adv Eng Technol Sci. 2024;11:86.
167. Leena NM, Kirti JM. Impact of biomedical waste on environment and human health: A review. Int J Zool Investig. 2022;8(2):484–489.
168. Ravindra K, Sareen A, Dogra S, Mor S. Appraisal of biomedical waste management practice in India and associated human health and environmental risk. J Environ Biol. 2023;44:541.
169. Meen T. Biomedical engineering, healthcare, and sustainability. In: IEEE Eurasia conference on biomedical engineering, healthcare and sustainability proceedings; 2019.
170. Mak T. Factors investigation for the development of medical devices towards a sustainable product. Proc Int Conf Ind Eng Oper Manag. 2019;2799–2810.
171. Kruijff S. Sustainable innovation with a green operation. Inaugural Lecture: Green Healthcare. 2024.

# Chapter 2
# Medical Devices and Instrumentation

This chapter provides a comprehensive exploration of medical devices and instrumentation, building on the foundational principles and applications of biomedical engineering. It begins by tracing the historical development of medical devices, highlighting key innovations that have shaped clinical practice and device design (Sect. 2.1). The section then examines technical characteristics, fundamental components (Sect. 2.2), and specialized devices, including imaging systems (Sect. 2.3), electrocardiographs (Sect. 2.4), blood pressure (Sect. 2.5) and patient monitors (Sect. 2.6), mechanical ventilators (Sect. 2.7), anesthesia machines (Sect. 2.8), pacemakers, defibrillators (Sect. 2.9), neonatal incubators (Sect. 2.10), and surgical instruments (Sect. 2.11). Each chapter discusses clinical applications, regulatory considerations, and safety standards, emphasizing their role in diagnostics, monitoring, therapy, and patient care. The section concludes by addressing emerging trends and innovations, including miniaturization, wearable technology, smart devices (Sect. 2.12), robotic systems (Sect. 2.13), implantable pumps (Sect. 2.14), and smart pills (Sect. 2.15), highlighting their potential to transform healthcare delivery and advance precision medicine.

## 2.1 Overview of Medical Devices

Medical devices play a fundamental role in modern healthcare, facilitating the prevention, diagnosis, treatment, and management of diseases and medical conditions. Medical devices have transformed patient care from basic tools like thermometers and stethoscopes to advanced technologies such as magnetic resonance imaging (MRI) scanners, robotic surgical systems, and artificial intelligence (AI) powered diagnostic platforms [1]. The increasing integration of biomedical engineering with digital technology, AI, and miniaturization has led to an unprecedented expansion in the range and capabilities of medical devices, making healthcare more efficient,



A. Badnjević et al., *Biomedical Instrumentation*, Series in BioEngineering,
https://doi.org/10.1007/978-3-032-10978-1_2

precise, and personalized [2]. The medical device industry is a critical component of the global healthcare sector, with billions of dollars invested annually in research, development, and manufacturing. As of today, medical devices encompass a vast array of innovations, including implantable devices, wearable health monitors, imaging systems, and therapeutic technologies. These devices improve the quality of life for millions of patients worldwide and reduce healthcare costs by enabling early diagnosis, minimally invasive procedures, and remote patient monitoring. Despite their immense benefits, the development and deployment of medical devices present significant challenges. Ensuring safety, efficacy, and regulatory compliance requires a robust framework that governs how devices are designed, tested, and approved for clinical use. Medical devices must undergo stringent regulatory evaluations to meet international standards, ensuring that they are safe for patient use while maintaining effectiveness. Regulatory agencies such as the U.S. Food and Drug Administration (FDA) and the European Medicines Agency (EMA) enforce guidelines to categorize and approve medical devices, ensuring that risks are minimized and benefits maximized [3].

While medical devices have transformed healthcare, their development and deployment have significant challenges. The high cost of research and development, complex regulatory approvals, and the need for extensive clinical trials can create barriers to bringing innovative devices to market. Additionally, the rapid pace of technological advancements presents concerns regarding cybersecurity, data privacy, and device interoperability. One of the most pressing challenges in medical device innovation is ensuring safety and efficacy. Unlike pharmaceutical drugs, which undergo rigorous testing in controlled clinical trials, medical devices often interact dynamically with the human body, requiring extensive real-world testing to evaluate their long-term effects. Device malfunctions, software errors, and biocompatibility issues can have severe consequences, making post-market surveillance a crucial component of regulatory oversight [4].

Cybersecurity is another primary concern in the medical device industry, especially with the increasing use of internet-connected devices. Implantable and wearable medical devices, such as insulin pumps and cardiac monitors, are vulnerable to cyberattacks, potentially endangering patient safety. Ensuring that these devices have robust security measures, such as encryption and authentication protocols, is essential to prevent unauthorized access and tampering [2]. Another challenge is the need for interoperability between medical devices and healthcare systems. As hospitals and clinics transition to electronic health records (EHRs) and digital healthcare ecosystems, seamless integration between devices and software platforms is critical [5, 6]. Standardization efforts, such as the adoption of Health Level Seven (HL7) and Fast Healthcare Interoperability Resources (FHIR), aim to address these issues by creating standard protocols for data exchange [7].

### 2.1.1 History

Medical equipment evolved over many centuries, beginning with simple devices like scalpels and trephines, which were employed in ancient societies for surgical procedures. Specific devices were created to treat injuries and diseases even from the Bronze and Iron Ages, paving the way for more complex innovations in the following eras. During the nineteenth and twentieth centuries, advances in anesthetics, aseptic techniques, and imaging technologies such as X-rays transformed surgical and diagnostic capabilities [8].

The twentieth century also witnessed the exponential expansion of electronic and implantable medical technology. The advent of cardiac pacemakers, prosthetic joints, and advanced imaging equipment revolutionized patient treatment. The development of semiconductors and digital systems in the mid-century culminated in biotelemetry equipment to monitor patients at a distance. Wireless technology expanded miniaturization and functionality in medical equipment, a practice continuing today [9, 10].

More recently, the COVID-19 pandemic has emphasized the critical role played by medical devices within health systems worldwide, ranging from diagnostic testing platforms to ventilators and telemedicine devices. It was a moment when there came an explosion in the development and regulation of AI-focused and connected medical devices, with consequent accelerated digital transformation of health care delivery. Experts call for establishing a dedicated academic discipline of medical device science to deal with the growing complexity and ensure safety, innovation, and ethical application [11, 12].

### 2.1.2 Technical Characteristics

Modern medical devices are notable for precision, connectivity, adaptability, and safety. Technical aspects of top priority include miniaturization, real-time processing, wireless transmission, and reliability under varying clinical conditions. The equipment must integrate seamlessly into a hospital's systems with strict safety and biocompatibility expectations. For example, hardware-software integration of diagnostic devices nowadays supports AI-enabled analysis and adaptive control, improving precision and operational efficacy [13]. In addition, the arrival of cloud computing and mHealth platforms has introduced flexibility and scalability that widened the scope of care delivery systems beyond clinical settings [14].

**Hardware**

Hardware components of medical devices include actuators, sensors, processors, power supplies, and user interfaces—each designed for ruggedness, precision, and real-time performance. The trend toward portable and wearable devices focuses on lightweight materials and battery optimization without compromising functionality. Hardware-software integration platforms are increasingly used in advanced systems such as diagnostic imaging, surgical robots, and remote monitoring kits. They support real-time signal processing and whole-scale testing, enhancing performance under dynamic clinical conditions [15, 16]. Investment in medical hardware remains essential to guarantee device reliability and innovation in complicated care settings [17].

**Software**

Software is increasingly the focal component of novel medical devices, enabling tasks like signal interpretation, patient monitoring, diagnostics, and decision support. Integrated into devices or utilized as stand-alone software (Software as a Medical Device or SaMD), medical software must also satisfy rigorous requirements like ISO 13485 and ISO 14971 for safety, effectiveness, and data integrity. Lifecycle processes include requirements gathering, risk analysis, and preclinical validation to establish clinical effectiveness and regulatory compliance [18, 19]. Advances in AI, cybersecurity, and real-time analytics are also transforming medical software into an efficient agent of personalized medicine and predictive healthcare [20].

In the following sections, we will explore the various types of medical devices, their roles in healthcare, and the regulatory frameworks governing their classification and approval. Understanding these aspects is essential for ensuring that medical devices continue to enhance patient care while adhering to the highest standards of safety and effectiveness.

### 2.1.3 *Types of Devices*

Medical devices encompass various instruments, equipment, implants, and software designed to diagnose, monitor, treat, or prevent medical conditions. These devices are integral to healthcare delivery, enabling precision medicine, minimally invasive procedures, and enhanced patient monitoring. The classification of medical devices is typically based on their intended use, risk level, and regulatory requirements, ensuring patient safety and efficacy [21].

### Diagnostic Devices

Diagnostic devices are crucial in identifying diseases and medical conditions, guiding clinical decisions, and facilitating early interventions. These devices range from basic point-of-care instruments to advanced imaging systems, significantly improving diagnostic accuracy and patient management. Technological advancements have made diagnostic devices more precise, portable, and accessible, enhancing early disease detection and reducing the burden on healthcare systems [22].

Medical imaging devices provide noninvasive methods for visualizing internal body structures. These technologies have revolutionized diagnostics, allowing for early disease detection and improved patient outcomes. Imaging techniques continue to evolve, integrating artificial intelligence for automated analysis and improving resolution for better visualization [23] (Table 2.1).

- X-ray Machines: Used primarily for detecting fractures, infections, and tumors, X-ray machines generate high-energy radiation that passes through the body to create images of bones and tissues. Digital X-ray technology has enhanced image quality and reduced radiation exposure, making it safer and more effective for repeated use [24].
- Computed Tomography (CT) Scanners: Provide cross-sectional images of the body, aiding in diagnosing cancer, internal injuries, and vascular diseases. Advanced CT scanners offer rapid imaging with lower radiation doses and can be used in emergency settings to assess traumatic injuries quickly [25].
- MRI Scanners: These scanners utilize magnetic fields and radio waves to produce detailed images of soft tissues, making them ideal for neurological and musculoskeletal conditions. Innovations in MRI technology, such as functional MRI (fMRI), allow researchers to study brain activity and neurological disorders in greater detail [26].
- Ultrasound Systems employ sound waves to visualize organs, blood flow, and fetal development. They are widely used in obstetrics and cardiology. Handheld ultrasound devices have expanded the reach of this technology, enabling bedside and remote diagnostics in resource-limited settings [27].
- Positron Emission Tomography (PET) Scanners: Detect metabolic activity and are particularly useful in oncology for identifying cancerous cells. PET-CT and PET-MRI hybrid systems combine metabolic and anatomical imaging, improving cancer diagnosis and treatment planning.

**Table 2.1** Various types of imaging devices

| X-ray | CT | MRI | PET | Ultrasound |
|---|---|---|---|---|
| 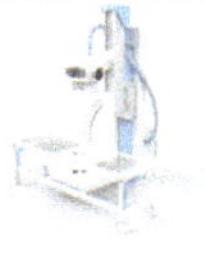 | 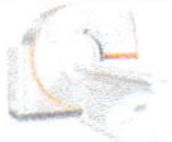 | 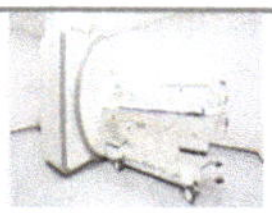 | 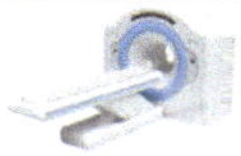 | 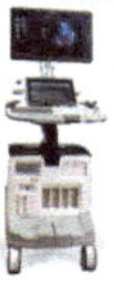 |

Laboratory diagnostic devices analyze biological samples to detect infections, genetic conditions, and biochemical imbalances. These devices play a critical role in personalized medicine, helping to tailor treatments based on individual genetic and biochemical profiles.

- Blood Analyzers: Measure blood cell counts, electrolyte levels, and biomarkers for diabetes and anemia. Modern analyzers can conduct multiple tests simultaneously, increasing efficiency and reducing diagnostic turnaround time [28].
- Molecular Diagnostic Systems: These systems detect genetic mutations and infectious diseases using polymerase chain reaction (PCR) and next-generation sequencing (NGS). These technologies enable early detection of conditions like cancer and hereditary diseases, leading to more effective treatment strategies [29].
- Point-of-Care Testing (POCT) Devices: These portable instruments, such as glucose meters and rapid antigen tests, enable immediate medical decisions. Advances in biosensor technology have made POCT devices more accurate and user-friendly, enhancing their application in home healthcare and remote settings [30].

Integrating machine learning and AI in diagnostic devices further transforms the field, allowing for automated image interpretation, predictive analytics, and personalized treatment recommendations. The continued development of diagnostic devices aims to enhance accessibility, affordability, and accuracy, ultimately improving global healthcare outcomes.

### Therapeutic Devices

Therapeutic devices support or replace physiological functions, aiding disease treatment and rehabilitation. These devices enhance patient outcomes through precision therapy and minimally invasive interventions. They encompass many technologies, from traditional surgical tools to highly sophisticated robotic-assisted systems and bioengineered implants that integrate seamlessly with human physiology [31].

Modern surgical devices range from simple handheld tools to complex robotic-assisted systems, improving the' precision, safety, and efficacy of medical procedures. Innovations in this field continue to minimize surgical risks, shorten recovery times, and enhance overall patient care [32] (Table 2.2).

- Endoscopic Instruments: Enable minimally invasive surgeries by inserting a thin, flexible tube with a camera and specialized surgical tools into the body through small incisions. This approach significantly reduces recovery times, postoperative pain, and surgical risks. Endoscopic techniques are widely used in gastroenterology, gynecology, and orthopedic procedures [33].
- Electrosurgical Units (ESUs): Use high-frequency electrical currents to cut, coagulate, or ablate tissue with minimal blood loss. These devices are commonly used in dermatology, gynecology, and general surgery to perform procedures

**Table 2.2** Advanced surgical devices and their applications

| Endoscopic instruments | Electrosurgical units | Robotic surgical system |
|---|---|---|
| 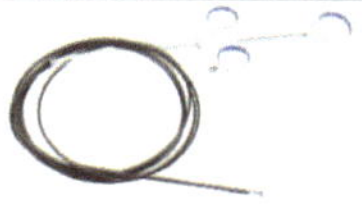 | 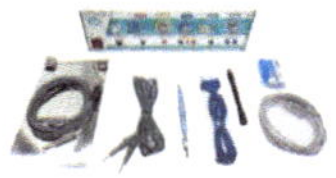 | 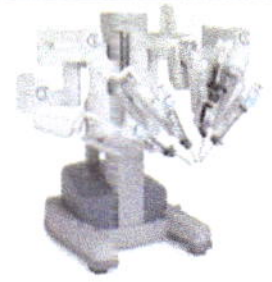 |

with precision and minimal thermal damage to surrounding tissues. Advanced models now incorporate real-time feedback mechanisms to optimize energy delivery and improve safety [34].

- Robotic Surgical Systems: The da Vinci Surgical System enhances precision and dexterity in complex cardiac, urological, and gynecological surgeries. These systems provide surgeons with enhanced visualization, increased range of motion, and greater accuracy, improving patient outcomes and reducing surgical complications. Integrating artificial intelligence in robotic-assisted surgery optimizes real-time decision-making and procedural efficiency [35].

Implantable devices are designed to replace, support, or enhance physiological functions within the body. These innovations restore mobility, organ function, and sensory perception, dramatically improving the quality of life for many patients.

- Cardiac Pacemakers and Defibrillators: These life-saving devices regulate heart rhythms and prevent sudden cardiac arrest. Pacemakers use electrical impulses to maintain a steady heart rate, while implantable cardioverter defibrillators (ICDs) monitor heart rhythms and deliver shocks when life-threatening arrhythmias occur. Modern pacemakers incorporate wireless connectivity for remote monitoring and adaptive algorithms that adjust therapy based on patient activity.
- Orthopedic Implants: Artificial joints, bone grafts, and spinal fixation devices restore mobility in patients with degenerative conditions such as osteoarthritis and osteoporosis. Advances in biomaterials, such as titanium alloys and biocompatible polymers, have enhanced implant longevity and integration with bone tissue. 3D printing technology has further revolutionized orthopedic implants, allowing for patient-specific customization and improved surgical outcomes [36].
- Cochlear Implants: Restore hearing in individuals with profound sensorineural hearing loss by bypassing damaged portions of the inner ear and directly stimulating the auditory nerve. Modern cochlear implants feature enhanced speech processing algorithms, wireless connectivity, and compatibility with external hearing devices, thereby improving auditory perception and communication abilities [37].

Beyond surgical and implantable devices, therapeutic technologies extend into drug delivery systems, prosthetic limbs, and neurostimulation devices, further broadening the impact of biomedical engineering on healthcare (Table 2.3).

**Table 2.3** Implantable therapeutic devices and their functionalities

| Cardiac pacemakers and defibrillators | Orthopedic implants | Cochlear implants |
|---|---|---|
| 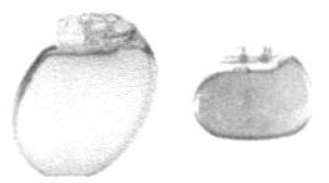 | 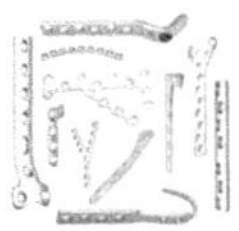 | 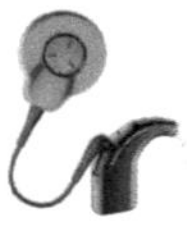 |

## Life Support Devices

Life support devices are critical components of modern healthcare, designed to sustain vital physiological functions and provide real-time data. These devices are essential in intensive care units (ICUs), operating rooms, emergency departments, and other critical care settings, where patients require continuous monitoring and intervention to stabilize their conditions. By assisting or completely taking over vital organ functions, life support devices play a key role in preventing complications and improving survival rates for critically ill patients [38–40].

Life support devices are used when a patient's body cannot maintain essential functions independently due to acute illness, injury, or chronic disease. These devices either [41, 42]:

1. Support or replace failing organ functions, such as mechanical ventilation for respiratory failure or dialysis for kidney failure.
2. Deliver essential medical interventions, such as infusion pumps that administer precise amounts of medication or defibrillators that restore heart rhythm.
3. Continuously monitor vital signs, such as patient monitoring systems that track heart rate, oxygen levels, and blood pressure, to detect early signs of deterioration.

Life support and monitoring devices can be categorized into several key groups based on their function:

### Respiratory Support Devices

These devices assist or replace natural breathing for patients with compromised lung function. They include mechanical ventilators, which provide controlled oxygenation, and extracorporeal membrane oxygenation (ECMO) systems, temporarily taking over lung and heart function in critical cases [43, 44].

### Cardiovascular Support Devices

Devices in this category help maintain or restore normal heart function. Defibrillators deliver electric shocks to correct life-threatening arrhythmias, while pacemakers regulate heart rhythm for patients with conduction abnormalities. Cardiac assist devices, such as intra-aortic balloon pumps and ventricular assist devices (VADs), provide temporary or long-term support for patients with severe heart failure.

Renal Support Devices

For patients with kidney failure, dialysis machines remove waste products, excess fluids, and toxins from the bloodstream when the kidneys can no longer perform this function. Dialysis is essential for patients with end-stage renal disease or acute kidney injury [45].

Drug and Fluid Administration Devices

Infusion pumps ensure the controlled and precise delivery of medications, fluids, and nutrients, critical in managing critically ill patients. These devices include volumetric pumps, syringe pumps, and patient-controlled analgesia (PCA) pumps, enhancing safety and therapeutic effectiveness [46] (Table 2.4).

### Patient Monitoring Devices

Patient monitoring devices are crucial in modern healthcare, as they continuously track vital physiological parameters, detect complications early, and facilitate timely medical interventions. These devices are used in hospitals, emergency care settings, home healthcare, and remote patient monitoring systems. They help clinicians assess a patient's condition in real-time, reducing the risk of undetected deterioration and improving overall patient outcomes [47]. The evolution of monitoring technologies has significantly expanded the capabilities of these devices, integrating wireless connectivity, artificial intelligence, and predictive analytics to enhance diagnostic accuracy and efficiency [48] (Table 2.5).

**Table 2.4** Life support devices and their functions in critical care

| Respiratory support | Cardiovascular support | Renal support | Drug and fluid administration |
|---|---|---|---|
| 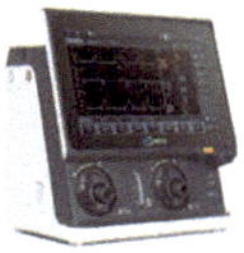 | 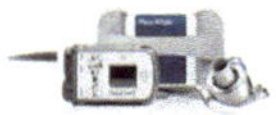 | 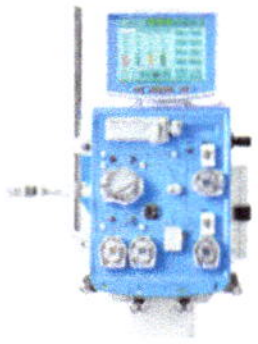 | 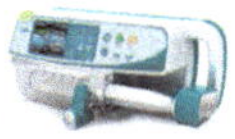 |

**Table 2.5** Monitoring devices and their functions

| Patient monitors | Heart monitors | Physical activity monitors | Respiratory monitors |
|---|---|---|---|
| 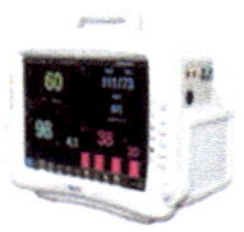 | 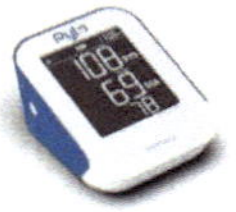 | 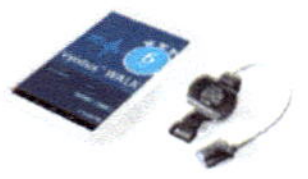 | 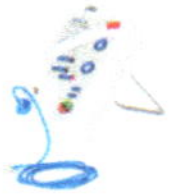 |

Patient monitoring devices serve several essential functions [49–51]:

1. Continuous Monitoring: Provides real-time tracking of vital signs such as heart rate, blood pressure, oxygen saturation, and respiratory rate.
2. Early Warning Systems: These systems alert healthcare providers to critical patient condition changes, reducing response time to medical emergencies.
3. Remote Healthcare Integration: Allows healthcare professionals to monitor patients from a distance, facilitating telemedicine and home-based care.
4. Preventive Healthcare: This approach encourages proactive health management through wearable technology that tracks fitness levels and early disease markers.

### Electrocardiogram (ECG) Monitors

ECG monitors track the heart's electrical activity and diagnose and monitor conditions such as arrhythmias, ischemic heart disease, and myocardial infarctions. These devices are available in various forms, including [52]:

- Bedside ECG Monitors: These are used in hospitals for continuous cardiac monitoring of critically ill patients.
- Holter Monitors: Portable devices worn for 24 to 48 hours to detect intermittent heart abnormalities.
- Implantable Loop Recorders (ILRs): Small, subcutaneous devices that provide long-term monitoring for patients with unexplained fainting or palpitations.

### Blood Pressure Monitors

Blood pressure monitoring is essential for detecting and managing hypertension, a significant risk factor for cardiovascular diseases. Devices range from [53]:

- Manual Sphygmomanometers: Used in clinical settings for precise blood pressure readings.
- Automated Digital Blood Pressure Monitors: These are common in hospitals and home healthcare for easy and frequent monitoring.
- Ambulatory Blood Pressure Monitors (ABPM): These are worn by patients for 24-hour readings to detect hypertension patterns, including nocturnal hypertension.

### Pulse Oximeters

Pulse oximeters measure blood oxygen saturation ($SpO_2$) and pulse rate, providing critical information for patients with respiratory conditions such as chronic obstructive pulmonary disease (COPD), asthma, and COVID-19. These devices can be [54]:

- Hospital-grade Pulse Oximeters: Used in intensive care units (ICUs) for continuous oxygen monitoring.
- Portable Finger Pulse Oximeters: Small, non-invasive devices for home use and outpatient monitoring.
- Wearable Oximeters: Integrated into smartwatches and fitness bands for continuous health tracking.

### Respiratory Monitors

Respiratory monitoring is vital for patients with lung diseases, anesthesia management and sleep disorders. Key devices include:

- Capnographs: Measure end-tidal carbon dioxide ($ETCO_2$) to assess ventilation efficiency in patients under anesthesia or mechanical ventilation.
- Spirometers: Evaluate lung function in conditions such as asthma and chronic bronchitis.
- Apnea Monitors: Detect pauses in breathing, particularly in neonates and individuals with sleep apnea.

### Temperature Monitors

Body temperature monitoring is crucial for detecting infections, inflammation, and fever-related conditions. Modern temperature monitoring includes:

- Digital Thermometers: These are used for routine temperature checks in clinical and home settings.
- Wearable Continuous Temperature Sensors: Provide ongoing monitoring for fever management, particularly in pediatric and post-surgical patients.

### Wearable Health Trackers

The rise of wearable technology has transformed preventive healthcare by providing continuous monitoring outside of clinical settings. These devices help track heart rate, activity levels, sleep patterns, and even stress levels, allowing users to make proactive lifestyle changes. Popular wearable monitoring technologies include [55]:

- Smartwatches with ECG and Heart Rate Monitoring: Detect abnormal heart rhythms and monitor physical activity.
- Biosensors: Small, adhesive patches that measure multiple biomarkers, including hydration, glucose, and body temperature.
- Smart Rings and Fitness Bands: These devices provide real-time sleep patterns, blood oxygen levels, and calorie expenditure data.

Advancements in artificial intelligence, cloud computing, and wireless technology are shaping the future of patient monitoring. AI-powered analytics can detect early signs of disease progression, while remote monitoring systems reduce hospital admissions by allowing physicians to manage chronic conditions from a distance. As these technologies evolve, patient monitoring devices will play an even greater role in personalized medicine, preventive care, and overall healthcare efficiency.

### Rehabilitation and Assistive Devices

Rehabilitation and assistive devices are crucial in enhancing mobility, communication, and independence for individuals with disabilities. These technologies support recovery from injuries, assist individuals with permanent disabilities, and improve the overall quality of life by restoring lost functions or compensating for impairments. Advances in robotics, artificial intelligence, and biomedical engineering have led to the development of highly sophisticated rehabilitation tools that adapt to user needs and provide greater autonomy [56, 57].

These devices serve several essential functions in healthcare and daily living [58–60] (Table 2.6):

1. Restoring Lost Functions: Advanced prosthetics and orthotics help individuals regain mobility and dexterity after limb loss or musculoskeletal impairments.
2. Enhancing Mobility: Devices such as exoskeletons and mobility aids support individuals with neurological or musculoskeletal conditions, allowing them to move more freely.
3. Supporting Communication: Assistive communication devices help individuals with speech and cognitive impairments interact more effectively with their surroundings.
4. Improving Sensory Perception: Hearing and visual aids enable individuals with sensory impairments to engage more fully in everyday activities.

**Table 2.6** Types of rehabilitation and assistive devices

| Rehabilitation and assistive devices | |
|---|---|
| 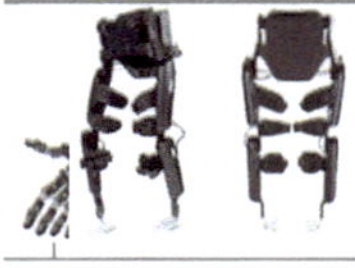 | 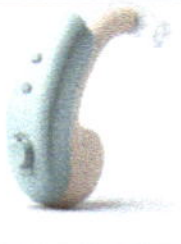 |

5. Facilitating Rehabilitation: Robotic and AI-powered rehabilitation tools help patients recover motor function after strokes, spinal cord injuries, and other neurological disorders.

### Prosthetic and Orthotic Devices

Prosthetics and orthotics provide functional support for individuals with limb loss, musculoskeletal disorders, or mobility impairments [61].

- Bionic Limbs: These advanced prosthetics use myoelectric sensors to detect muscle signals and translate them into natural limb movements, allowing users to perform everyday tasks more easily.
- Smart Prosthetics: AI-integrated prosthetics adapt to user movement patterns, providing a more intuitive experience.
- Orthotic Braces: Spinal braces, ankle-foot orthoses (AFOs), and knee braces provide stability and support for individuals with musculoskeletal conditions.

### Exoskeletons and Mobility Aids

Exoskeletons and mobility assistive devices enable individuals with physical impairments to regain movement, maintain independence, and improve rehabilitation outcomes [62].

- Powered Exoskeletons: Wearable robotic devices assist individuals with spinal cord injuries, stroke recovery, and neurological disorders in walking and performing movements.
- Wheelchairs and Mobility Scooters: These devices provide essential mobility for individuals with severe movement impairments. Innovations such as smart wheelchairs with AI navigation further enhance accessibility.
- Canes, Walkers, and Crutches: Traditional mobility aids support balance and stability for individuals recovering from injuries or with chronic conditions affecting mobility.

### Speech and Communication Aids

For individuals with speech impairments caused by conditions such as ALS, cerebral palsy, or stroke, assistive communication devices enable verbal expression and social interaction.

- Speech-generating devices (SGDs): These devices convert text or symbol-based input into synthesized speech, allowing nonverbal individuals to communicate effectively.

- Eye-Tracking Communication Systems: These systems enable individuals with severe motor impairments to control communication devices using eye movements.
- Text-to-Speech Software: Used in mobile applications and computers, these programs help individuals with speech difficulties communicate through digital platforms.

Hearing and Vision Assistive Devices

Sensory impairments can significantly impact an individual's ability to interact with their environment. Assistive devices for hearing and vision help enhance perception and improve daily functioning [63].

- Hearing Aids: These devices amplify sound for individuals with hearing loss, using advanced noise reduction and speech enhancement technologies.
- Cochlear Implants: These surgically implanted devices bypass damaged parts of the ear and stimulate the auditory nerve directly, restoring partial hearing for individuals with severe hearing loss.
- Visual Aids: Technologies such as screen readers, braille displays, and electronic magnifiers help individuals with visual impairments read and access digital information.

AI-Powered Rehabilitation Tools

Recent advancements in artificial intelligence and robotics have revolutionized rehabilitation therapies, providing personalized recovery programs and real-time feedback [64].

- Robotic Rehabilitation Devices: These systems assist patients in regaining movement after strokes or injuries by guiding limb movements and enhancing muscle reactivation.
- Virtual Reality (VR) Rehabilitation: VR-based training programs immerse patients in interactive environments to improve coordination and cognitive function.
- AI-Assisted Therapy: Machine learning algorithms analyze patient progress and adjust rehabilitation exercises based on real-time data, optimizing recovery outcomes.

The rehabilitation and assistive devices field continues to evolve with advancements in neuroscience, bioengineering, and AI. Future developments will focus on enhancing device integration with the human nervous system, improving personalization through adaptive AI algorithms, and expanding accessibility through cost-effective solutions. As technology progresses, these innovations will further empower individuals with disabilities, enabling greater independence and participation in everyday life.

### Emerging Technologies in Medical Devices

The landscape of medical devices is evolving rapidly, driven by breakthroughs in artificial intelligence, nanotechnology, and personalized medicine. These innovations transform healthcare by improving diagnostic accuracy, enabling real-time patient monitoring, and enhancing treatment outcomes. As medical technology becomes more intelligent and interconnected, it is ushering in a new era of precision healthcare that is proactive rather than reactive.

Artificial intelligence is one of the most significant advancements shaping the future of medical devices. AI-powered diagnostic systems are redefining medical imaging by detecting anomalies more accurately than traditional methods. Deep learning algorithms analyze X-rays, MRIs, and CT scans to identify early signs of diseases such as cancer, reducing the chances of misdiagnosis and expediting treatment decisions [65]. Beyond imaging, AI is also enhancing patient monitoring through predictive analytics. By continuously analyzing vital signs and other health metrics, AI algorithms can detect subtle changes that may indicate an impending medical emergency, such as cardiac arrest or sepsis. This allows for earlier intervention, improving patient outcomes and reducing hospital admissions [66, 67].

Wearable technology is another transformative force in modern healthcare, enabling remote monitoring and early disease detection. Continuous glucose monitors (CGMs) have revolutionized diabetes management by providing real-time glucose readings without frequent finger-prick tests. Patients can track fluctuations in their blood sugar levels with greater precision, leading to more effective and personalized treatment plans. Similarly, smart contact lenses equipped with biosensors are being developed to monitor ocular health, detecting early signs of diseases like glaucoma and diabetic retinopathy before symptoms become severe [68, 69].

Integrating AI with wearable devices becomes more seamless as the field advances, creating innovative health ecosystems that provide continuous monitoring and real-time feedback. Patients can receive personalized alerts and recommendations, while healthcare providers gain access to comprehensive datasets that enhance clinical decision-making. The shift toward AI-driven, data-rich medical devices is paving the way for a future where diseases are detected earlier, treatments are more precise, and patient care is more efficient.

Beyond AI and wearables, nanotechnology is pushing the boundaries of what medical devices can achieve. Researchers are developing nanoscale sensors that can travel through the bloodstream, enabling the identification of disease markers at the molecular level. These tiny yet powerful devices have the potential to revolutionize diagnostics, enabling the early detection of cancer, infections, and neurological disorders long before they are evident in traditional tests. Additionally, implantable nanodevices are being designed to deliver targeted drug therapies, reducing side effects and improving the efficacy of treatments.

The future of medical devices is also closely linked to the rise of personalized medicine, where treatments are tailored to an individual's genetic profile, lifestyle, and real-time health data. Advances in genomics and biotechnology enable the development of smart implants and bioengineered devices that adapt to the unique physiological characteristics of each patient. For example, AI-powered pacemakers can adjust heart rhythms dynamically based on real-time data, optimizing performance and reducing complications. Similarly, bioresorbable implants dissolve after their therapeutic function is complete, eliminating the need for surgical removal [70].

As these emerging technologies evolve, the medical device industry is shifting toward a more interconnected and intelligent healthcare ecosystem. Integrating AI, nanotechnology, and personalized medicine is not just improving patient care but redefining how we prevent, diagnose, and treat diseases. The future holds the promise of more intelligent, more responsive medical devices that empower patients and healthcare providers, ultimately leading to a more efficient and proactive healthcare system.

### 2.1.4 Clinical Applications

Medical devices are at the center of modern clinical practice, supporting diagnosis, therapy, and monitoring of patients across a wide range of healthcare settings. From simple devices to AI-powered diagnostics, these technologies are crucial in enhancing outcomes, minimizing errors, and facilitating personalized medicine. Medical devices, such as cardiovascular monitors, smart insulin pumps, and neurostimulators, deliver real-time therapy and continuous data feedback, enabling clinicians to respond rapidly to changes in patient conditions [71, 72]. Medical devices, including those used in cardiology, neurology, and oncology, among others, have enabled a shift toward more targeted and preventive care.

Technology has accelerated the use of embedded systems and Internet of Things (IoT)-connected devices in remote and home care. These smart devices continuously capture and transmit patient data to clinicians, enabling distant diagnosis, identification of complications at an early phase, and preemptive intervention. It is essential to treat chronic conditions like diabetes, hypertension, and respiratory disease, where wearable monitors and mobile applications enhance care outside the hospital [73, 74]. These applications have been beneficial in the COVID-19 pandemic for monitoring recovering or quarantined patients at home.

Medical devices now face rigorous examinations in regulatory approvals and clinical trials, similar to pharmaceuticals but with device-specific considerations. Clinical trials establish safety, usability, and performance, especially for high-risk or implantable devices. These trials often consider daily use, patient variation, and long-term outcomes [75, 76]. Integrating advanced medical devices into clinical practice revolutionizes healthcare delivery, improves diagnostics, simplifies therapies, and improves patient quality of life.

## 2.1.5 *Regulatory Considerations*

Medical devices play a crucial role in modern healthcare, and ensuring their safety and effectiveness is a priority for regulatory agencies worldwide. Because these devices interact with patients—sometimes in life-sustaining or invasive ways—governing bodies have established rigorous approval processes to mitigate risks and ensure that every product meets strict standards before reaching the market. Two of the most widely recognized regulatory frameworks are the FDA and the European Union's CE marking system, which classify medical devices based on their risk level and intended use. While these regulatory systems share the same overarching goal of patient safety, their approaches differ [77, 78]. The FDA follows a centralized and structured regulatory process in which medical devices undergo classification and evaluation based on risk level, intended use, and complexity. Meanwhile, the CE marking system relies on a decentralized network of Notified Bodies, independent organizations that assess devices for compliance with EU regulations [79]. Despite their differences, both systems require manufacturers to provide substantial evidence of a device's safety, reliability, and performance before approval, particularly for high-risk products.

**Medical Device Classification in the U.S.: The FDA Framework**

In the United States, the FDA classifies medical devices into three categories based on their level of risk to patients and the type of regulatory controls necessary to ensure their safety and effectiveness [80].

1. Class I (Low Risk): These devices pose minimal potential harm to patients and are subject to the least regulatory oversight. Examples include surgical instruments, elastic bandages, and examination gloves. Most Class I devices do not require premarket approval and are exempt from extensive clinical testing. However, they must adhere to general controls, including good manufacturing practices, proper labeling, and reporting requirements for adverse events [81].
2. Class II (Moderate Risk): These devices are more risky than Class I and require additional controls to ensure safety. Examples include infusion pumps, powered wheelchairs, and diagnostic imaging equipment. Class II devices must comply with special labeling requirements and performance standards. They often require a 510(k) premarket notification, in which manufacturers must demonstrate that their device is substantially equivalent to an already legally marketed device [82].
3. Class III (High Risk): These are the most complex and high-risk devices, often critical to sustaining life or preventing severe health conditions. Examples include implantable pacemakers, artificial heart valves, and deep-brain stimulators. Because they pose the highest potential risk, Class III devices must undergo the rigorous premarket approval (PMA) process, requiring extensive clinical trials, laboratory testing, and scientific evidence to prove safety and effectiveness before marketing [83].

The FDA also enforces strict post-market surveillance requirements for all medical devices, particularly high-risk ones. Manufacturers must continuously monitor and report adverse events, device malfunctions, and safety concerns, ensuring that medical products remain safe even after widespread clinical use [84] (Figs. 2.1 and 2.2).

## Medical Device Classification in the EU: The CE Marking System

The European Union follows a different regulatory approach under the Medical Device Regulation (MDR) framework, which replaced the earlier Medical Device Directive (MDD). Unlike the FDA, which directly regulates medical devices, the EU relies on Notified Bodies—independent organizations authorized to assess whether medical devices meet the required safety and performance standards before they receive a CE mark [85].

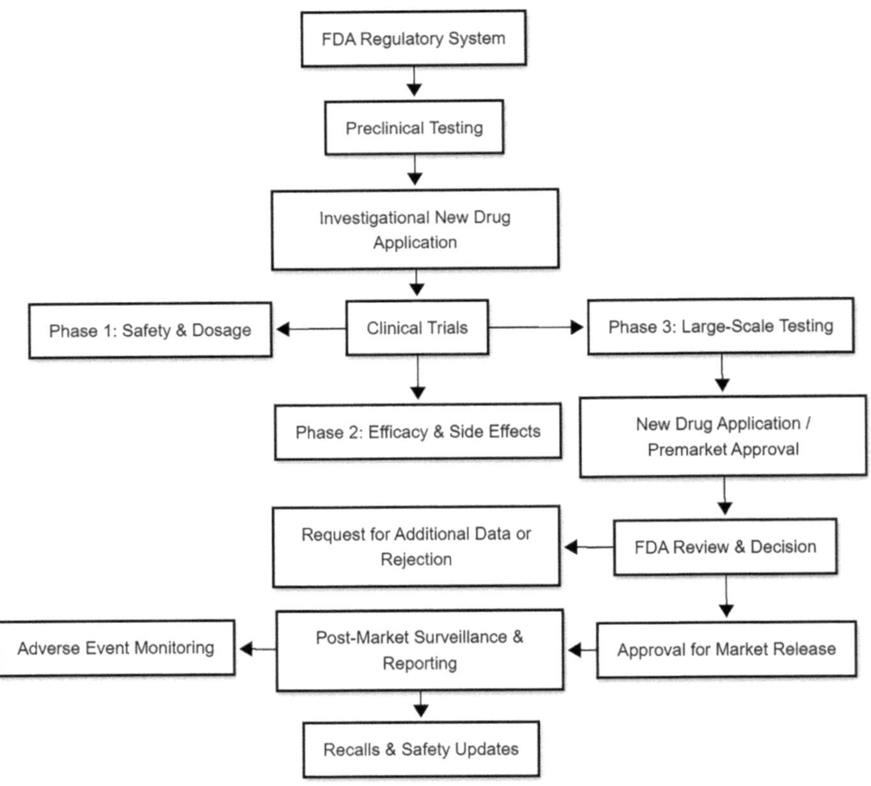


**Fig. 2.1** Flowchart of the FDA system

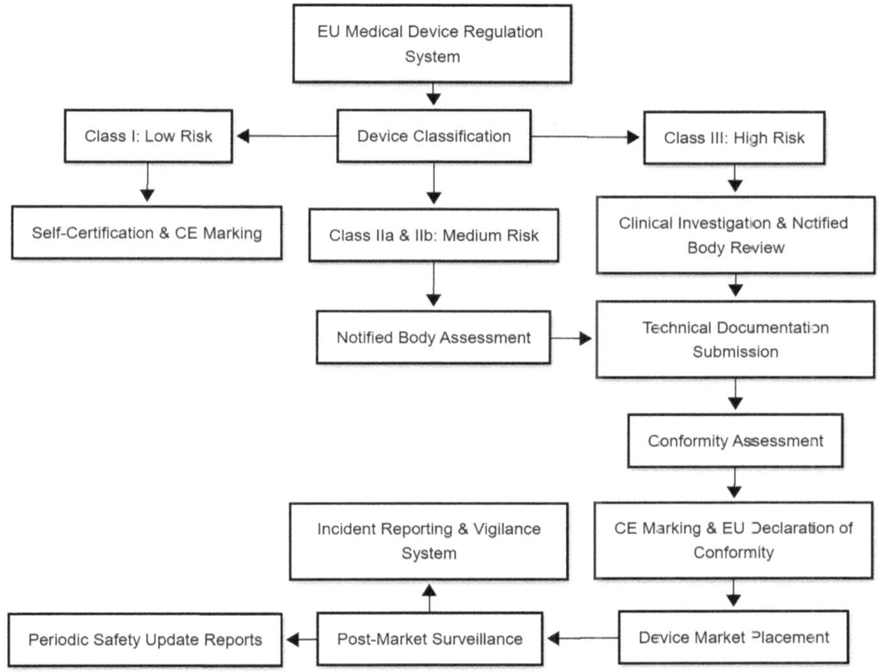


**Fig. 2.2** Flowchart of the EU MDR system

The EU classifies medical devices into four risk-based categories [86, 87]:

1. Class I (Low Risk): Similar to the FDA's Class I, these devices include basic tools such as stethoscopes, bandages, and surgical scissors. Manufacturers of Class I devices can often self-certify compliance with safety standards without the involvement of a Notified Body.
2. Class IIa (Medium-Low Risk): Devices such as hearing aids, dental fillings, and ultrasound machines fall into this category. These products require some external assessment to ensure compliance with EU regulations.
3. Class IIb (Medium-High Risk): Class IIb includes more complex and riskier devices, such as ventilators and infusion pumps. These devices require detailed performance evaluations and the approval of a Notified Body before being marketed.
4. Class III (High Risk): Equivalent to the FDA's Class III category, this includes life-sustaining or highly invasive devices such as implantable defibrillators, heart valves, and artificial organs. Before being approved, these products undergo the most stringent regulatory scrutiny, including clinical trials and comprehensive risk assessments.

A key feature of the CE marking system is that medical devices can be sold across all European Union member states once approved. Unlike the FDA's centralized control, CE certification relies on Notified Bodies, which assess medical devices on behalf of manufacturers. Once a device passes evaluation and earns a CE mark, it can be freely distributed within the European Economic Area (EEA).

### Comparing FDA and CE Marking Approaches

While both regulatory frameworks aim to ensure patient safety and device efficacy, there are significant differences in how they operate [88, 89] (Table 2.7):

1. The FDA follows a centralized regulatory process, meaning that all medical devices must be reviewed directly by the agency before they are approved for the U.S. market. In contrast, CE marking relies on Notified Bodies, independent organizations that assess device compliance before granting certification.
2. The FDA requires premarket approval (PMA) for high-risk devices, involving extensive clinical trials and scientific validation. The EU's Class III devices also require extensive clinical testing, but the process is handled through Notified Bodies rather than a single regulatory authority.
3. Post-market surveillance requirements differ between the two systems. The FDA enforces strict post-market monitoring, including mandatory adverse event reporting. At the same time, the EU's MDR has strengthened post-market surveillance, requiring continuous reassessment of device safety and performance even after approval.

**Table 2.7** Comparison of FDA and EU frameworks

| Aspect | USA | EU |
|---|---|---|
| Regulatory authority | U.S. Food and Drug Administration | European Medicines Agency & Notified Bodies |
| Regulatory framework | Federal Food, Drug, and Cosmetic Act | Medical Device Regulation |
| Device classification | Class I, II, III based on risk | Class I, IIa, IIb, III based on risk |
| Approval process | 510(k) Premarket Notification, Premarket Approval | CE marking via conformity assessment by Notified Bodies |
| Clinical evidence requirement | Stringent for high-risk devices, it can require clinical trials | Requires clinical data for all but low-risk devices |
| Post-market surveillance | Mandatory post-market reporting and monitoring | Strict post-market surveillance and periodic safety updates |
| Labeling requirements | Detailed requirements, including Unique Device Identifier (UDI) | Harmonized labeling, including language requirements |
| Timeline for approval | Typically 6 months—2 years, depending on device class | Typically 6 months—3 years, depending on device class |
| CE mark vs. FDA approval | FDA approval is required before marketing | CE marking allows market access across the EU |

4. The CE marking process is often faster than FDA approval because manufacturers can work with different Notified Bodies rather than a single centralized agency. However, recent updates to the MDR have introduced more stringent clinical evaluation requirements, making the EU's approval process more rigorous than before.

### 2.1.6 Future Perspectives

The future of medical devices is shaped by emerging technologies such as artificial intelligence, nanotechnology, 3D printing, and regenerative medicine. AI-driven diagnostics, for example, enable faster and more accurate detection of diseases by analyzing medical images, genetic data, and electronic health records. Machine learning algorithms are also used to predict patient outcomes, optimize treatment plans, and personalize medical interventions based on individual risk factors [90, 91]. Nanotechnology holds immense promise for developing next-generation medical devices, particularly in drug delivery and biosensing applications. Nanoscale materials and devices can target specific cells and tissues, improving the efficacy of treatments while minimizing side effects. Smart implants, capable of releasing drugs on demand or responding to physiological changes, are paving the way for more personalized and responsive medical treatments [92].

3D printing technology is revolutionizing the production of medical devices, offering customizable solutions for prosthetics, implants, and surgical tools. The ability to create patient-specific devices on demand reduces costs and improves compatibility, leading to better clinical outcomes. Additionally, 3D bioprinting is making strides in tissue engineering, with researchers exploring the possibility of printing functional organs for transplantation [93]. Regenerative medicine and bioengineering are also pushing the boundaries of medical device innovation. Advances in stem cell therapy, tissue engineering, and biomaterials are leading to the development of bioresorbable implants and artificial organs. These breakthroughs have the potential to address critical shortages in organ transplants and improve treatment options for conditions such as heart disease, spinal cord injuries, and neurodegenerative disorders [94].

As medical technology advances, the FDA and CE regulatory systems evolve to accommodate innovations such as AI-powered medical devices, wearable health technologies, and personalized medicine solutions. Artificial intelligence and machine learning algorithms, in particular, pose unique regulatory challenges because they continuously evolve after deployment. To address this, the FDA has introduced a Software as a Medical Device (SaMD) framework, which outlines specific guidelines for AI-driven diagnostic and monitoring tools. Similarly, the EU's MDR has expanded its regulatory scope to include software-based medical devices and digital health technologies [95, 96]. The global harmonization of medical device regulations is becoming increasingly important, as companies seek to bring their products to multiple markets. Efforts such as the International Medical

Device Regulators Forum (IMDRF) aim to align regulatory standards across different regions, making it easier for manufacturers to navigate multiple approval pathways while maintaining high safety standards [97].

Understanding these regulatory requirements is essential for successful market entry for medical device developers. Compliance with FDA or CE regulations ensures product safety and determines market access and commercial success. As technology continues to push the boundaries of innovation, regulatory agencies will continue to adapt, ensuring that new medical devices meet the highest standards of quality, reliability, and patient care [98, 99].

## 2.2 Basic Components and Functions

Electronics has long made an undeniable and valuable contribution to medicine. New medical electronic devices are based on available medical knowledge combined with electronics technologies. Electronics in medicine have many applications, from diagnostics to therapy, always aiming to provide new tools to improve the population's well-being [78, 100].

Nowadays, miniaturization and integration technologies are driving the development of new electronic medical devices that should be portable, wearable, and unobtrusive, but with controlled costs. Regardless of the technologies involved, the primary goal of such devices is typically to measure physiological variables for use in diagnostics, monitoring, and therapy [48, 101].

Therefore, this chapter begins by describing several commonly recorded signals, the corresponding electronics and sensing mechanisms used, and the problems associated with such acquisition systems, with a focus on wireless and wearable devices. It ends with examples of developing electronic devices, essentially for remote health monitoring. This chapter aims to present to the reader those aspects that are common and specific to many medical electronic devices, and to give an overview of what is required and the challenges faced when designing electronics in this field, as well as provide examples under development.

### *2.2.1 History*

From our perspective, electronics in medicine encompass all electronics that address the challenges encountered when using electronics to understand or solve medical problems, not necessarily restricted to humans [16]. Electronics in medicine encompass the study of the electrical behavior of the human body and its response to electrical stimuli. Those stimuli may be voltages, electric currents, or magnetic fields. In this case, electronics are used as a model to represent such behavior.

Electronics may be used to describe biological activities, as with the widely used Hodgkin-Huxley models for a neuron cell, to help restore lost electrical activity, as with pacemakers or Parkinson's disease, to help replace full body parts, for diagnostics, therapy, or monitoring.

In this sense, it is difficult to write a chapter that includes all the aspects, difficulties, and aspects associated with electronics in medicine. Moreover, there are various perspectives and views when examining medical electronics, encompassing electrical engineering, chemical engineering, ethical considerations, security and privacy issues, physics, and medicine, among others. However, it is possible to identify two different sides of the same coin: electronics and medicine. On the electronics side, no one is very interested in knowing what is going on behind the electronic system under development. Rather, the system is purely developed to fulfill the requirements [102]. From the medical side, what is important is how the system can help to solve an existing problem and how the system can be used. Fortunately, these two worlds are converging, and many great advancements are expected in the field of electronics in medicine.

Since this field encompasses numerous applications, ranging from magnetic resonance imaging (MRI) to electrocardiogram (ECG) recording, through biosensors and DNA chips, it is a very broad field, and it is impossible to include and describe all the electronics used in medical applications. Therefore, this chapter introduces the reader to several key issues that must be addressed when developing electronic devices for medical applications. Many problems must be tackled and solved when using electronics in medicine. Of course, some of these problems, fortunately, are also shared by other application fields.

## 2.2.2 *Technical Characteristics*

### Hardware

The design of electronics for medical applications implies the fulfillment of a set of requirements due to the nature of their operation. Such electronics must be designed to be small and capable of being integrated into the environment where they will operate. Another important aspect is that these systems may be required to operate in very harsh environments (inside the stomach, where lots of substances are prepared to digest almost everything), using only a single battery, with no possibility of replacement during tests, and many times only possible using surgical procedures. This requires low-power design techniques, biocompatibility, and long-term usage capability [16].

Since in many applications, the electronics are required to interface with the human body, in order to record signals or to deliver signals or drugs, or to monitor their effect on the human body, one feature of such electronic devices is the ability to register very small variations of the variables under measurement, and many times it is necessary to record many signals at the same time, leading to challenges in terms of analog-to-digital conversion [103]. Most electronics that are used in medicine are designed to sense and transmit a variable, or to control an actuator. In this way, most of the developed solutions have their roots in instrumentation or communication electronics.

Electronic devices in the medical field are usually based on state-of-the-art technologies in order to maximize benefits. They use the latest developments in terms of micro/nanoelectronics, micro/nanosensors, smart material technologies, device integration, device packaging, intelligent systems, etc. However, beyond all the electronics, most intelligent devices will only succeed if they are also designed to comply with the requirements of the software agents that are used to monitor, detect, and provide alerts based on the measured health condition [74].

Another important requirement is the ability to operate as a clinical tool. Many electronic devices being developed that claim potential use in the medical field are far from this goal, because there is a big difference between developing a device to monitor the heart rate while jogging versus use in a clinical application [104]. Before clinical use, a long certification process has to be completed. Simultaneously, many such electronics must also be reliable for operation inside a clinical environment, such as a hospital. As is well known, mobile phones are certified electronic devices, but they are not allowed inside many clinical facilities [105]. This is also the situation for many wireless technologies.

Beyond the certification requirements, which are more demanding than in other fields of electronics, the development of electronics for medicine poses its own technical challenges, due to the various operating constraints. Also, legal and cultural aspects, which differ from country to country, have to be dealt with. Moreover, since the developed solutions are usually for use by medical doctors, it is also necessary to break the acceptance barrier for some new technologies, despite the certification. Finally, and no less important for many applications, the proposed electronic solutions must gain user acceptance, in particular if they are for use outside the clinical environment.

#### Medical Electronics Specific Requirements

At first glance, the field of medical electronics may not seem as challenging as it is. Signal amplitudes and frequency ranges are not that demanding, the operating range is not that large, the operating voltages and currents are, in general, normal, etc. This leads us to the use of standard amplifiers, filters, analog-to-digital converters (ACDs), digital-to-analog converters (DACs), microprocessors, microcontrollers, etc. [100]. So, what are the problems when designing medical electronics? The problem lies, as in all electronic fields, in the combination of the requirements specific to such devices.

The Fig. 2.3 shows a schematic of the electronics involved in a typical solution for a biomedical device. This represents a solution for an advanced device, meaning that only the most sophisticated devices require all the modules represented. In other cases, only a subset of such modules will be required; for example, not all electronic modules used in medicine require a microcontroller or a bidirectional wireless link.

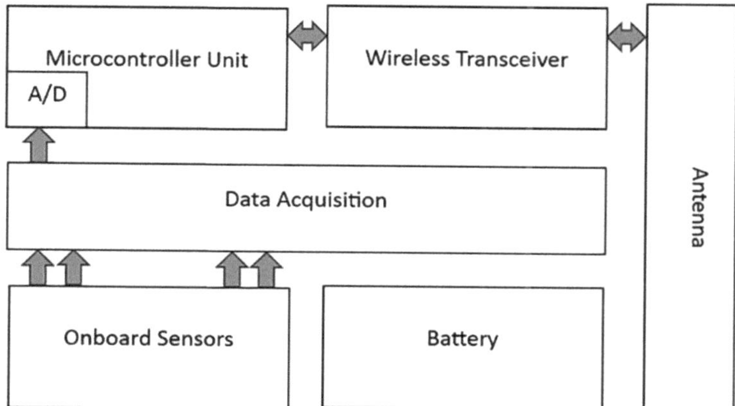


**Fig. 2.3** Main electronic components required for advanced clinical data acquisition

Considering the discussion above, a set of challenges may be identified when developing electronics for medicine. These challenges may be found in data acquisition, filtering, power autonomy, and communications. Furthermore, for AAL applications, it is desirable that devices may be easily worn by the user, leading to miniaturization and wearability requirements. This has also implications in the fashion field, because many people do not like to use electronic devices because they are not fashionable.

The challenge at the data acquisition level results from the combination of a set of requirements particular to this type of system. The frequency range of interest encompasses the 50/60 Hz alternating current (AC) voltage, which introduces a powerful oscillating component into the supplied power. This interfering component may easily become larger than the signal to be measured, and the minimum measurable signal amplitude will increase. To avoid this, either a meticulous power supply design is required, or a battery is used as the power supply. Since many systems are designed for use on or in the body, the battery solution addresses many of these issues. However, power lines may also be coupled to the human body, and when measuring biopotentials, interference is still a problem even when using batteries as the power supply [102]. It is easy to have a few millivolts superimposed on the measured biopotential due to the power lines, which are of the same order of magnitude as the biopotential. One possible solution is to use a notch filter to remove this component. However, this is a challenge because the signal components of interest are around this frequency and must also have a high attenuation factor. An attenuation of 30–40 dB is sufficient for most applications. Although some may benefit from values up to 70–80 dB. However, this high attenuation introduces a new challenge, namely, how to obtain such devices with a very low noise factor.

Another problem during signal acquisition is associated with subject activity, which has frequency components inside the frequency band of interest, introducing so-called movement artifacts. Since these slow components are within the band of interest, they cannot be simply removed by standard low- or high-pass filtering. More complex filters, such as adaptive filtering, must be used to remove these components [106].

At the acquisition level, we have another important aspect, especially for biopotentials, which is the well-known amplifier standard mode rejection ratio (CMRR). Since the subject under measurement is at a different potential with respect to the power supply, often the output signal may be a few millivolts, even when both inputs are at the same potential. The standard solution is to connect the subject to a reference potential, thereby lowering the standard mode voltage and reducing its effect on the recorded signal. However, this solution requires the use of an additional electrode, which also necessitates extra space to accommodate it, which is undesirable when designing miniaturized devices [107].

Power autonomy is also a critical issue and is easy to understand when considering other power-limited devices, such as mobile phones. When dealing with medical electronics, this issue becomes more complicated, as some devices are required to operate inside the human body for an extended period, as is the case with pacemakers. In terms of power autonomy, we can divide the systems into three categories: systems designed to be inserted into the body (such as endoscopic capsules), systems that operate within the human body (such as pacemakers), and systems that operate on the body (such as wearable devices for AAL). Usually, when recording a single channel (EEG, ECG, etc.), it is not difficult to find a solution that operates on a small battery for a few days.

The problem arises when it is necessary to record multiple channels or when it is also required to actuate another device to obtain the necessary reading. When readings from many channels are required, one option is to design all the electronics based on low-power approaches. The other option, also valid for situations where actuators are present, is to integrate energy harvesting or scavenging technologies. Despite some promising proposals, such approaches are not yet available as solutions to fully power a complete system. However, they may be a potential solution to extend the autonomy of existing systems, and in the near future it is expected that they may replace batteries in some applications [108].

We have also to consider communications, in which regard the desirable solution is usually to use wireless communications. However, this introduces new challenges, as this subsystem is typically the most power-hungry. To reduce the power consumption of this subsystem, an efficient power amplifier design must be used, and antennas should also be selected as efficiently as possible. The challenge regarding antenna design results from the operation of wireless systems in low frequency bands in order to decrease the power required for transmission, but this degrades antenna efficiency because they must be electrically small to fit inside the space available in the device.

### Health Condition Monitoring

Health condition monitoring requires the use of a set of sensors to monitor a wide variety of signals, either clinical or environmental, forming a sensing component, for example, surface electrodes to measure bioelectric signals, together with the acquisition electronics. The measured signals can be classified according to their nature and/or type of monitoring (Table 2.8).

Physiological signals include bioelectric events and other biochemical and physical parameters that are crucial for assessing the user's state of health. They can be detected using biosensors, a specific category of wearable sensors that monitor biological properties and processes. Each signal is important for capturing the entire status of the subject and the surrounding environment. On top of such an acquisition system, use of intelligence is usually required so that the system can automatically detect any relevant health condition and, based on that, trigger alarms or send warnings to healthcare providers or the patient being monitored [73].

### Biosignals and Transducers

Biosignals offer an interface between the human body and electronic systems. They are directly related to the physiology and function of organs and organ systems, allowing evaluation of a subject's health condition through their acquisition and monitoring. An electronic system is used to measure physiological signals. Those signals may be electrical, or if not, they are translated to electrical signals using one of various transducers or translation methods [109].

### Power Supply

All electronics and sensors require a power supply for operation. Electronic devices in medicine must have a very small form factor, including the power supply. In this regard, it is necessary to use batteries with very high charge density. However, despite all the solutions available, there is always a need to recharge the batteries. Batteries for wireless wearable devices may operate for 1 day or for 1 week, but, as for cellular phones, recharging will always be required for system operation. Several wireless ALL solutions for monitoring have been proposed in the past few years. Most of them are based on standards for communications on wireless local-area and sensor networks, such as Wi-Fi, Bluetooth, and ZigBee, because of the availability of commercial modules that can be customized for any wireless application. However, a few solutions that make use of other unlicensed industrial, scientific, and medical (ISM) bands exist.

Since wireless monitoring is required, these systems must operate on battery power or utilize an energy harvesting scheme. Either way, system power consumption must be kept as low as possible. This leads to the design of systems where power consumption must be optimised. This is done by selecting the most

**Table 2.8** Categories and types of possible biosignals measured to infer an individual health condition

| Sensing modality | Typical measurement | Sensing site |
|---|---|---|
| Electrocardiogram (ECG) | Heart rate (variability) and ECG-waveform segments | Thorax |
| Electrodermal activity (EDA) | Skin sweat level and fluctuations | Palm, foot, and wrist |
| Electroencephalogram (EEG) | Brain waves (alpha, beta, and theta) | Scalp |
| Electromyogram (EMG) | Muscle tension, facial expressions, and eye blink rate | Upper back and face |
| Electrooculogram (EOG) | Eye movement and blink rate | Near the eye |
| Impedance cardiogram (ICG) | Heart rate, heart stroke volume, and pre-ejection period | Thorax and neck |
| Inductive plethysmography (RIP) | Respiration rate and tidal volume | Thorax |
| Near-infrared spectroscopy (NIRS) | Blood oxygen saturation | Scalp |
| Photoplethysmogram (PPG) | Heart rate, blood oxygen saturation, and blood pressure | Finger and ear |
| Sphygmomanometer | Blood pressure | Upper arm and finger |

power-efficient components available. If energy is consumed carelessly, the wireless acquisition system may become completely useless due to lack of available power. To prevent such failure, energy should be carefully saved using different approaches; for example, if the patient is in the normal state, then the sampling rate of sensors can be reduced to save power, or if the battery charge becomes low then its energy should be reserved for more vital tasks; i.e., the monitoring activity should adapt by the patient's clinical state to save energy [104, 110]. It should be recognized that to conserve further energy, communication protocols should be simplified, and data should be aggregated, compressed, and transmitted in efficient packets, as computation demands significantly less energy than transmission. However, attention must be paid to the delay, which tends to increase linearly with packet length.

### Battery Power Budget Considerations

Since the battery is the main power source for wireless devices, it should be selected to fit the requirements of the electronics which it will supply. The main requirement is its ability to power the electronic device for as long as possible, always considering a minimum period that is acceptable for operation. In many applications this minimum period should not be less than 1 day. After battery autonomy, and many times as important, come the issues of battery dimensions, format, and conformability.

However, other factors must also be considered when making this selection. One consideration is the recharging time, which must be suitable for the application, as many devices utilize embedded batteries that are difficult to replace. This time is usually acceptable if it is below 3 h, the time during which the device may not be used. Also, due to battery lifetime, often it is convenient to use a battery with a protection circuit, which prevents the voltage from dropping below a safe value. In this way, recharging is faster at lower currents, and the device will have an increased lifespan. Another parameter that is used for battery selection is its nominal current [107]. However, its ability for peak currents also must be taken into account. Higher current values may be required, for example, when a module has wireless communication capabilities. When the wireless link is in transmission mode, peak currents may be required. Finally, the operating temperature also interferes with battery lifetime. Notwithstanding attempts to follow the previous guidelines, battery selection may be a hard task to accomplish, first because often it may not be easy to know beforehand the real power consumption of the device. Power consumption depends, for example, on the data rate, operating mode (sleep, standby, transmission, reception), error rate, antenna efficiency due to antenna positioning, and transmission power level. This implies that tests must be carried out under real-world scenarios, or that the battery must be overspecified.

Another problem is that it is only possible to determine the power consumption accurately when the system is already assembled and ready for operation, where predicted values of system autonomy may diverge from those expected [111]. This may be due to several factors, including incomplete manufacturer specifications, the consideration of only standalone power consumption, and the dependence of power consumption on factors such as sampling rates and clock frequency. The measured values of the ZigBee module were similar to the values specified in the datasheet. The ZigBee module presented higher consumption than the proprietary module but lower than the Wi-Fi module. The measured current consumption of the proprietary module was slightly higher than the value specified in the product information. The proprietary module had the lowest power consumption, and the measured power consumption was close to the predicted value [112] (Table 2.9).

From the power measurements, it is also evidence that it may be worthless to design extremely low-power acquisition electronics, sometimes sacrificing acquisition performance, when the main power consumption may be due to the wireless subsystem that, even for the lower-power solution, is one order of magnitude higher. Finally, it was verified that all the devices were able to work on a tiny battery for periods of 1–3 days, which we believe is acceptable for AAL solutions. The Wi-Fi device, as expected, is more power-hungry; however, it transmits at much higher power levels, and the data rate is also significantly higher. Since all microcontroller units have similar power consumption, it is expected that reducing the RF power consumption will significantly reduce the overall Wi-Fi system consumption of this device.

### Wireless Power

Most medical electronic devices requiring the use of batteries will need to be recharged. The most desirable solution would be one where the user does not need to pay too much attention to its use. The most straightforward approach is to use a wireless power link, and even more interesting would be that the device can be recharged without needing to be taken out. This is desirable because it is uncomfortable to remove and replace the device, or because continuous monitoring is required. Another benefit of such solutions is power cable removal, allowing for easy fulfillment of requirements such as devices without connectors or that are completely sealed. Moreover, it allows the development of innovative solutions, such as recharging devices that are inside the body, or recharging devices that we use while we sleep. For short distances, two solutions may be used for wireless recharging:

**Table 2.9** Wireless modules used for autonomy testing

| WiFi | ZigBee | Proprietary |
|---|---|---|
| 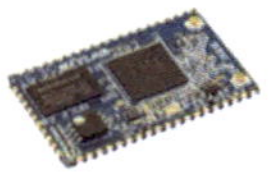 | 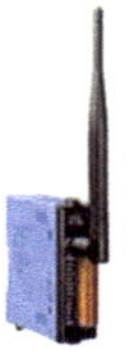 | 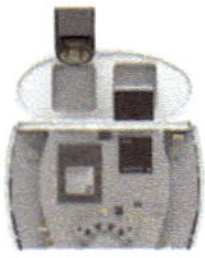 |

capacitive or inductive. It is also possible to use microwave links or optical links, or other forms of energy, but these options lie outside the scope of this chapter.
From basic transformer theory, we know that the voltage and current available at the receiver depend on the voltage and current at the transmitter. The inductive solution for wireless power transmission uses two inductors: the primary and the secondary. On the transmission side, a power amplifier drives the primary inductor. This power amplifier must be matched to the inductor in order for the available power to be transmitted to the inductor and the maximum power to be obtained in the secondary. The inductor acting as a receiver at the secondary side is connected to a power rectifier, followed by a circuit to control the battery charge. To obtain maximum efficiency, the receiving inductor should also be matched to the load [113]. However, as the battery charges, the current usually decreases and the load presented to the inductor also changes. This implies that, for continuous matching, the matching circuit should change during the charging period.

### Wireless Communications

As in many other scenarios, wireless communication is a desirable solution for sensors used for data acquisition in biomedical applications. It is possible to distinguish three main situations: communication between devices inside the human body (intrabody), communication between devices on the body, and communication between devices on the body and the outside world (body to air).
Several aspects should be considered when implementing wireless communication for these various situations. For devices inside the human body, the available power of those devices is very limited, it is challenging to recharge them from outside, and RF losses are very high since the wireless medium is highly conductive. This implies that the link must be made at low frequencies (kHz to MHz). This is a problem because, at these frequencies, antennas tend to be very large or, if their size is reduced to fit inside the devices, antenna efficiency drops [48].

For devices on the body, one main characteristic is that the operation of the device is very close to a highly conductive medium. This has implications for antenna design and signal propagation. Antennas must be designed so that the signal propagates close to the human body; otherwise, power is wasted, and it may be required to operate in the antenna near field, as opposed to the standard operation in the far field. It is challenging to predict where devices should be placed to establish an efficient wireless link. In the latter two scenarios, a module with limited power may be used if easily rechargeable. The main challenge is to hide the antenna in the user environment while maintaining device operation. Solutions such as placing monopole antennas on the user's hat, which may work, are not desired since they are not fashionable. Many small modules are already sold with small antennas attached, and they seem to be very convenient for direct use [105]. However, these antennas are designed to operate in free air. When they are placed close to the human body, their operating frequency and bandwidth, as well their radiation diagram, will be modified.

When dealing with wireless communication, one main problem is to guarantee that data are delivered with sufficient quality of service (QoS) for the desired purpose. It is already possible to find many devices that transmit the measured data wirelessly, but it is tough to find one that can be used for clinical applications. One problem is the lack of solutions to guarantee QoS for biomedical wireless links. Since data are not to be used for clinical decisions, they must be obtained through solutions that guarantee that acquired data are correct and complete, otherwise, patient health may be at risk.

#### Energy Harvesting

Another option available to power wireless devices is the use of some form of energy harvesting. Any form is valid, since it is possible to use that energy to charge a supercapacitor or a battery. Many forms of energy conversion may be used to benefit from the available energy sources: thermal, electric, mechanical or chemical. Despite the main proposed solutions, they still cannot provide sufficient power to drive complete medical electronic devices continuously. Devices already exist that operate on this kind of power source. However, they tend to work in particular conditions and for very specific situations. The amount of power that can be obtained from these solutions is still below the requirements. Moreover, they require very advanced electronic solutions. All required electronics must be based on low-power designs, and wireless transmission must occur at low-power levels. However, and notwithstanding these limitations, this may be a potential solution as an extra power source to help increase battery lifetime.

### Software

#### Signal Amplitude

Bioelectric signals are relatively easy to measure from this perspective. When searching for non-electrical signals, it is also observed that both signal amplitudes and their dynamic ranges are not particularly challenging.

One main problem related to signal amplitudes is that different signals fall within the same range of amplitudes and frequencies. That is a problem since some signals tend to act as interference to others, thus appearing as so-called artifacts. For example, electrocardiography (ECG) or electrooculography (EOG) signals often appear overlapped with electroencephalography (EEG) signals. Even simple patient movement, which occurs on the order of a few Hertz, interferes with signals such as ECG, respiration rate, and blood pressure [114] (Table 2.10).

**Table 2.10** Description and properties of commonly monitored biosignals

| Biosignal | Range | Frequency | Sensor type |
|---|---|---|---|
| Blood flow | 1–300 mL/s | 0–20 Hz | Electromagnetic or ultrasonic |
| Blood pressure | 0–400 mmHg | 0–50 Hz | Cuff or strain gage |
| Blood oxygen saturation | 95–99% | 0–50 Hz | Paired infrared LED and photodiode |
| Cardiac output | 4–25 L/min | 0–20 Hz | Fick, dye dilution |
| Electrocardiogram (ECG) | 0.5–4 mV | 0.05–150 Hz | Skin electrodes |
| Electroencephalogram (EEG) | 5–300 μV | 0.5–150 Hz | Scalp electrodes |
| Electrooculogram (EOG) | 10–100 μV | 0–10 Hz | Skin electrodes |
| Electromyogram (EMG) | 0.1–5 mV | 0–10 kHz | Needle electrodes |
| Electroretinogram (ERT) | 0–900 μV | 0–50 Hz | Contact lens electrodes |
| Action potentials | −80–80 mV | 10–10 kHz | Neuronal electrodes |
| Local field potentials | 0.1–1 mV | 0.1–500 Hz | Neuronal electrodes |
| pH | 3–13 pH units | 0–1 Hz | pH electrode |
| $pCO_2$ | 40–100 mmHg | 0–2 Hz | $pCO_2$ electrode |
| $pO_2$ | 30–100 mmHg | 0–2 Hz | $pO_2$ electrode |
| Pneumotachograph | 0–600 L/min | 0–40 Hz | Pneumotachometer |
| Respiration rate | 2–50 | 0.1–10 Hz | Impedance, electroactive |
| Temperature | 32–40 °C | 0–0.1 Hz | Thermistor |
| Activity | | 0–100 Hz | Accelerometer, GPS, Wi-Fi |
| Body weight | 0–150 kg | 1 time/day | Weighing machine |
| Glucose | 70–180 mg/dL<br>3–8 mmol/L | 0–5 times/day | Glucose meter |

## Signal Frequency

From this perspective, physiological signals are also relatively easy to measure. The maximum frequency is on the order of a few kHz. However, since many of them are in the same frequency band, as mentioned above, they tend to interfere with one another. Another common problem is electromagnetic fields coming from power lines (operating in the frequency range 50–60 Hz), which are easily coupled through the power source (that may also introduce a 100 Hz component due to the use of full-wave rectifiers), or because the human body acts as an antenna for those fields. Sometimes the coupled signal may have higher amplitude than the biosignal being measured.

One solution is to use batteries to power some electronic devices, avoiding interference from the power supply. To remove the effect of interference picked up by electromagnetic coupling, the solution is to use an instrument amplifier not with an input impedance as high as possible but instead designed to kill the 50/60 Hz component. However, the bioelectric signal has limited power. Another problem due to the low frequencies involved, is the requirement for high capacity values, leading to large capacitors for filtering blocks. This has implications for device dimensions and response times during the transitions of such systems.

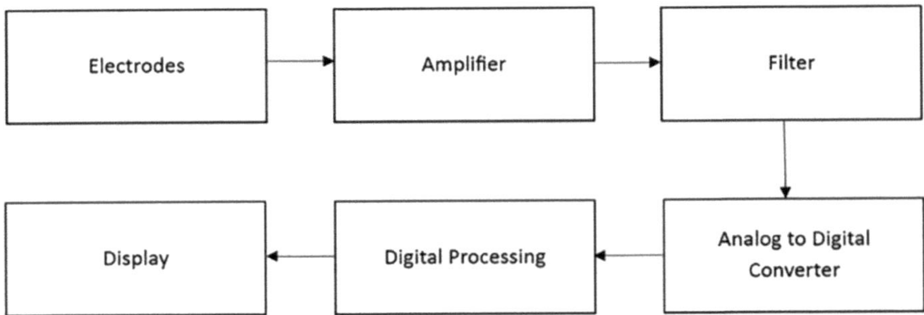


**Fig. 2.4** Typical acquisition system for bioelectric signals

### Signal Power

Many of the important signals that need to be measured are biosignals that originate from body electrical activity. One characteristic of such signals is their small amplitude. However, that is not the main problem with their acquisition; the main problem is their low power (Fig. 2.4).

Since the source current is an order of pA, the available power is also very small. This is a problem when implementing the proposed solution for power line noise cancellation. The interference is canceled, but the biosignal is also attenuated. This means that any small current flow to the instrumentation amplifier will lead to a voltage drop on the electrodes, which will make the available voltage even smaller and more difficult to measure.

### Signal Translation

When the biosignal to be measured is not an electrical signal, it is necessary to use a transducer to obtain an electric signal proportional to the physical variable being measured. Oximetry provides a signal obtained from measurements of light, while spirometry results in a signal obtained from temperature variation or by abdominal volume variation. These are only a few examples but one key aspect may be highlighted: most of these devices also require an actuator and they tend to be bulky. In this way, measurements become more difficult when portable devices are required, and even more difficult when wearable devices are considered. When portable or wearable devices are required, often it is difficult to find a solution that is reliable enough and at the same time acceptable for use by the patient [115].

### Data Acquisition

Acquisition of biosignals from the human body requires similar instrumentation and methods as for any other signal which requires transducers. However, biosignals, namely those that are electrical, typically have small amplitudes and bandwidths and are therefore very susceptible to interference or artifacts, which can easily be superimposed on the biosignal being monitored. Moreover, part of the information contained in the biosignal may not be readily available from the raw signal, requiring further analog or digital processing for feature extraction. Therefore, the design of acquisition electronics for biosignals must contain suitable instrumentation to ensure the integrity of the information contained in the biosignal, while any forms of interference or artifacts must be minimized, so that the acquired biosignal is useful for health condition monitoring or diagnostics, since a corrupted signal could provide misleading or meaningless information.

Sensors represented in the first block are responsible for converting clinically relevant physical quantities into an electrical output that can be processed by electronic instrumentation. Different sensor types are used according to the physical quantity associated with the biosignal (Fig. 2.5).

For electrical biosignals, it might be presumed that sensors would not be required since an electrical property, namely current flow on the human body, is measured. However, transducers are indeed required for acquisition of electrical biosignals, since the current flow on the human body is due to ion transport whereas current flow in the acquisition instrumentation is due to electron movement. This conversion is provided by biopotential electrodes, which are placed on the surface of the human body, as close as possible to the organ that generated the biosignal, such as the heart (ECG) or brain (EEG). For non-electrical biosignals, various types of sensors are used depending on the nature of the biosignal, such as mechanical or thermal devices, and the locations of sensor placement vary according to where the signal is strongest or the measurement most accurate.

Following the sensor stage, the signals obtained are usually weak in amplitude and may have considerable levels of added interference, as mentioned above. Thus, analog processing, featuring low-noise amplification and filtering, is required to increase the amplitude of the acquired signal, match the input range of the ADC, and limit its bandwidth to the range of interest of the monitored biosignal. Care must be taken when designing or choosing amplifiers for analog processing of biosignals. Desirable features for a biosignal amplifier include high input impedance, low output impedance, high differential gain, high common-mode rejection ratio, and frequency response temperature stability. Filtering of the biosignal is usually required, since biosignals are susceptible to interference and artifacts. Filtering of

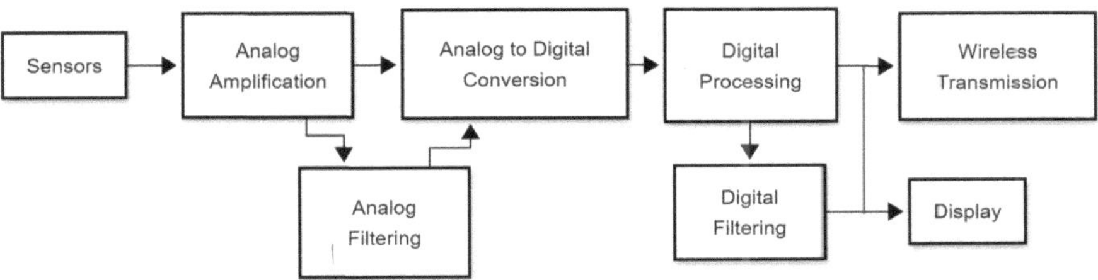


**Fig. 2.5** Typical block diagram of the necessary instrumentation for biosignal acquisition

biosignals can be performed in either analog or digital fashion. Analog filters are implemented using modified amplifier stages that attenuate unwanted frequency components from the acquired biosignal while providing gain to those which are relevant, thus contributing to removal of low and high frequency noise [116]. If necessary, electromagnetic interference from power lines may be further attenuated using notch filters centered at 50 or 60 Hz. Additionally, analog filtering is used to limit the bandwidth of the monitored signal according to the ADC's sampling frequency, thereby avoiding aliasing. Although analog filters are essentially used to remove undesirable signal features, their design must ensure that the filter itself does not cause distortion of the relevant frequency components of the monitored signal. To minimize signal distortion, analog filters should be designed to provide a constant modulus and linear phase frequency response over the pass band.

After the analog filtering stage, the monitored signal is converted to digital format using standard sampling and quantization methods such as sigma-delta or successive approximation. In digital format, biosignals can be handled by digital processors, such as microcontrollers or microprocessors, and be further processed using digital filtering techniques. Digital filters offer advantages over analog filters, as they can be easily modified by changes in programming code, as opposed to changing components in analog designs, and they do not suffer from component tolerances or environmental influences such as temperature. Still, digital filtering and processing techniques require that the processor has enough available computational power, depending on the complexity of the algorithms to be executed by the processor. This may not be the case when the processor is already performing other tasks, such as control of acquisition or communications. Lastly, the biosignal can be displayed to physicians and users, as is common in hospital instrumentation, or, in wireless health monitoring systems, sent wirelessly to a remote location, either in real-time or offline, to allow observation and monitoring.

As described above, signal acquisition appears to be a straightforward procedure. However, many problems can arise when acquiring data from biomedical devices for use in clinical applications. Many of these problems are because the subject under observation is moving, particularly when considering wireless devices. This causes changes in the measurement conditions. These measurement conditions include registering positioning of the transducer and changer in body impedance due to movement, chest movement due to arm movement, as well as breathing. For clinical applications, data acquisition may often be conditioned by the requirement that the measurement device must be applied by a caregiver, and not by someone without medical training [117]. Otherwise the signals have no clinical significance.

Signal acquisition may also be conditioned by requirements from the medical side and not from the signal side. In this way, it is a practice to show the acquired signal to a medical doctor and check if the signal is good enough for diagnostics and not look at the time and spectral content of the signal and decide all the details based on that. It is difficult to find specifications for the desired characteristics of signal acquisition. For many biosignals, it is therefore hard to specify the sampling frequency, number of bits for digitalization, resolution, signal latency, delay between signals, etc.

### System Integration

When developing electronic devices to give mobility to patients, it may be attempted to achieve different degrees of mobility. A system may allow the patient to move inside a clinical facility. In this case, the device must be designed to be portable, so the patient can move around the facility. Alternatively, the system may allow the patient to be monitored at home. This is similar to the previous case, but with additional requirements. Such a system must have a set of alarms to inform the patient that something is not right. Moreover, since the user may be required to place the equipment himself, it should be planned in such a way that the patient is able to place it without the need for caregiver assistance, otherwise the equipment will not be used or will be used improperly. Also, since the equipment may be required to stay at the patient's home for some time, it must be designed so that it can be cleaned at his home. Also, it must be resistant to potential crash accidents. Another approach is to design the electronic device so that the patient can wear it as if it were just another piece of clothing.

Regarding wearable devices, a few different approaches may be adopted. One solution is based on discrete modules that are placed at different locations where signals need to be measured. However, for some applications, this may not be desirable; for example, to record an ECG, it is necessary to have physical connections between the different leads and the instrument's amplifier, and this solution implies the use of a few wires on the patient's body. Moreover, with this solution, it is difficult to clean and control placement of the different measuring devices. The other solution is to design the sensors to be integrated with clothes, with the electronics to be attached to those sensors at a convenient location. This implies integration of wires with textiles and the development of interconnection technologies to interface wires and electronic devices on textiles [78]. Another approach is to embed all the electronics, wires, and sensors on a polymer foil, leading to a smart sheet of material with the ability to record the desired signals. Still using the integration approach, instead of electric methods, optical fibers with optical sensors may be integrated, thereby reducing the problem of integrating wires and electronics.

For wearable devices, the system should be developed taking into account that the user must be able to apply it himself. No help will be provided from any health professional. In this way, it must be developed in such a way that, after putting it on as any regular piece of clothing, the system should only require intuitive adjustments to achieve correct operation. Moreover, since it is something to wear, it must be able to undergo the same cleaning processes as regular clothing.

### 2.2.3 Types of Devices

Medical electronic devices encompass a broad spectrum of devices intended to monitor, diagnose, and enhance human health, from traditional clinical instruments to advanced wearable technologies. Conventional equipment such as electrocardiogram (ECG) and electroencephalogram (EEG) machines are used routinely to monitor cardiac and brain functions, respectively, while implantable devices such as pacemakers and defibrillators are vital in the control of chronic ailments by replacing or complementing missing physiological processes [78]. These devices are being made smaller and more integrated to allow long-term, minimally invasive health monitoring.

Over the years, developments have expanded medical electronics applications to include wearable technology and Ambient Assisted Living (AAL) systems. Wearables, such as health bands and smartwatches, can be used to continuously monitor heart rate, oxygen saturation, and activity levels. AAL systems, on the other hand, place sensors within home settings to monitor activity levels of old persons, supporting them in real time and adding to safety and independence [69]. These technologies are designed to address the challenges posed by an aging population and the increasing burden of chronic diseases.

Furthermore, medical electronics increasingly facilitate human enhancement technologies, such as brain-computer interfaces (BCIs) and exoskeletons, that enhance cognitive or physical capabilities. BCIs provide immediate interaction between the brain and external devices, with emerging prospects for assisting individuals with severe motor disabilities. Exoskeletons are increasingly used for rehabilitation and mobility assistance, enabling patients to rehabilitate or regain motor capabilities. Additionally, smart textiles using sensors and conductive yarn in clothing enable gentle, unobtrusive tracking of vital signs, blurring the line between healthcare and wearable fashion. Such technologies collectively showcase the range and growing importance of electronic devices in reshaping healthcare provision and quality of life.

### 2.2.4 Clinical Applications

Electronics in medicine may include many applications, as mentioned above; for example, ultrasound and MRI imaging systems are often used in diagnostics, as are ECG recording systems, all of which look very different at a high level. However, upon closer examination, all of them are designed to sense physical variables to aid in clinical diagnosis. In this way, in most medical electronic devices, the requirement is to design adequate instrumentation electronics to interface with a transducer that is used to convert a physical variable of interest into an electrical signal, which is finally used to help in the diagnostics [101].

The success of electronics in medicine relies on their ability to help medical doctors determine a set of parameters that are compared against a range of values considered healthy. After beating the challenge of determining which parameter is important to measure, and in which range it must be, it is up to the medical electronics to provide solutions to perform these measurements reliably and in a solution that can be easily deployed. In this way, instrumentation is a very important field when dealing with medical electronics. Many medical devices measure specific variables, which may be chemical, physical or electrical [118, 119]. These measurements are supported by appropriate electronics and a transducing mechanism to convert, e.g., an ionic concentration to a voltage stage, proportional to it.

Some recordings may be obtained by direct measurements, such as when a temperature sensor is used for measuring body temperature. Alternatively, they may be obtained by indirect measurements, such as breathing rate using a temperature sensor, where temperature changes of air flow are measured to determine the breathing rate. In this way, sensing techniques and sensors are also important when dealing with medical electronics. They are essential because without sensors, there is no medical information to process, analyze, transmit, or store.

### Electronics for Wireless Health Monitoring

Wireless health monitoring systems (WHMS) are among the most promising applications of wireless communication technology, and they have been a very active research topic with considerable advances during the last decade. These systems consist of groups of wireless-enabled sensors attached to the human body in a non-invasive or minimally invasive fashion, together forming a wireless body area network to acquire diverse physiological signals (also known as biosignals) and transmit them via radio to a remote location, for display or monitoring to enable assessment of the user's health condition.

The development of WHMS envisions improving the quality and efficiency of healthcare, which is currently facing increasing demand and, consequently, increasing global costs. The tendency for increasing healthcare demand is mainly motivated by the aging of the world population, which is expected to cause an increase in the incidence of chronic diseases and physical disabilities. According to the United Nations, the world population is currently enduring an unprecedented and irreversible ageing process, which will cause a growth in the proportion of elderly people (over 60 years old) to a third of the population in developed countries, and to 22% of the total world population by the year of 2050. Therefore, there is a growing need for health monitoring solutions to provide more efficient use of healthcare resources to caregivers and better quality of life to the elderly or diseased, relieving excessive pressure on healthcare demand and costs.

Wireless technology in healthcare provides new means for close observation of patients' health conditions. Typically, observation of a patient takes place when he feels some sign of illness and reactively seeks healthcare. Alternatively, his health condition may be followed by a caregiver, requiring the patient either to visit a healthcare facility or to stay there in case of prolonged examination or intervention. This leads to time and location constraints for the patient and can only provide limited periods of observation of his health condition, which may mean that diagnosis of health complications or pathologies may be late or overlooked. Moreover, conventional health monitoring equipment uses wired connections to the patient, hindering the activity of monitored patients.

On the other hand, WHMS inherently provides mobility to patients, allowing them to be monitored virtually, anytime, and anywhere within the wireless network. Hence, WHMS allows patients to be monitored in a convenient location, typically at home, which reduces disturbance to their daily activities, helping them adopt a healthier lifestyle and improving their quality of life and independence. In addition, WHMS also offers the possibility of continuous health monitoring. Following the current trends towards miniaturized and low-power-consumption electronics development, WHMS can be used for extended periods (e.g., 24 h), providing approximately continuous evaluation of the health condition of a subject. Furthermore, continuous health monitoring is a very useful feature for the enhancement of preventive care and quality of treatment. By monitoring a subject continuously, any slight changes in health condition about the long-term circadian pattern can be detected early by the caregiver, allowing for better decision-making and anticipating severe health complications. Thus, continuous health monitoring offers better treatment possibilities for patients suffering from chronic diseases or enduring rehabilitation processes. Subjects without illness may also be continuously monitored to receive feedback on their activities and modify their behavior to prevent illness by promoting a healthier lifestyle.

### Requirements for Wireless Devices

Even though WHMS have the potential to provide significant benefit in healthcare, they have not yet matured to a point of general use, as a considerable number of application and user requirement issues, including the following, hinder their application to real-life situations and acceptance by caregivers and patients:

#### Ergonomics and Wearability

A WHMS needs to be as small and lightweight as possible so that the user feels comfortable using it over long periods, and it should not affect the patient's daily activities. Ideally, the WHMS should go unnoticed by both the user and others, as the users of WHMS may become stigmatized if it is perceivable. An appropriate solution is the integration of the WHMS into textile garments, resulting in wearable or smart-textile monitoring systems.

#### Low Power Consumption

WHMS, as a mobile application, is required to include its own power source, which is typically a battery, although energy harvesting solutions appear as a possible alternative in the future. The power sources of these devices can only offer limited operation time, and therefore, it is essential to reduce the power consumption to minimal levels to ensure appropriate monitoring periods [118].

### Quality of Service (QoS)

The wireless communication protocol implemented on the WHMS must include a proof mechanism to ensure that the biosignal data is reliably delivered to the base station, especially for continuous monitoring, and if an emergency is detected.

### User Friendliness

In order to achieve user acceptance, WHMS operation should be autonomous but perceivable by the system's user, either the patient or healthcare personnel. It should also require as little maintenance as possible.

### Privacy and Security

The health condition of a patient must be regarded as private information. Therefore, data encryption methods and protection against unauthorized access should be implemented [120]. WHMS are expected to be a valuable tool to address the effects of population ageing on healthcare. They benefit both patients and caregivers, enabling improved quality of life and independent living for patients and improved efficiency and better use of healthcare resources for caregivers. However, the design of such systems is challenging, and solutions that can be widely accepted by patients and caregivers have yet to be implemented.

### Wireless Power Link Analysis

A wireless link was implemented and analyzed to understand the losses expected from this antenna solution. An external (transmitter) subsystem consisting of a Collpitts oscillator generated an AC signal to feed the power amplifier. The implanted (receiver) subsystem has an AC-DC converter for power recharging purposes, and a notch filter for power link rejection precedes the data link path. This way, it is possible to power the receiver and receive wirelessly transmitted data. The wireless link was implemented using two coins in parallel, with the following dimensions: width, 2 cm; length, 4 cm; and thickness, 0.254 mm. Four capacitors were used as the matching network for the inductors, two in series (4.7 nF) and the other two in parallel (2.2 nF), to avoid losses due to power mismatch in the wireless link. The matching network was optimized using a simulation to enhance the efficiency of the wireless link. The wireless link was designed to operate at a distance of 3 mm between the two inductive coils. Measurements, simulations, and analytical models were used to investigate the link performance. Measurements were made for the inductive wireless link and compared with simulation results. The link efficiency was computed and compared with the efficiency obtained from analytical models for other antenna solutions. Return loss measurements were performed

using a vector network analyzer, enabling efficiency measurements. On the other hand, all simulations were done using Ansoft Designer SV software.
First, the inductive wireless link was characterized without any matching network and compared with the simulation results. The results showed high losses, but they were intended to provide a means of designing the matching network and validating the previously performed simulations. Using the measured results as input for the simulator, it was possible to design the corresponding matching network and compute the capacitance required for matching.

Wireless Power Charger

Despite the losses expected when using wireless power transmission, there are situations where implementing this option is necessary. With the developed wireless link, recharging the three modules takes approximately 2.5 h. For their planned application, the modules have an autonomy of approximately 20 h. The solution, despite being effective, requires removing the wearable device for recharging. A desirable solution would be the ability to recharge such devices while the user is performing an activity, close to a location where it is possible to place the charger. One solution that may be adopted is using a charger format that may be transformed into a power pillow or a power mattress.
Another solution is to place chargers on equipment at the gymnasium, or on a desk or desk chair. The idea behind these concepts is to provide a solution for recharging wearable devices without the need to remove them from the body. Using this concept, power is transmitted to the system's battery while the user is lying in bed, whether sleeping or undergoing diagnostics or treatment at the hospital. However, these kinds of solutions, beyond the technical problems that must be solved before their implementation, also require a more profound understanding of the potential effects that the recharging electromagnetic field may have on user health.

Despite the many benefits envisaged by this technology, it still has a long way to go before it can be widely deployed. This technology suffers from several problems, which are challenging to resolve, with link efficiency being one of the most significant. Very special conditions must be met to achieve efficiencies of 70–80%. Regular links will not exceed 50% of the total transmission distance, even for short distances. However, this solution may be very interesting for applications where the charging device and wireless module may be placed close together.

## Impact of Integrated Electronics on Medicine

Healthcare presents a singular opportunity to improve the quality of life in our society through technology. In modern medical practice, the premier diagnostic and monitoring tools are electronic instruments, as illustrated by the X-ray and electrocardiograph. An electronic prosthesis, the implantable cardiac pacemaker, is essential to life for many patients. In medical research, a myriad of electronic instruments

ranging from electron microscopes to pinpoint-size microelectrodes contribute enormously to the prevention, identification and treatment of disease.
The ideal diagnostic instrument provides definitive data on the patient's condition, causes no harm or discomfort, and is convenient, reliable, and economical for the physician or their medical associates to use. A monitoring instrument imposes the additional stringent requirement of virtually total freedom from the need for a human operator. Because of their noninvasive character, transcutaneous instruments such as computer-aided tomographic X-ray scanners, electrocardiographic monitoring units with automatic arrhythmia detection, and ultrasonic imaging and blood flow meter systems offer the most incredible possibilities of fulfilling these idealized specifications [121]. However, given the limitations of noninvasive techniques in medical research involving animal models of human disease, invasive instruments such as subcutaneously implanted telemetry systems for measurement of blood flow and pressure are invaluable in their ability to collect physiological data that would otherwise be unavailable.

### 2.2.5 Regulatory Considerations

Incorporating wearable technology into the healthcare sector presents several regulatory challenges, particularly regarding data privacy, security, and device interoperability. With the devices constantly logging sensitive health information, it becomes necessary to comply with standards such as HIPAA and GDPR. One of the most significant concerns is the lack of standardized data protocols, which can slow the integration of wearable data into electronic health records (EHRs) and clinical decision-making systems [122]. Regulations must evolve to ensure patient safety and protect health data transmission.

Device certification and clinical validation are the other challenges. Unlike traditional medical devices, most wearable health devices initially exist as consumer electronics, subject to less stringent clinical assessment. Wellness devices often blur the lines and are not easily separable from medical tools, potentially leading to misinterpretation or improper usage. The lack of adequate regulatory control can have false findings or an overstated feeling of protection for both consumers and clinicians [79, 123].

To counter these issues, harmonized global standards and more comprehensive guidelines from regulatory bodies such as the FDA and EMA are increasingly in demand. Regulators increasingly recognize the potential of wearables in-home monitoring and are crafting adaptive, risk-adjusted approaches to approval. The success formula, however, rests on interdisciplinary collaboration between engineers, clinicians, and policymakers to ensure wearable devices are safe, effective, and ethical while driving innovation [124].

### 2.2.6 *Future Perspectives*

The future of wearable technology in medicine is rapidly moving towards proactive and personalized medicine. The ongoing monitoring enabled by smartwatches, biosensors, and textile-based systems facilitates the early detection of physiological abnormalities and the management of chronic diseases outside traditional clinical settings [125]. These devices will be at the center of preventive care systems, facilitating timely interventions before serious symptoms manifest.

Emerging technologies, such as artificial intelligence (AI), smart textiles, and energy harvesting, will revolutionize the capabilities of wearable devices. Intelligent interpretation of real-time health data through AI integration will enhance diagnostic accuracy and facilitate adaptive treatment regimens. Improvements in battery life, wireless charging, and biodegradable materials will also enhance comfort and sustainability, making wearables more comfortable and environmentally friendly [126].

In the long term, wearable health technology is expected to play a crucial role in developing equitable and affordable healthcare systems. By enabling remote care, especially in underserved communities, pressure on hospital infrastructure should be reduced, and healthcare disparities bridged. In the future, innovations must consider ethical issues such as data ownership, informed consent, and equitable access to technology by all [127]. The next decade will witness a revolution in healthcare, with wearable electronics at its core.

## 2.3 Imaging Devices

The evolution of imaging devices has fundamentally transformed healthcare, reshaping the landscape of medical diagnostics and treatment. From early mechanical systems to cutting-edge digital technologies, imaging devices have played a pivotal role in detecting diseases, monitoring patient conditions, and guiding therapeutic interventions. In today's healthcare environment, imaging devices are indispensable, allowing clinicians to visualize internal structures, detect abnormalities, and make informed decisions that significantly improve patient outcomes. These devices have revolutionized how clinicians approach everything from routine check-ups to complex surgeries, enhancing diagnostic accuracy and contributing to more effective, personalized treatments.

The rapid progress of imaging technology has been fueled by the convergence of several scientific disciplines, including biomedical engineering, computer science, and artificial intelligence. The integration of advanced data analytics, automation, and imaging modalities like X-ray, computed tomography (CT), magnetic resonance imaging (MRI), and ultrasound has made it possible to detect diseases at earlier stages, track the progression of chronic conditions, and assist in minimally invasive interventions. These devices provide real-time visual insights into the body's internal structures and physiological processes, offering non-invasive methods to assess conditions that once required invasive procedures or surgeries [128].

At the heart of modern diagnostic capabilities are imaging modalities that allow clinicians to peer inside the body with unmatched precision. X-ray imaging remains a staple for diagnosing fractures and detecting diseases such as pneumonia and cancer. MRI, with its ability to produce detailed images of soft tissues, plays a crucial role in neurological and musculoskeletal imaging. Ultrasound, on the other hand, provides real-time visualization for monitoring pregnancy, assessing heart function, and guiding biopsies. These imaging technologies allow clinicians to make more accurate diagnoses, tailor treatments, and reduce the need for exploratory surgeries.

In addition to diagnostic imaging, therapeutic imaging technologies play a crucial role in guiding procedures such as radiation therapy and minimally invasive surgeries. For instance, real-time imaging guidance, such as fluoroscopy and CT scans, enables surgeons to navigate delicate operations with precision, thereby minimizing risks and enhancing patient safety [22]. Imaging devices also assist in monitoring the effectiveness of treatments, allowing healthcare providers to assess changes in a patient's condition over time and adjust interventions as needed.

One of the most significant advancements in imaging technology is integrating artificial intelligence (AI) into diagnostic imaging. AI algorithms are now being employed to enhance the interpretation of imaging data, automate the detection of abnormalities, and provide predictive analytics that can identify health risks early. AI-powered imaging systems can help reduce human error, expedite the diagnostic process, and enhance the accuracy of interpretations, particularly in complex cases.

Furthermore, portable imaging devices transform healthcare delivery by allowing remote diagnostics and patient monitoring. Compact devices like handheld ultrasound machines and mobile X-ray units enable healthcare professionals to assess patients in diverse settings, from rural clinics to emergency rooms. These portable technologies help bridge the gap in healthcare access, making it easier for clinicians to provide timely care, regardless of location.

As the demand for more accessible, efficient, and personalized healthcare continues to grow, the role of imaging devices in both diagnostic and therapeutic contexts is expected to expand. With the increasing integration of digital health solutions, remote monitoring, and telemedicine, imaging devices will be crucial in delivering high-quality care to underserved populations and those in remote areas.

The future of imaging technology holds great promise, with advancements in AI, machine learning, and data analytics poised to revolutionize the field further. These innovations will not only enhance diagnostic precision and treatment outcomes. However, they will also help address challenges in healthcare delivery, ensuring that imaging devices remain at the forefront of medical advancements. The following sections will delve deeper into specific imaging modalities, exploring their principles, applications, and impact on patient care.

### 2.3.1 History

X-ray imaging is one of modern medicine's most fundamental and widely used diagnostic tools. Since its discovery by Wilhelm Conrad Roentgen in 1895, it has revolutionized how physicians diagnose and monitor medical conditions. By providing a non-invasive means of visualizing internal structures, X-ray technology has enabled early detection of diseases, guided treatment decisions, and improved patient outcomes in various medical specialties.
The principle of X-ray imaging relies on the ability of X-ray radiation to pass through the body and create contrast based on the density of different tissues. Dense structures, such as bones, absorb more X-ray radiation and appear white on the resulting image, while soft tissues allow more radiation to pass through and appear in shades of gray. This ability to differentiate between tissues makes X-ray imaging particularly useful for identifying fractures, infections, tumors, and other abnormalities (Fig. 2.6).

Over time, X-ray technology has evolved from simple radiographs to more advanced techniques such as CT, fluoroscopy, and digital radiography, each offering improved image resolution and diagnostic capabilities. With digital imaging and

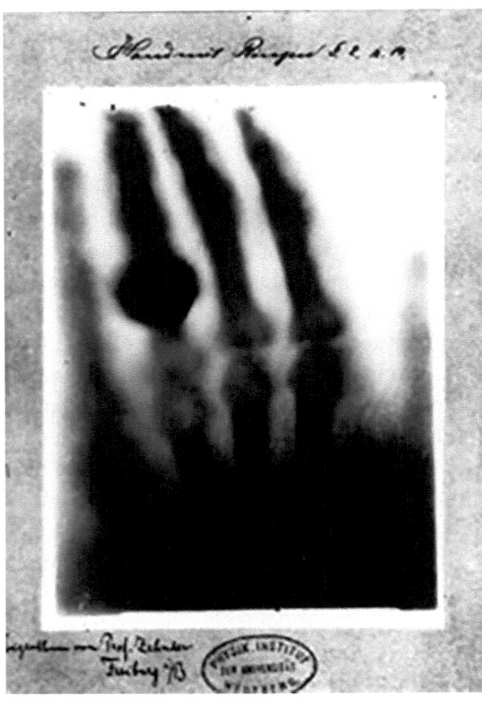

**Fig. 2.6** Wilhelm Roentgen's first X-ray image of his wife's hand (1895) (https://commons.wikimedia.org/wiki/File:First_medical_X-ray_by_Wilhelm_R%C3%B6ntgen_of_his_wife_Anna_Bertha_Ludwig%27s_hand_-_18951222.gif)

artificial intelligence integration, modern X-ray systems provide faster, safer, and more accurate diagnoses while minimizing radiation exposure.

X-ray imaging is based on the interaction between electromagnetic radiation and human tissues. When an X-ray beam is directed toward the body, it travels through different tissues at varying rates. The differences in how much radiation each tissue absorbs create the characteristic contrast seen in X-ray images. The X-ray tube is at the core of an X-ray system, which generates high-energy X-ray photons. This tube consists of a cathode that emits electrons and an anode that receives them. When a high voltage is applied, the electrons accelerate toward the anode, colliding with a metal target—typically tungsten—producing X-ray radiation. This radiation is then directed toward the patient's body, interacting with tissues to produce an image on a detector.

The resulting image is a radiograph formed based on the X-rays' absorption pattern. Denser structures like bones absorb more X-rays and appear bright, while less dense structures, such as muscles and lungs, allow more X-rays to pass through and appear in darker shades. This ability to differentiate between various tissues makes X-ray imaging a valuable diagnostic tool.

The early adoption of X-ray technology in the medical field was swift, with physicians using it to visualize fractures, detect foreign objects in the body, and diagnose certain diseases. The ability to see inside the body non-invasively revolutionized how doctors approached diagnosis and treatment. The first applications were primarily focused on skeletal imaging, as X-rays could reveal broken bones or dislocations with remarkable clarity. However, the early days of X-ray imaging were not without challenges. The technology was still in its infancy, and many unknowns surrounded the effects of exposure to ionizing radiation. Initially, neither physicians nor patients knew of the potential health risks associated with frequent X-ray examinations. Early radiologists and technicians often experienced skin burns and other radiation-related injuries due to prolonged exposure.

Despite these risks, the therapeutic potential of X-rays was undeniable, and the field continued to evolve rapidly. The development of the fluoroscope in the early twentieth century allowed physicians to observe real-time images, providing dynamic insight into the functioning of internal organs. This ability to view moving structures within the body, such as the motion of the heart or the gastrointestinal tract, further expanded the clinical applications of X-rays (Fig. 2.7).

As the twentieth century progressed, X-ray technology continued to undergo significant advancements. The introduction of contrast agents, which could enhance the visibility of blood vessels and soft tissues, made it possible to visualize previously indistinct structures within the body. Innovations such as angiography, which involves injecting a contrast medium into blood vessels to visualize their structure, have become integral to diagnosing cardiovascular diseases. Modern X-ray imaging has advanced significantly with the introduction of digital radiography, which replaces traditional film-based X-rays with electronic sensors. This enables faster image acquisition, improved contrast enhancement, and the ability to manipulate images for enhanced diagnostic accuracy.

In the post-World War II era, the widespread use of X-ray machines in hospitals and medical centers accelerated, spurred by advances in electronics and materials

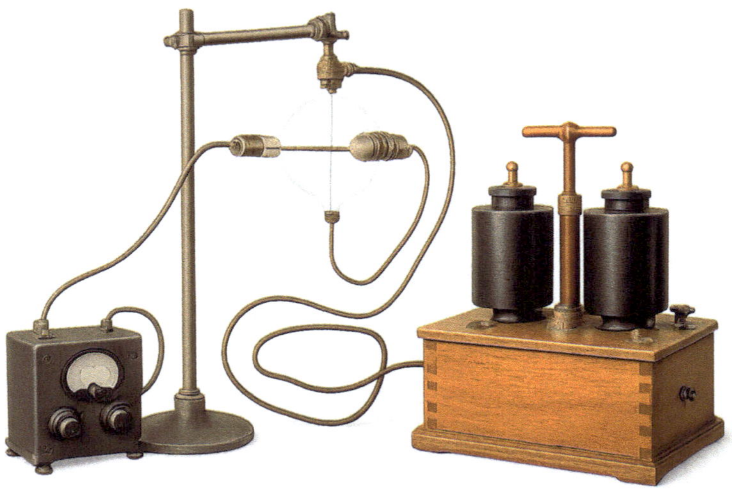

**Fig. 2.7** Early X-ray machine setup from the late nineteenth century

science. Developing more reliable and efficient machines allowed for greater accessibility and accuracy. However, alongside these advancements, the dangers of radiation exposure became increasingly evident. It became clear that while X-rays were invaluable for diagnosing medical conditions, their misuse or overuse posed significant health risks, especially for both patients and healthcare professionals. Over the years, various X-ray imaging techniques have been developed to address specific medical needs. These techniques range from basic radiography to more complex imaging systems that allow real-time visualization of internal structures.

Conventional Radiography remains the most commonly used form of X-ray imaging. It is widely employed for diagnosing fractures, detecting infections, and evaluating lung conditions such as pneumonia. Chest X-rays, skeletal X-rays, and abdominal X-rays are the most frequently performed radiographic examinations. Another significant advancement is fluoroscopy, which provides real-time moving images of internal structures. This technique is beneficial in procedures such as angiography, gastrointestinal studies, and catheter insertions, where continuous monitoring is required. Using contrast agents, fluoroscopy enhances the visibility of blood vessels, the digestive tract, and other soft tissues (Fig. 2.8).

Computed Tomography (CT) scanning, a more advanced form of X-ray imaging, utilizes multiple X-ray beams and computer processing to generate cross-sectional images of the body. CT scans provide greater detail than conventional X-rays and are particularly valuable in detecting tumors, internal bleeding, and complex fractures [25]. Advancements in digital radiography have further improved image quality and efficiency. Unlike traditional film-based X-rays, digital X-rays allow immediate image viewing, reduced radiation exposure, and better storage capabilities through hospital digital imaging systems. These images can be easily shared among healthcare providers, enhancing collaboration and patient care.

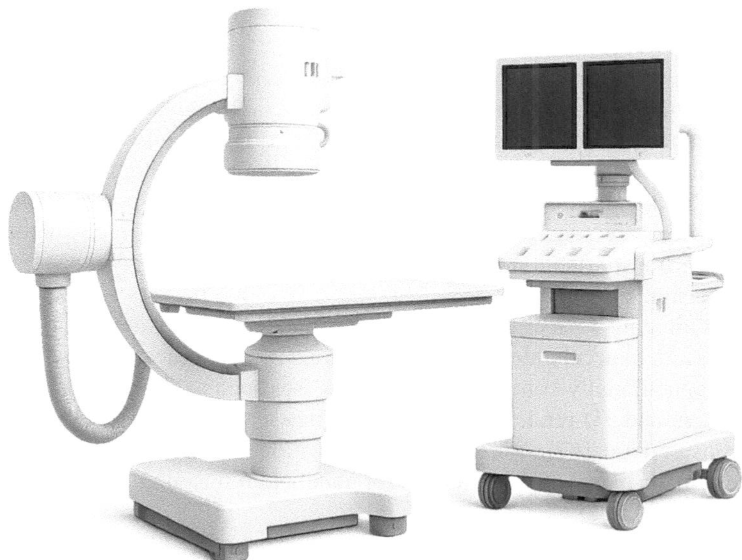

**Fig. 2.8** A fluoroscope

## 2.3.2 Technical Characteristics

Medical imaging devices use advanced electronics, mechanics, and computer science systems to produce high-resolution images of the human body's interior. These systems must meet stringent performance, accuracy, and safety standards while being easy to use and cost-effective. The requirements for high-resolution imaging call for advanced detectors, high-speed signal acquisition, and strong data processing chains capable of managing large datasets in real time. System responsiveness and image quality depend heavily on minimizing noise, optimizing spatial resolution, and carefully calibrating optics and sensors.

In the last several years, imaging systems' key performance indicators have focused on accuracy, speed, energy efficiency, and portability. Embedded computing and low-power architecture are increasingly favored to facilitate point-of-care and mobile imaging solutions, especially in underserved or remote areas. Additionally, imaging modalities must comply with biomedical safety standards, particularly when employing ionizing radiation or electromagnetic fields, requiring ongoing technical innovation in shielding, control systems, and compliance with standards.

To meet these diverse technical requirements, modern imaging platforms increasingly utilize hybrid designs of analog and digital systems, integrated circuits, high-speed ADCs, and smart software frameworks. The systems must also be interoperable with hospital information systems and EHRs, thus embracing open communication standards such as DICOM and HL7. Collectively, the technical characteristics of imaging systems determine their reliability, diagnostic utility, and clinical impact.

### Hardware

The hardware of medical imaging devices is core to their operation, enabling accurate signal detection, processing, and image display. The most important hardware elements include radiation sources (e.g., X-ray tubes), detectors (e.g., scintillators, semiconductor arrays), mechanical positioning systems, and high-level microprocessors. In MRI and CT devices, among other subdevices, high-power magnets and cooling devices are required to ensure image integrity. With more demand for lighter, more transportable units, manufacturers are prioritizing compact, modular hardware design.

Today's imaging devices incorporate high-efficiency digital detectors and multicore processors to accelerate imaging and reconstruction times. GPUs and FPGAs handle computationally complex parallel processes such as noise reduction, image segmentation, and 3D rendering, which yield massive improvements in speed and power consumption [67]. Wireless communication modules and touch-sensitive interfaces enhance usability, especially for handheld ultrasound and digital radiography devices.

New hardware developments also aim at improved accessibility. Battery-powered handheld imaging tools and AI-enabled edge computing platforms are being developed for deployment in remote and emergency settings. These developments allow clinicians to perform high-quality imaging without depending on fixed, large-scale infrastructure. Ultimately, continuous optimization in hardware development facilitates the move toward more efficient, scalable, and patient-focused diagnostic equipment.

### Software

Software is the intelligent layer of medical imaging platforms, governing everything from image acquisition and reconstruction to data management and diagnostic interpretation. Imaging software with high performance synchronizes the timing, control, and visualization processes to enable real-time feedback and automated adjustments during scanning [129]. It also guarantees images meet clinical standards for clarity, contrast, and accuracy in various types of patients and diagnostic goals.

Advances in machine learning and artificial intelligence in the last decade have enormously expanded the functionality of imaging software. AI-based applications can now assist with detecting tumors, quantifying organ size, marking abnormalities, and even predicting patient outcomes based on imaging biomarkers. Software platforms are becoming cloud-enabled to a large extent, and therefore, remote access, automated reporting, and interfacing with telemedicine platforms and EHRs are all feasible. These innovative solutions boost productivity, enhance diagnostic consistency, and reduce radiologist fatigue.

Apart from this, modularity and scalability of software architectures enable imaging systems to be updated regularly without hardware replacement. Software development kits and open-source toolsets enable software developers and clinicians to customize applications for specific use cases, such as cardiology, neurology, or oncology. As imaging becomes increasingly data-intensive and precision-driven, the role of software in enabling clinical insights and operational flexibility will continue to grow.

### 2.3.3 *Types of Devices*

#### MRI Imaging

Magnetic Resonance Imaging (MRI) is a powerful, non-invasive imaging technique that is pivotal in modern medicine. Unlike X-ray or CT, MRI does not rely on ionizing radiation, making it a safer option for various diagnostic purposes. Since its introduction in the 1970s, MRI has become one of the most essential diagnostic tools in the medical field, providing detailed images of soft tissues in the body with exceptional clarity. MRI's versatility and non-invasive nature have revolutionized the diagnosis and monitoring of numerous medical conditions, particularly those involving the brain, spine, muscles, and joints (Fig. 2.9).

The underlying principle of MRI imaging is based on the behavior of hydrogen nuclei in the body when exposed to a magnetic field. These hydrogen nuclei, primarily found in water and fat, align with the magnetic field. When exposed to a radiofrequency (RF) energy pulse, these nuclei are temporarily displaced from their alignment. Returning to their original state, they emit RF signals detected by the MRI scanner, which are used to create detailed images of the internal structures.

MRI is particularly useful in visualizing soft tissues, making it invaluable in detecting neurological disorders, musculoskeletal injuries, cardiovascular conditions, and certain cancers. The ability to create highly detailed images without invasive procedures has made MRI a cornerstone of modern medical diagnostics. MRI

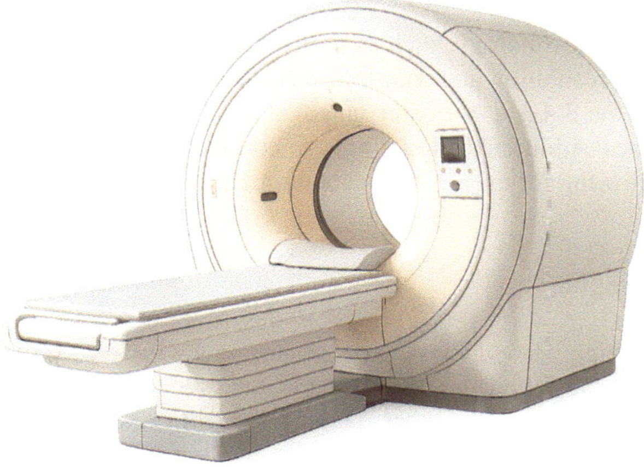

**Fig. 2.9** MRI machine

works by taking advantage of the magnetic properties of hydrogen atoms, which are abundant in the human body, particularly in water and fat. The MRI scanner generates a powerful magnetic field, which aligns the hydrogen nuclei in the body. A radiofrequency (RF) pulse is applied, causing the hydrogen nuclei to absorb energy and become temporarily misaligned. When the RF pulse is turned off, the nuclei return to their original alignment, releasing energy.

The MRI scanner detects this released energy, which varies depending on the tissue type, and uses this information to create detailed images of internal structures. Different tissues in the body, such as muscles, fat, and organs, have unique magnetic properties that allow them to be distinguished from one another in the resulting images. For instance, fat produces a high signal, making it appear bright on an MRI scan, while water-based tissues, such as muscles and organs, generate a lower signal, appearing darker.

#### Techniques in MRI Imaging

Various MRI techniques have been developed to enhance the ability of the system to visualize specific tissue types or anatomical areas. These techniques include:

- T1-weighted imaging: Provides detailed images of anatomical structures and is commonly used to visualize soft tissues, such as the brain and muscles.
- T2-weighted imaging: Highlights tissues with higher water content, such as fluid-filled cavities and edema, making it useful for detecting inflammation and tumors.
- Diffusion Tensor Imaging (DTI) is a specialized technique for mapping and characterizing the white matter in the brain, often used in the study of neurological disorders.
- Functional MRI (fMRI): Measures brain activity by detecting changes in blood flow, offering insight into brain function, and is used in pre-surgical planning for brain surgery or for studying cognitive processes.

Advances in MRI technology, such as high-field MRI scanners, have significantly improved image resolution and speed. Modern MRI systems use stronger magnetic fields, often in the 3 Tesla or higher range, allowing for more explicit images and faster scan times. Additionally, advances in coil technology have improved signal acquisition, allowing for even better resolution and signal-to-noise ratios.

### Ultrasound Imaging

Ultrasound imaging, also known as sonography, is a widely used diagnostic tool in medicine that employs high-frequency sound waves to create images of the internal structures of the body. Unlike other imaging modalities, such as X-rays and MRI, ultrasound does not require ionizing radiation, making it a safe, non-invasive option for many diagnostic applications. It is particularly valuable for real-time imaging of soft tissues and organs, offering a dynamic and versatile method for assessment in clinical practice.

The ultrasound system consists of a transducer, which emits high-frequency sound waves and detects the echoes that return from tissues in the body. Various tissues reflect these sound waves differently depending on their density and composition. The ultrasound machine processes the returning echoes, which generate an image based on the time it takes for the sound waves to return.

Ultrasound imaging has become a standard tool in many medical fields due to its non-invasive nature, real-time capability, and relatively low cost. It is commonly used to visualize organs, monitor pregnancies, assess blood flow, and guide specific medical procedures, such as biopsies or injections (Figs. 2.10 and 2.11).

The fundamental principle behind ultrasound imaging is the reflection and transmission of high-frequency sound waves. These sound waves travel through the body at varying speeds depending on the tissue they encounter. When the sound waves hit different tissues or interfaces, some sound is reflected to the transducer, while the rest continues to pass through the tissue.

The time it takes for the sound waves to return to the transducer helps create an image, with denser tissues (such as bone) reflecting more sound waves and creating bright areas on the image. In contrast, less dense tissues (like fluids) reflect fewer sound waves, appearing darker on the ultrasound image. These varying reflections help to distinguish between different types of tissues in the body. Ultrasound images are created in real-time, allowing clinicians to observe the structure and movement of tissues, blood flow, and organs as they happen. This real-time imaging is

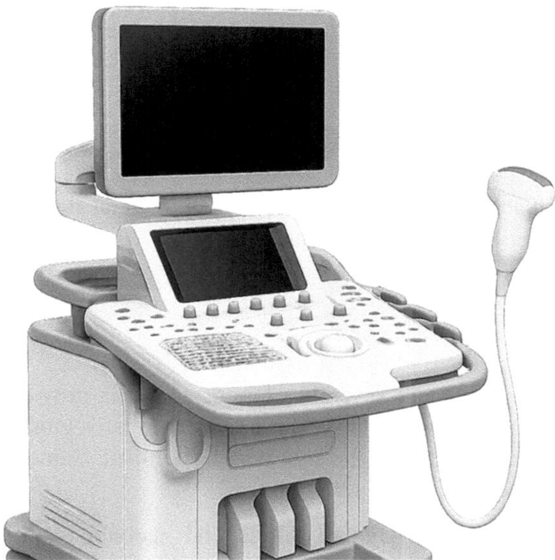

**Fig. 2.10** Ultrasound machine with a transducer for an abdominal scan

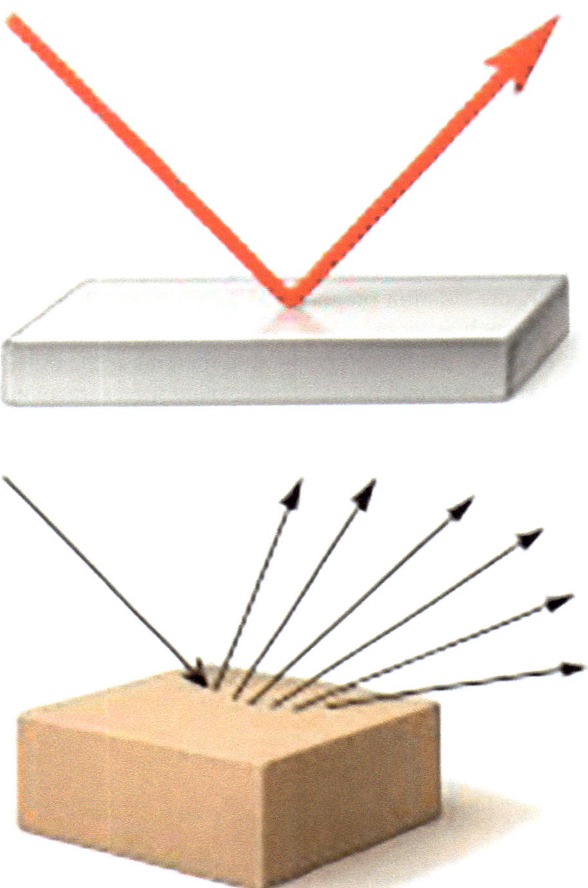

**Fig. 2.11** Specular vs. diffuse reflection

particularly valuable in monitoring heart function, fetal development, and blood flow during surgeries or other procedures.

### Techniques in Ultrasound Imaging

Ultrasound imaging includes several techniques that can provide detailed views of anatomical areas and organ systems. These techniques are commonly used based on the patient's clinical needs and the area being examined. Some of the most widely used ultrasound techniques include (Fig. 2.12):

- 2D Ultrasound: This standard ultrasound technique produces flat, two-dimensional images of internal organs and structures. It is commonly used in obstetrics to monitor pregnancy and in cardiology to evaluate the heart.

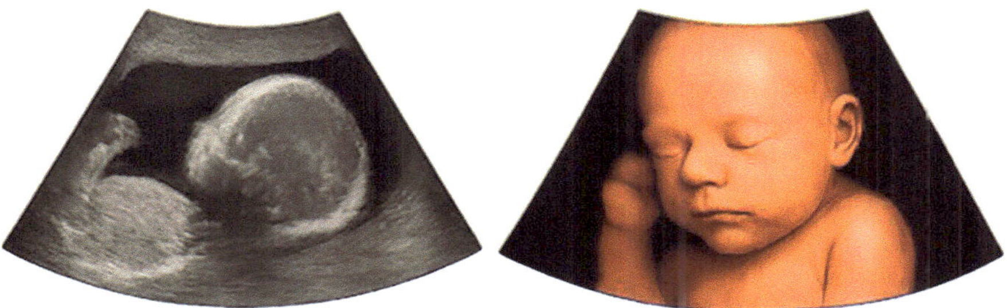

**Fig. 2.12** 2D vs. 3D ultrasound images

- 3D and 4D Ultrasound: These techniques offer three-dimensional and real-time, moving images (4D), respectively, and are often used in obstetrics for viewing the fetus. 4D ultrasound provides a dynamic image of the fetus in the womb, allowing for the assessment of fetal movements.
- Doppler Ultrasound: This technique measures and visualizes the flow of blood through vessels. Doppler ultrasound provides information about blood flow velocity by measuring the change in frequency of the sound waves as they bounce off moving red blood cells. It helps diagnose conditions such as blood clots or heart defects.
- Elastography is a newer ultrasound technique that measures tissue stiffness. It helps assess the presence of tumors, liver fibrosis, and other pathologies by evaluating how tissues respond to external pressure.

In addition to these specific techniques, ultrasound imaging can be performed using different approaches depending on the area being examined, including:

- Transabdominal ultrasound: This is the most common approach, in which the transducer is placed on the abdomen to examine organs such as the liver, kidneys, and reproductive organs.
- Transvaginal ultrasound: A more invasive technique where the transducer is inserted into the vagina, providing higher-resolution images of the uterus and ovaries, often used in early pregnancy or gynecological assessments.
- Transesophageal ultrasound: This is used to assess the heart. The transducer is placed in the esophagus to obtain clearer images of the heart, particularly in patients with certain heart conditions.

## *2.3.4 Clinical Applications*

### Clinical Applications of X-Ray Imaging

X-ray imaging has become an indispensable tool in nearly every branch of medicine. One of its most common applications is in orthopedics, where it is used to diagnose fractures, joint dislocations, and degenerative bone diseases such as

osteoporosis. X-ray scans provide critical information about bone alignment and healing progress, allowing physicians to make informed treatment decisions.
In pulmonology, chest X-rays are essential for diagnosing lung conditions such as pneumonia, tuberculosis, chronic obstructive pulmonary disease (COPD), and lung cancer. The ability to visualize lung structures and detect abnormalities quickly makes X-ray imaging a first-line diagnostic tool in respiratory medicine. In cardiology, X-ray-based techniques, such as angiography, allow for the visualization of blood vessels and the assessment of conditions like arterial blockages and heart disease. During angiographic procedures, a contrast dye is injected into the bloodstream, and X-ray images are taken to identify areas of restricted blood flow.

Dentistry also heavily relies on X-ray imaging for diagnosing cavities, gum disease, and impacted teeth. Dental X-rays provide detailed images of the teeth and jawbone, assisting in treatment planning for conditions such as orthodontic corrections and implant placements. Beyond these fields, X-ray imaging is widely used in gastroenterology, urology, and trauma medicine, making it one of the most versatile diagnostic tools in healthcare.

## Clinical Applications of MRI Imaging

MRI imaging has widespread applications across various medical disciplines, due to its ability to provide detailed images of soft tissues and organs. Some of the key clinical applications include (Fig. 2.13):

- Neurology: MRI is invaluable in diagnosing brain and spinal cord disorders, such as multiple sclerosis, Alzheimer's disease, stroke, and brain tumors. It is the preferred imaging modality for evaluating neurological conditions due to its superior soft tissue contrast.

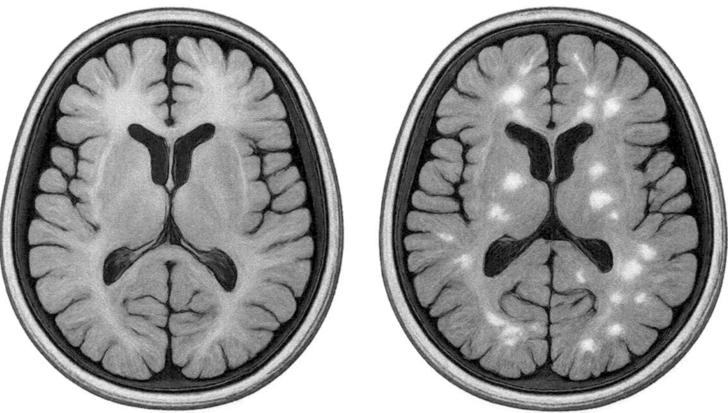

**Fig. 2.13** Brain MRI images showing normal tissue versus areas affected by multiple sclerosis

- Orthopedics: MRI is often used to assess joint injuries, tears in ligaments or tendons, and conditions such as arthritis or degenerative disk disease. It is particularly effective in visualizing the soft tissue components of the musculoskeletal system.
- Cardiology: Cardiovascular MRI (CMR) is used to assess heart function, detect myocardial infarctions, and evaluate conditions like cardiomyopathy. It can provide detailed images of the heart's anatomy and blood flow.
- Oncology: MRI is crucial in detecting and monitoring cancers, particularly in organs like the brain, liver, and prostate. It helps in tumor localization, staging, and evaluation of treatment response.
- Obstetrics and Gynecology: MRI evaluates the uterus, ovaries, and fetal development, offering an alternative to ultrasound in certain cases where more detailed images are required.

### Clinical Applications of Ultrasound Imaging

Ultrasound imaging is a versatile tool used in various clinical specialties because it provides real-time, dynamic imaging without ionizing radiation [119]. Some key applications include:

- Obstetrics and Gynecology: One of the most well-known uses of ultrasound is in pregnancy monitoring. It allows clinicians to visualize the developing fetus, assess fetal growth, and check for abnormalities. It is also used to assess the health of the ovaries, uterus, and fallopian tubes and guide fertility treatments.
- Cardiology: In cardiology, ultrasound assesses the heart and blood vessels. Echocardiography, a type of ultrasound, helps evaluate heart function, detect structural heart defects, and monitor conditions such as heart failure or valve disease.
- Musculoskeletal Imaging: Ultrasound is frequently used to examine muscles, tendons, ligaments, and joints. It is helpful in diagnosing sprains, tears, and other musculoskeletal conditions and can guide the placement of needles for injections or biopsies.
- Abdominal Imaging: Ultrasound is routinely used to assess organs in the abdomen, including the liver, kidneys, spleen, and gallbladder. It helps detect conditions such as tumors, cysts, stones, and fatty liver disease.
- Vascular Imaging: Doppler ultrasound is often used to assess blood flow in the arteries and veins. It is a valuable tool for diagnosing deep vein thrombosis (DVT), varicose veins, and arterial blockages.
- Oncology: Ultrasound helps identify and assess tumors in various organs. It is commonly used for breast cancer screening, guiding biopsies, and monitoring the progression of tumors in the liver or other areas.

### 2.3.5 Regulatory Considerations

#### Regulatory Considerations of X-Ray Imaging

Despite its invaluable role in medicine, X-ray imaging involves exposure to ionizing radiation, which has the potential to cause cellular damage. While the radiation doses used in medical imaging are generally low and considered safe, it is essential to minimize unnecessary exposure (Fig. 2.14).

Healthcare professionals adhere to the ALARA principle (As Low As Reasonably Achievable) to ensure that radiation doses remain minimal while obtaining high-quality diagnostic images. Protective measures such as lead aprons, thyroid shields, and collimation techniques help reduce radiation exposure to patients and healthcare workers.

Pregnant women and young children are susceptible to radiation, and extra precautions are taken when imaging these populations. In many cases, alternative imaging modalities such as MRI or ultrasound may be preferred when repeated imaging is required [79]. Recent advancements in low-dose X-ray systems and AI-driven image enhancement techniques have significantly reduced radiation exposure while maintaining high diagnostic accuracy. The ongoing development of radiation-free imaging options continues to improve patient safety in diagnostic radiology.

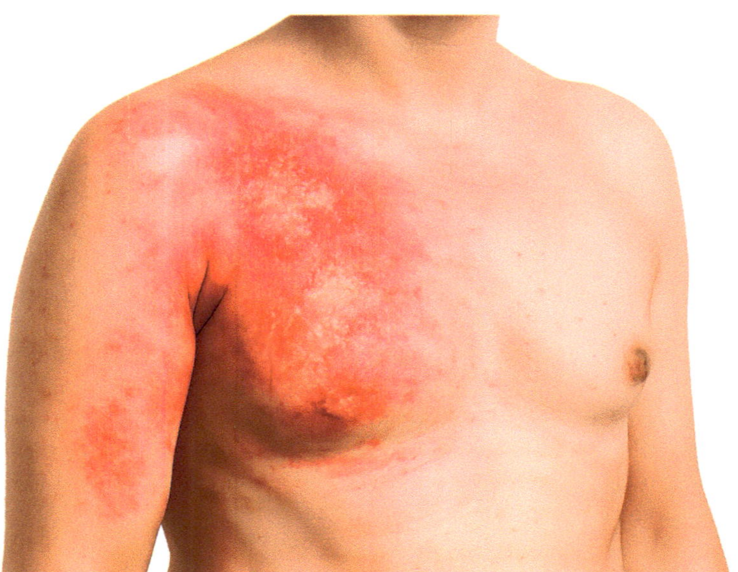

**Fig. 2.14** Radiation burns

**Table 2.11** MRI safety symbols for metal implants and medical devices

| MR safe | MR conditional | MR unsafe |
|---|---|---|
| MR | MR | MR |
| An item that does not present recognized risks in any MRI setting | An item that has been proven not to pose identified MRI setting | An item that is recognized as causing risks in any MRI setting |

### Regulatory Considerations of MRI Imaging

MRI is a safe imaging technique when appropriate guidelines are followed, particularly due to the absence of ionizing radiation. However, safety precautions are necessary due to the strong magnetic fields involved in the procedure. Patients with implanted medical devices, such as pacemakers or metal implants, may not be suitable candidates for MRI scans, as the magnetic field could interfere with these devices or cause harm (Table 2.11).

Additionally, MRI can cause discomfort in some patients, especially those with claustrophobia, due to the enclosed nature of the MRI machine. To mitigate this, open MRI machines have been developed, which provide a less confined space for patients who experience anxiety during scans.

### Regulatory Considerations of Ultrasound Imaging

One of the primary advantages of ultrasound imaging is its safety profile. Unlike X-ray and CT scans, ultrasound does not involve ionizing radiation, making it suitable for repeated use and imaging sensitive populations such as pregnant women and young children [48]. However, certain precautions should be followed to ensure patient safety and the quality of the images.

While ultrasound is generally considered safe, it is essential to use it judiciously to avoid prolonged exposure to high-intensity sound waves, which may have an unknown impact, particularly during pregnancy. However, there is currently no conclusive evidence to suggest that ultrasound poses significant risks to patients or their unborn babies when used properly by trained professionals (Fig. 2.15).

## *2.3.6 Future Perspectives*

### Future of X-Ray Imaging

In recent years, the field of X-ray imaging has seen the integration of artificial intelligence (AI) and machine learning techniques, which have the potential to revolutionize diagnostic radiology. AI algorithms can now assist radiologists by automating

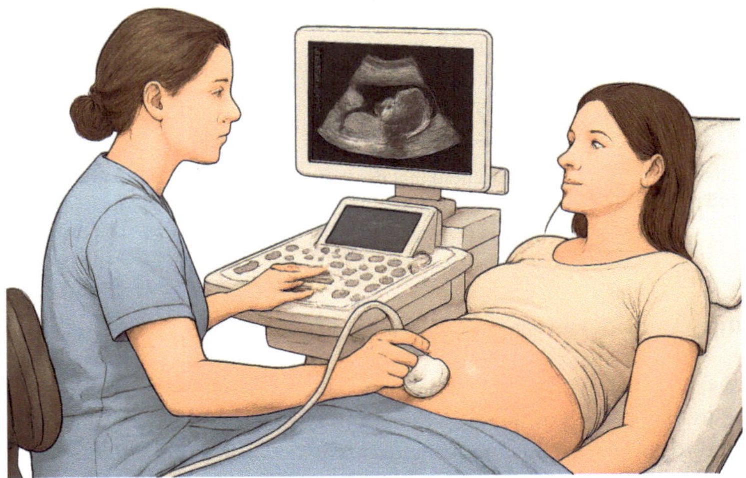

**Fig. 2.15** A sonographer performing a routine pregnancy ultrasound

the interpretation of X-ray images, detecting subtle abnormalities that human eyes may miss. These tools have shown great promise in improving diagnostic accuracy, particularly in early cancer detection and bone fractures.

AI's role in X-ray technology also extends to improving the efficiency of healthcare systems. Automated systems can help prioritize urgent cases and even assist in managing large volumes of images. With the increasing demand for medical imaging, AI-driven platforms are becoming an indispensable tool for enhancing the capacity of radiology departments [25, 69] (Fig. 2.16).

Moreover, AI has the potential to optimize X-ray imaging itself. Machine learning algorithms can enhance image quality by reducing noise, improving resolution, and compensating for poor imaging conditions. These innovations promise to make X-ray imaging faster, more accurate, and safer for patients.

While the advances in X-ray technology have been transformative, challenges remain. Radiation exposure, although reduced over the years through innovations in dose reduction and shielding techniques, continues to be a concern, particularly for vulnerable populations such as children and pregnant women. Additionally, the increasing reliance on AI and machine learning in X-ray imaging raises questions about the potential for algorithmic bias and the need for human oversight [117].

Looking ahead, the future of X-ray technology will likely see further integration with other imaging modalities to create hybrid systems that offer the best of both worlds. Hybrid imaging technologies, such as PET/CT and PET/MRI, are already being used to provide both functional and anatomical data in a single scan, enhancing diagnostic precision and enabling better treatment planning.

Moreover, as the field of personalized medicine continues to evolve, the role of X-rays in tailoring medical interventions will become even more critical. Personalized imaging techniques, aided by AI, may allow for more targeted approaches to treatment, reducing unnecessary procedures and improving patient outcomes.

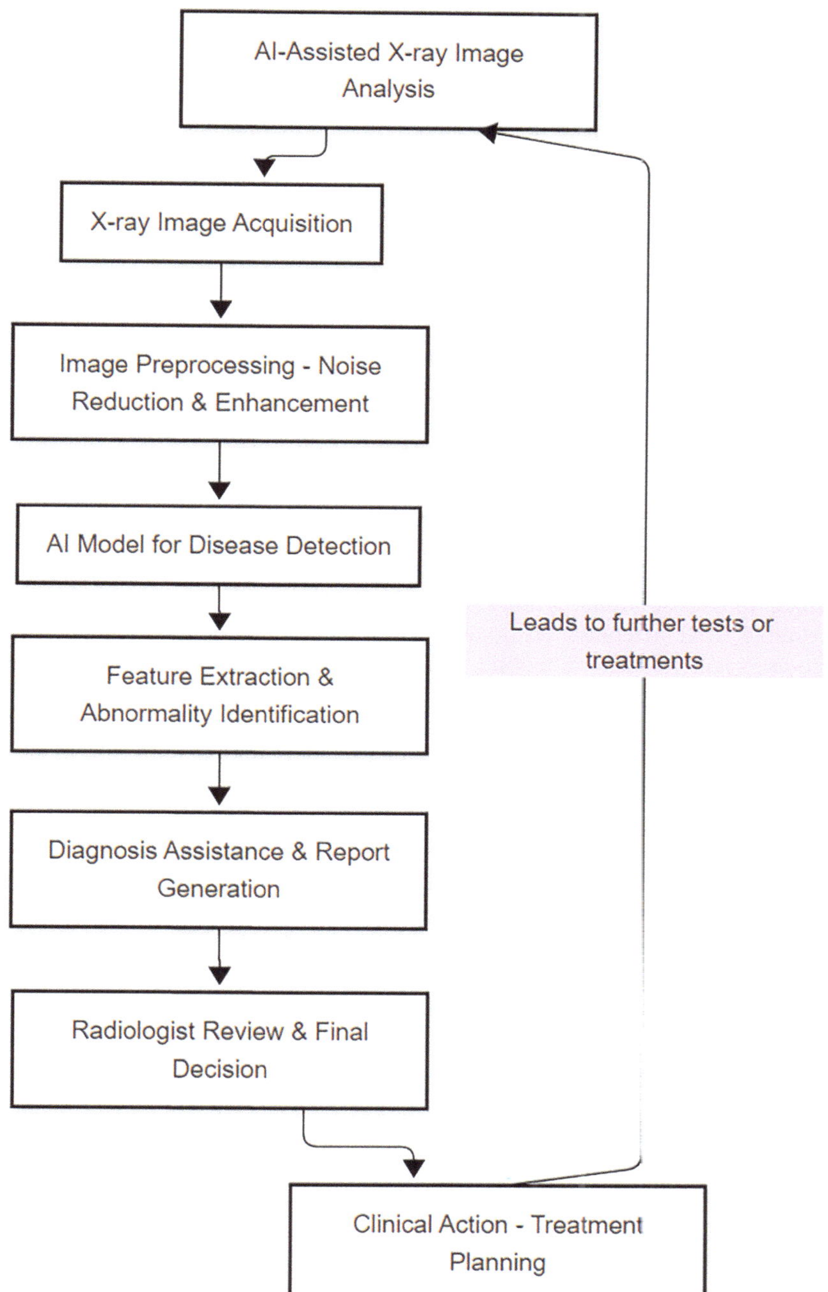


**Fig. 2.16** Flowchart of AI-assisted X-ray image analysis

One exciting frontier is the potential of portable and mobile X-ray systems. These devices, which offer compact and mobile alternatives to traditional machines, promise to expand access to medical imaging in remote or underserved areas. With the rise of telemedicine, there may also be an increased ability to share X-ray images remotely, enabling consultations and diagnoses from specialists worldwide.

### Future of MRI Imaging

Due to ongoing technological advancements, the future of MRI imaging holds exciting possibilities. The integration of artificial intelligence (AI) in MRI analysis is one area that promises significant improvements in diagnostic accuracy. AI algorithms can assist radiologists in detecting subtle abnormalities that may be missed by the human eye, improving early diagnosis, particularly in complex cases like cancer or neurological disorders.

Furthermore, MRI technology continues to advance in terms of speed and resolution. The development of ultra-high-field MRI, with magnetic fields stronger than the standard 3 Tesla, will allow for even more detailed images, particularly at the microscopic level [130]. This is expected to significantly enhance the diagnosis and treatment of diseases at the cellular level, especially in oncology and neurology.

Portable MRI machines are another exciting development. These machines, which are smaller and more mobile, could provide greater access to MRI imaging in rural or underserved areas, where traditional MRI facilities may not be available. As personalized medicine evolves, MRI will be increasingly important in tailoring treatment to individual patients, ensuring that medical interventions are more targeted and effective. The future of MRI imaging looks promising, with advancements in technology and AI opening new frontiers in medical diagnostics. MRI imaging has revolutionized how clinicians diagnose and monitor various medical conditions, offering detailed, non-invasive views of soft tissues and organs. With ongoing advancements in imaging technology, AI integration, and the potential for portable MRI systems, the future of MRI looks poised to improve patient outcomes further and expand the reach of high-quality medical imaging.

### Future of Ultrasound Imaging

The future of ultrasound technology is rapidly advancing, with several exciting developments on the horizon. Integrating artificial intelligence (AI) into ultrasound systems is expected to improve image quality, automate image interpretation, and assist clinicians in making quicker and more accurate diagnoses. AI algorithms can help detect subtle abnormalities, which may improve early detection and treatment outcomes, particularly in complex conditions like cancer or heart disease.

Portable ultrasound devices also advance, allowing point-of-care imaging in remote or underserved areas. These devices are smaller, lighter, and more affordable, making them accessible for use in various settings, including rural clinics, emergency rooms, and even in the field for military or disaster relief operations.

Additionally, 3D and 4D ultrasound technology is improving, offering higher resolution images and real-time imaging further to enhance the understanding of complex anatomical structures and functions. As ultrasound technology evolves, it is expected to play an even more significant role in personalized medicine, enabling clinicians to tailor treatment based on real-time, high-quality imaging data. Ultrasound is poised to remain a critical tool in medical diagnostics, particularly as it becomes more integrated with emerging technologies [100].

Ultrasound imaging has become an indispensable tool in the medical field, providing detailed, real-time images without ionizing radiation. Its versatility, affordability, and safety make it a popular choice for various diagnostic applications, from monitoring pregnancy to evaluating heart function and musculoskeletal conditions. As technology advances, the integration of AI and portable devices, along with improvements in 3D and 4D imaging, will likely continue to expand the utility and reach of ultrasound in clinical practice, providing enhanced diagnostic capabilities for clinicians and better outcomes for patients.

## 2.4 Electrocardiographs

Electrocardiography (ECG) is a method of recording electrocardiograms, which record the temporal and spatial profiles of the electrical excitation processes in the myocardium in the form of waves, peaks, and lines, and performing diagnostic analyses of these electrocardiograms (Fig. 2.17).

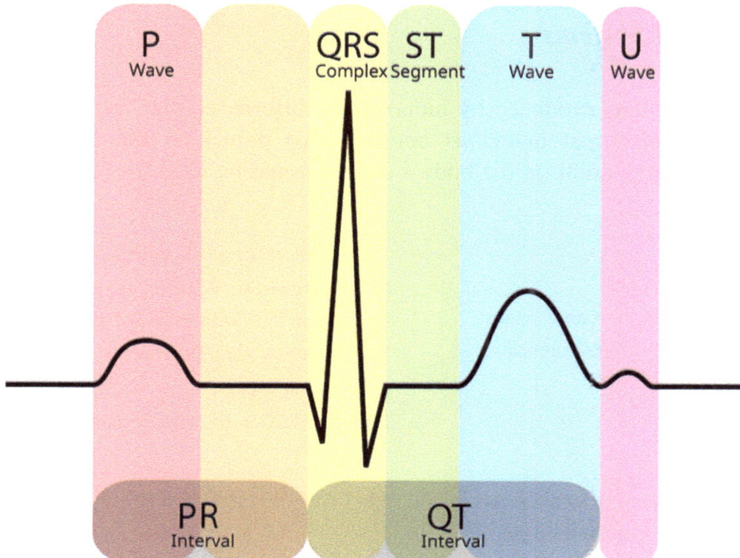


**Fig. 2.17** Nomenclature of the electrocardiogram (https://commons.wikimedia.org/wiki/File:ECG_Complex.svg)

Every instance of depolarization through cardiac fibres is the source of an electric potential. These noninvasive measurements generally measure potential differences that occur across an electric field on the body's surface, which make up only a fraction of the potential generated by the heart. The heart is thus interpreted as a source of potential. Hence, the ECG ultimately provides an image of the generation of electricity (potential shift) and reflects the excitation processes in the measurement selected.

### 2.4.1 Operating Modes

A fundamental distinction is drawn between manual and automatic operating modes. Automatic programs, such as standard ECGs with 12 leads, ergometry, and arrhythmia, are typical modern cardiographs that can be programmed by the user [131]. The lead mode, formatting, baseline, calibration, and sensitivity are, for the most part, automated. Alternatively, registration can be performed manually at any time.

### 2.4.2 ECG Methods (Fig. 2.18)

### 2.4.3 Lead Systems

The action currents produced by biopotential differences that vary with time are measured as electrical potentials between two points on the body's surface. Theoretically, any point on the body's surface could be used for this purpose, but

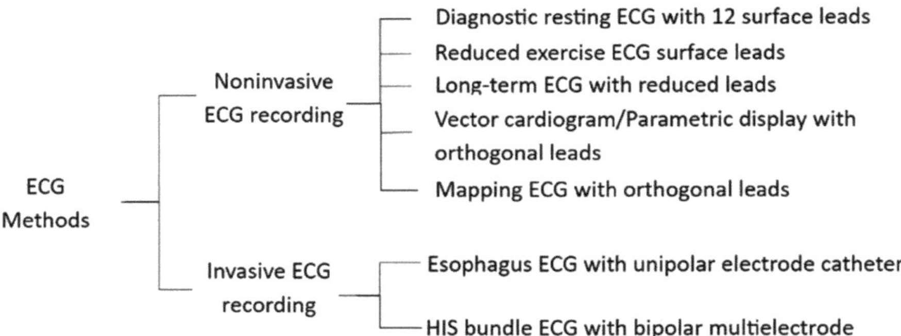


**Fig. 2.18** Noninvasive and invasive ECG methods

specific electrode sites have developed in practice, and the respective leads are defined according to these sites. The leads differ substantially in terms of recording technique and spatial arrangement.
Leads between two points are described as bipolar leads. In contrast, in unipolar leads, the different electrodes are connected to a zero electrode. This collector electrode is created by connecting limb leads via high-impedance resistors. The limb leads provide a spatial view of the frontal plane, and the chest leads provide a spatial view of the horizontal plane [132].

## 2.4.4 Standard Leads

The standard leads are the three bipolar limb leads known as Einthoven's leads, the three unipolar limb leads constructed from these three bipolar limb leads (Goldberg's leads: aVR, aVL, aVF), and six unipolar chest leads known as Wilson's chest leads [133].

### Einthoven's Bipolar Limb Leads

For these, the potential difference is measured between two electrodes (Fig. 2.19):

R: right arm = red connector
L: left arm = yellow connector
F: left foot = green connector
N: right foot = black connector (earth)

The three leads lie in the frontal plane and form what is known as Einthoven's triangle.

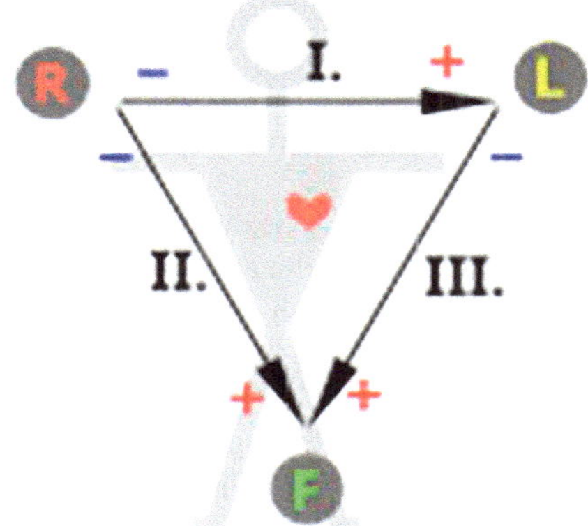


**Fig. 2.19** Einthoven's triangle (https://upload.wikimedia.org/wikipedia/commons/e/eb/ECG-Einthoven-triangle.svg)

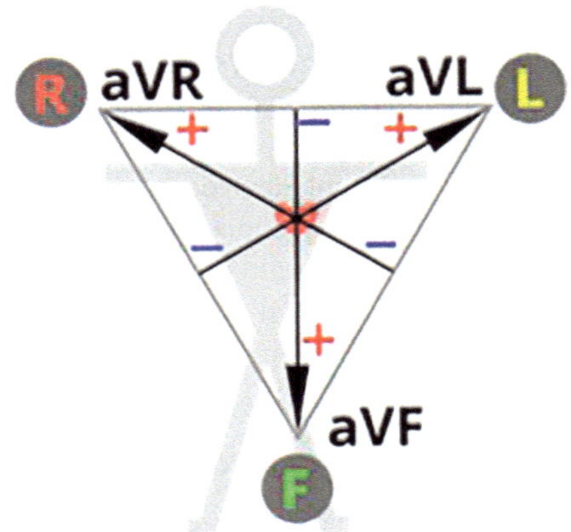


**Fig. 2.20** Goldberger's lead system (https://upload.wikimedia.org/wikipedia/commons/5/5e/ECG-Goldberger.svg)

### Goldberg's Unipolar Limb Leads

For these, the potential difference is determined between each electrode on the limb and an electrical zero, which lies at the central potential between the two other limbs (Fig. 2.20).

aVR: R − L + F/2
aVL: L − F + R/2
aVF: F − L + R/2

### Wilson's Unipolar Chest Leads

The chest electrodes are placed at six defined points on the thorax. The three limb leads are combined via a high-impedance resistor to form a collector electrode. Wilson's central terminal forms the electrical zero point. As a result of the proximity to the heart, the amplitudes of the chest leads are greater than those of the limb leads [134] (Fig. 2.21).

### Cabrera's Lead Sequence

Cabrera's circle is a hexaxial system that can be used, among other things, as an aid when determining the axis deviation. The circle includes leads of the frontal plane, each rotated through 30 degrees with respect to one another. The leads form Einthoven's triangle are shifted parallel such that lead I assumes an angle of zero, lead II 60 degrees, and lead III 120 degrees. The Goldberger leads are also included in this system, with angles of aVR −150, aVL −30, and aVF +90 degrees [135, 136]. By flipping the aVR lead through 180, we get -aVR at 30. The axis deviation

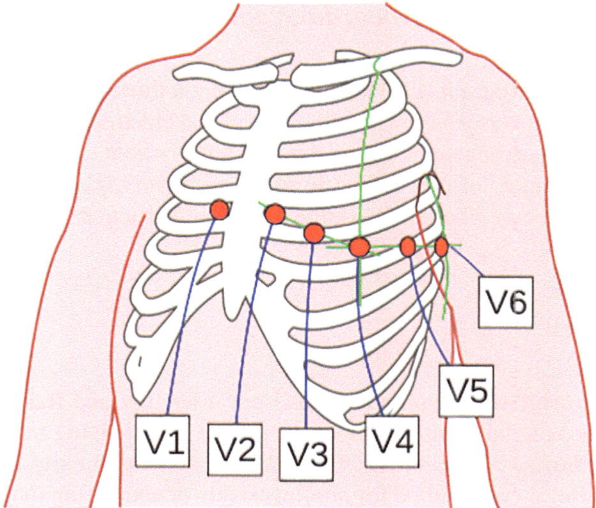


**Fig. 2.21** Unipolar chest leads according to Wilson (https://commons.wikimedia.org/wiki/File:Precordial_Leads_3.svg)

can be determined simply by determining the highest R amplitude from the leads. The angular space allocated to the leads determines the axis's deviation.

### 2.4.5 *Augmented and Reduced Leads from the Surface of the Body*

Augmented leads include the corrected orthogonal leads of Frank and the additional unipolar chest leads of Wilson. The Frank leads are based on a theoretical model in which the heart is at the center of a square three-dimensional coordinate system consisting of a lateral axis x, a longitudinal axis y, and a sagittal axis z. The excitation processes can therefore be registered as vector loops [137]. Reduced leads include ECG monitoring, long-term ECG, and ergometry leads.

### 2.4.6 *Invasive Leads*

#### Unipolar Esophageal Leads

An electrode catheter is inserted via the esophagus to just above the cardia when using esophageal leads. The aim is to obtain a precise assessment of the proximal potentials of the posterior myocardial wall and the left atrium [138].

### 2.4.7 HIS Bundle Electrocardiography

An intracardiac electrogram (EG) is obtained using a three-pole electrode catheter. This investigation is performed with radiological and electrocardiographic monitoring. The particular advantage of this lead is that it is possible to precisely investigate the proximal potentials of the right atrium, the right ventricle, and the conductive system, and in this case, the HIS-Purkinje system in particular [139].

### 2.4.8 History

Electrocardiograph (ECG) equipment has been a lengthy and transformative process, beginning as a rudimentary diagnostic device and evolving into a cornerstone of modern cardiovascular medicine. ECGs began to be used early in the twentieth century, providing a new method for non-invasively documenting the heart's electrical function. ECG technology progressively transitioned from bulky analog machines to portable, small devices with high-resolution recording and analyzing capabilities. Today, ECGs are commonplace in hospital and outpatient practice and are utilized as a matter of course for screening, monitoring, and diagnosing a wide range of cardiac disorders.

Perhaps the most significant development in ECG technology was the transition from analog to digital systems. Digital ECGs improved signal quality, data processing, and automation. They enabled the integration of functions like automatic analysis, digital media storage, and wireless communication. This type of digitalization paved the way for PC-based ECG systems (PC ECGs), which separate the sensor module and the processing unit, enabling mobility, remote diagnosis, and easy sharing of data over secure networks [128, 140].

In the last several years, PC ECG modules have kept cardiological diagnostics up to date with affordable, low-cost, and easy-to-use solutions. These systems eliminate mechanical printouts, are paper-saving, and enable real-time telemonitoring. Although they introduce new challenges such as potential signal artifacts from digital interference, their benefits in clinical workflow efficiency and patient accessibility have moved them into widespread adoption [141]. The evolution of ECG equipment keeps tracing the path of wireless technology, artificial intelligence, and cloud-based data management innovations, making ECGs an essential tool in contemporary medicine.

### 2.4.9 Technical Characteristics

ECG systems are low-noise differential amplifiers; in other words, they consist of a strongly coupled DC amplifier with a high amplification factor and inverting (reversed) and noninverting inputs. The output voltage is a multiple of the voltage present at the input terminals. It is the differential voltage of the two voltages at the same pole. Particularly high requirements are set for an ECG preamplifier compared to usual amplifier technology: interfering high-frequency AC voltages are attenuated using a high-frequency filter upstream of the preamplifier input, so that no overamplification or self-excitation can occur. Likewise, Extreme interference voltages are blocked by discharge sections and antiparallel diodes. A relatively high input resistance keeps the input currents very low [142].

Capacitively coupled mains-frequency AC voltages are eliminated through high common-mode rejection. Following a 20 to 30-fold preamplification, a high-pass filter separates the ECG signal from the direct current. The time constant of this filter is 1.5 or 3.2 s. Whereas the processed ECG signal is fed to the respective channel amplifiers via a lead selector in analogue ECG equipment, this step is omitted in digital ECG equipment. The recorded signals are instead connected to 12 leads, amplified, and fed to a processor system via multiplexers and A/D converters. The system software processes all of the digitized input signals, interpolates the individual measurement readings to give continuous curves, controls equipment processes, and communicates with the operator via the keypad, display and print out; it prepares text outputs, displays the time, produces a QRS trigger signal, and evaluates the remote start ergometer input. Output occurs via the thermal comb's digital recording system [143]. In an analogue ECG equipment, following further amplification to near 1–2 V using the respective channel amplifier, the ECG signal is output via a power amplifier stage (final amplifier) and a mechanical recording system [141].

ECG measurement, the signal path, and signal processing resemble a measurement chain, from the test object (patient) via transducer or sensors and the transfer of measurement readings to signal processing, signal evaluation, and documentation. The recording electrodes or the intracardiac electrode on the body's surface receive the ECG signal and transmit it via a cable to the input amplifier of the cardiograph. There is a galvanic potential between the skin and the metal section of the electrode, which is substantially influenced by the electrode material, the composition of the electrolytes, and the condition of the electrode/electrolyte interface. This electrochemical contact potential can be up to 300 mV.

The transmitted input signal from the amplifier consists of four different fractions:

1. The proper signal with an amplitude of 50 μV to approximately 1 mV, and
2. A DC voltage component of up to 300 mV that is superimposed on the sound signal
3. Interfering signals of up to 100 mV and
4. Extreme interference voltages of up to 3000 V can also occur.

To ensure that the patient is galvanically isolated from the mains voltage, the power supply and the output signal are galvanically decoupled [144]. To promote reproducibility, the ECG signal processing, recording, and measuring process is standardized (Frequency 0.05–100 Hz, ECG amplitude 2.5, 5, 10, 20 mm/mV. Times 10,25, 50, and 100 mm/s).

### Hardware

ECG recorders are mainly classified according to the number of channels of the device and the equipment technology used (Fig. 2.22).

A new generation of ECG systems has evolved from analog to digital systems with integrated recording components, known as PC ECGs. The recorded analogue signals are amplified, digitized, and supplied to data transmission equipment in an external module. The data can be transmitted to a connected computer using a USB microcontroller or wireless data transmission technology. Whereas the USB port is also used to supply power to the module, the Bluetooth method makes mains-independent operation possible with an accumulator battery. The transmitted data is processed and prepared on the computer using the installed ECG application programs. In addition to the visual image on the computer display or external monitor, ECG graphs and interpretations can be printed on a connected printer and plain paper for documentation purposes [145] (Fig. 2.23).

The PC ECG has practical advantages over conventional ECG equipment: the ability to save any desired ECG sequences at any time, the comprehensive availability of the data, the considerable reduction in the consumption of expensive ECG paper and therefore financial savings, the lack of mechanical equipment components, the ability to back up data on common storage media, the capacity for mobile use with mains-independent operation, as well as the possibility of interactive data exchange via the internet [140]. A disadvantage is the restricted data exchange

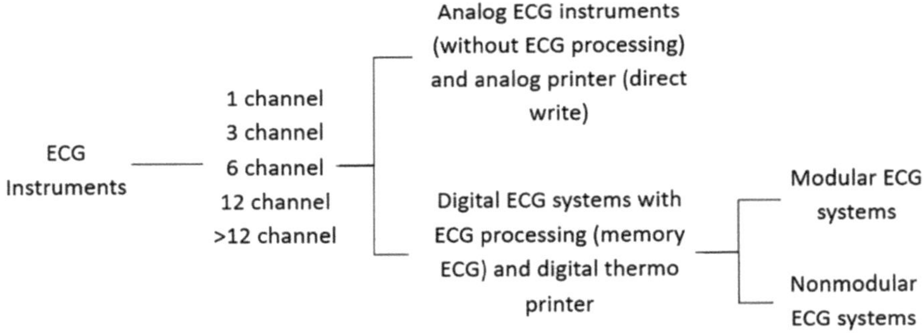


**Fig. 2.22** Overview and differentiation of ECG recording equipment

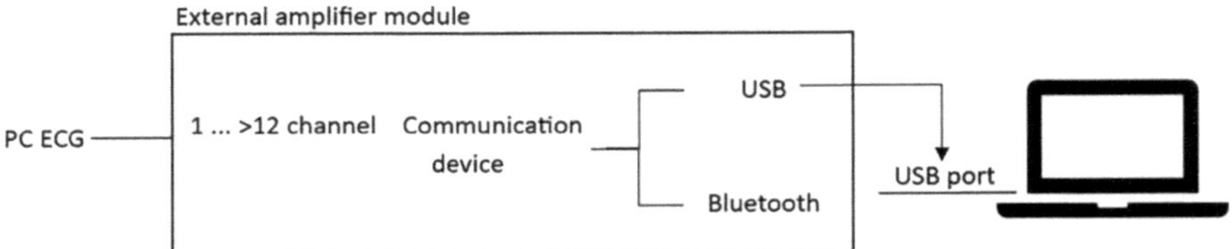


**Fig. 2.23** PC ECG module

possible via data carriers or over the internet, as data can only be exchanged with an application program compatible with the PC ECG software. An artefact characteristic of PC ECG equipment, and probably a result of computer electronics, leads to interference in the sensitive ECG analysis.

### Recording Systems

Recording systems can be considered to have various technical possibilities for recording components. The digital thermal array recording method is currently the state of the art. Thermal comb recordings have high resolution and a low susceptibility to interference from the recording system, and they allow optimum reproduction of the recorded and processed ECG signal.

### Electrode Technology

The electrodes fundamentally influence the recording and transmission of the ECG signal from the body's surface and the quality of this signal. They represent a junction between the electrode surface's ionic conduction and the transmitting cable. There is, therefore, an electrical potential between the body and the electrode, which is dependent on three factors in particular:

1. Electrode material
2. Composition of the electrolytes
3. Condition of the electrode-electrolyte interface

Electrochemical contact potentials of up to 300 mV can occur at these interfaces. The electrode impedance—the sum of the electrode and skin impedances and also the resistance of the contact medium, which is dependent on the current density—is the result of the current state of the skin, body, contacting agent, and electrode material [146]. For this reason, electrode pastes or gels are used to reduce transfer impedance.

Unwanted polarization voltages may occur, particularly in the case of polarizable electrode material. These spontaneous voltage fluctuations are superimposed on the ECG signal and lead to signal instabilities in the recording [147, 148].

## Software

Electrocardiographs (ECG devices for short) and PC ECG modules are diagnostic devices for recording, amplifying, storing, processing, analysing, and documenting (registering) an electrocardiogram. Noninvasive electrocardiography has been a standard procedure for several decades, and ECG equipment is therefore as good as mandatory in hospitals and small private practices [149].

### System Properties

The following properties represent the performance spectrum and the same time for the requirements for modern ECG systems [128]:

- Simultaneous display of the 12 standard leads in a time frame of 15 s
- Various alphanumeric recording options
- High operational convenience and programmability
- Digital signal processing
- Automated control together with programs
- Interfaces for communication with other systems
- A high-resolution recording system without mechanical parts

An upgradable system has the advantage of being able to perform more functions than just one ECG registration. The ECG device has these so-called multifunctional system properties when equipped with additional functions such as spirometry, arrhythmia monitoring, Doppler ultrasound, etc. Data communication with a PC and networking with other systems are also standard [150]. Therefore, the conditions for the use of medical EDP statistics, ECG data management, and ECG software libraries are satisfied.

### Computer-Based Assessment

The nature and number of events within a certain time interval provide insight into cardiac arrhythmia. At the beginning of the analysis, there is a learning phase for the program: the QRS complex that is typical of this particular patient is calculated, and the QRS morphology is learnt and considered the normal curve shape to distinguish the QRS morphology from deviating QRS complexes and artefacts.
The arrhythmia program uses the detection area for the QRS complex to draw a rhythmological distinction between physiological and pathological cardiac actions [151]. The polarity of the R wave, the amplitude, the QRS area and position, the offset of the QRS from the baseline, and the slope of the R wave are calculated and determined as particular features for each QRS complex.

The individual parameters are used at various points in the analysis for decision-making purposes. Thus, for example, the height of the complex provides an additional criterion when validating a QRS complex. This feature determination enables morphological and individual complex assessment, ultimately leading to a conclusion regarding arrhythmia (Fig. 2.24).

The cross-correlation method is a continuous comparison between the current QRS complex and the learnt QRS. The classification of each QRS complex forms the basis of arrhythmia monitoring. The complex's shape and time of occurrence are considered for this purpose.

If the typical QRS shape of this patient is found after a learning phase, the next complex will be compared with the stored reference complex by superimposing the two complex shapes and checking point-for-point for a match. When there is a low

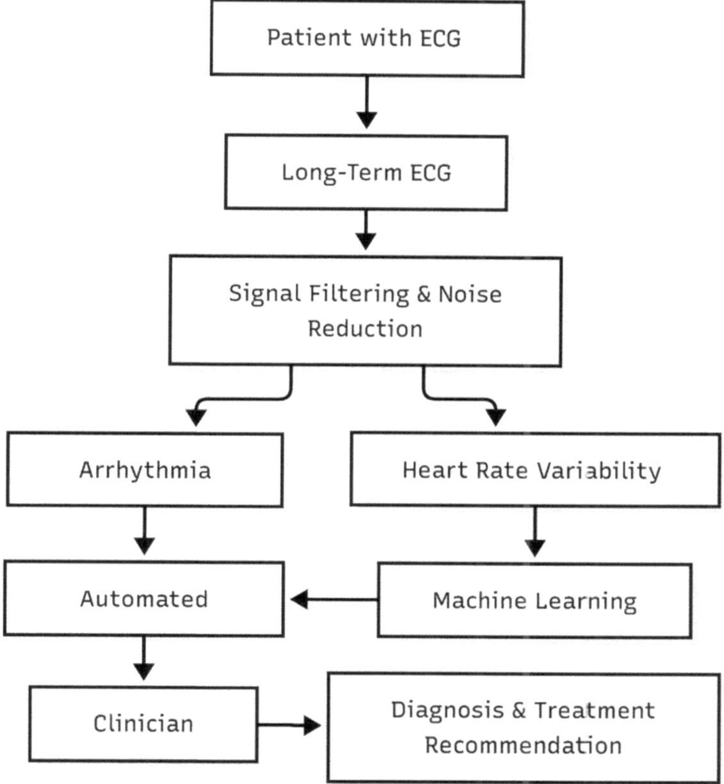


**Fig. 2.24** Flow diagram of a computer-based assessment of the long-term ECG

percentage of deviation, the complexes are defined as identical in shape and are used as the reference complex for subsequent shape comparisons. If there is no match, this is stored in what is known as a QRS class memory [152]. In order to qualitatively assess diagnostic effectiveness and analytical accuracy, it is necessary to test analytical programs with equipment-specific algorithms against recognized and evaluated ECG databases and compare the results (validation).

### *2.4.10 Types of Devices*

#### Long-Term ECG

Long-term ECG, also known as Holter monitoring, ambulant ECG, or ambulatory monitoring, is a noninvasive routine ECG procedure that is central to primary diagnosis and the therapeutic monitoring of cardiac arrhythmias. As its name suggests,

in this procedure, the ECG is recorded and analysed over a relatively long period of time, during everyday stress.
Whereas other electrocardiographic investigation procedures, such as resting or exercise ECGs, only allow a diagnostic statement to be made over a limited period of time under specific conditions, the long-term ECG follows the various physical and emotional stresses that occur over at least 1 day/night period.

#### Leads

To date, there is no uniform agreement on the best electrode positions for long-term electrocardiography. Efforts are being made towards standardization to ensure better comparability of the results obtained. The electrodes must be placed on the thorax at sites where there is little muscle, the patient's freedom of movement must not be restricted, and the amplitude of the R wave in relation to the P and T waves must be sufficient for computer-based ECG analysis of the recordings [153].

As a general rule, right and left precordial leads are chosen. Preference is given to the following bipolar chest leads: MC5, MX, and CC5. In addition to the leads mentioned here, modified leads are recommended by various authors in order to optimize the sensitivity of detection [154].

#### Long-Term ECG Systems

Long-term ECG systems consist of a portable recording device with 2–3 channels that registers and stores the ECG signals, a computerized playback device, and a high-performance analysis unit. Using FFT, application programs enable frequency analysis for artefact recognition, automatic evaluation according to various criteria, accelerated analysis, or batch processing [155]. If we consider the recording technology, a distinction can be drawn between continuous and discontinuous recording of long-term electrocardiographic systems in which the data carrier of the recording device is either a tape cartridge or solid-state memory [156, 157]. In continuous recording, the ECG potentials are stored for between 24 and 72 h. In addition to real-time analysis, high-quality devices also make it possible to evaluate highly amplified ECG, long-term blood pressure, heart rate variability, and other functions on the unit in parallel.

Discontinuous system-based ECGs are plotted according to the recording device's limited storage capacity. Following a continuous recording analysis, only time-limited ECG information and results are stored and documented. With these so-called event recorders, the patient can activate the recording via an activator or remote control unit if symptoms occur. Loop recorders have memory on a loop; in this case, ECG information remains stored for a limited period of time.

Only ECG sequences marked by the patient using the activator remain stored. A further development of the event recorder is the subcutaneous implantable loop recorder, which is used particularly in the case of symptomatic cardiac arrhythmias that occur infrequently. The device, which generally has an operating time up to 2 years, is implanted subcutaneously in the region of the left sternum using local anesthetic. The continuously recording bipolar electrogram is evaluated in the implant. ECG episodes that deviate from programmed ECG criteria are recorded [158]. Here, too, the patient can also mark and store symptoms or events that occur using a remote control.

With so-called simple sampling recorders, ECG sections are recorded only in specific time segments, without the recording being triggered by cardiac arrhythmias and without being influenced by the patient. This intermittently recording system, which stores information only randomly and nonspecifically, leads to recordings with limited informative value regarding the complete day/night rhythm. The transmission of stored ECGs and complete long-term ECG data records via telephone to a computer in the hospital or a private practice is increasingly gaining significance [159]. Telecommunications developments enable ECGs to be transmitted using mobile phones, thus permitting online diagnosis.

Prognostic indicators such as heart rate variability (HRV) and heart rate turbulence can be calculated from a long-term ECG recording. Whereas HRV provides information on the variations in heart rate over a relatively long period, heart rate turbulence refers to the variations in the interval between two heartbeats following the occurrence of a ventricular extrasystole. In order to assess the heart rate variability, the standard deviation of the RR intervals recorded throughout 24 h is ascertained [160].

The range of indications for performing a long-term ECG has changed. The most important indication is an investigation where there is suspicion of underlying cardiac arrhythmias. Other indications are risk stratification achieved by recording ventricular arrhythmias and monitoring an antiarrhythmic therapy. The guidelines of the American College of Cardiology (ACC), the American Heart Association (AHA), and the European Society of Cardiology (ESC) provide further possible applications [153].

The long-term ECG is of great significance for primary cardiological diagnosis, the monitoring of therapy for arrhythmias, and the diagnosis of ischemia. Resting and exercise ECGs usually do not allow a reliable judgement to be made on the frequency and nature of cardiac arrhythmias since they record only a small period. A significant advantage of the long-term ECG is the continuous recording of the ECG over a relatively long period [161, 162]. In addition, the analysis results can be quantitatively measured, documented, or passed on for further data processing.

#### The Exercise ECG

Ergometry, the most commonly used exercise tolerance test in clinical and outpatient cardiology, is a noninvasive routine procedure in cardiovascular diagnostics. By providing additional information to the resting ECG, ergometry yields essential insights into current cardiopulmonary performance and limitations on performance that may result from coronary heart conditions.

Ergometry refers to generating a defined and reproducible stress with an ergometer per unit time, and the subsequent monitoring of the ECG, heart rate, blood pressure, and oxygen consumption, and more on recording electrocardiographic changes during and after the period of exertion. Conventional ergometry generally does not include oxygen consumption and saturation measurements, whereas such measurements are essential in ergospirometry [163].

### Physical and Technological Principles

The work performed by the test subjects during the exercise period at various stress stages is the product of force and distance. Including the time component, the output generated can be measured in Newton meters per second.

If we now consider a bicycle ergometer, a force must be expended over a distance when the bicycle pedal is rotated. The speed at which the bicycle pedal is rotated equals the time this output is generated. As the bicycle pedal rotates, the output is thus calculated from 2pi x rotational speed x torque. The torque is calculated from the force with which the pedals are rotated multiplied by the length of the pedal cranks [164, 165]. In the process, it becomes clear that the performance changes depending on the force or rotational speed applied.

### Ergometry Measuring Station

In order to avoid standalone systems and restrictions on the range of equipment that can be used, complete systems known as fully automatic ergometry measuring stations are currently available. These measuring stations consist of a 3, 6 or 12 channel ECG device, an ergometer or treadmill, a 1, 3, 6 or 12 channel cardioscope, a defibrillator, a noninvasive blood pressure meter, an electrode application system and a portable equipment trolley that carries this equipment and thus enables flexible transportation of it. When new equipment is acquired, conventional ECG devices are usually replaced with PC ECGs. The advantage of these systems is that they allow data storage and transfer [166] (Fig. 2.25).

## Types of Ergometers

Regarding technology and apparatus, there are three main types of ergometers: bicycle ergometers used in the sitting position, recumbent bicycle ergometers, and treadmill ergometers.

In bicycle ergometers dependent on rotational speed, the output can be increased by increasing the braking resistance and pedaling frequency. If a particular braking action that predefines the force is set, a specific rotational speed must be maintained to determine the output precisely. In practice, this situation is rather challenging to

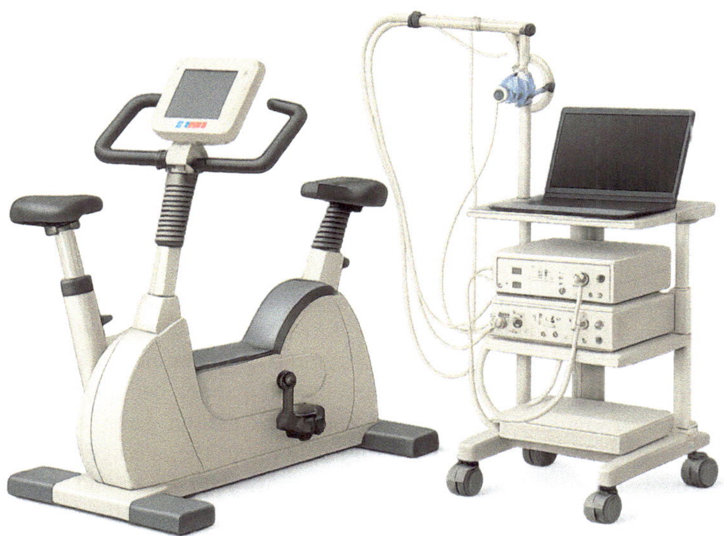

**Fig. 2.25** Ergometry measuring station with bicycle ergometer

implement. This is why bicycle ergometers, which depend on rotational speed, are unsuitable for ergometry. The use of these devices for medical investigations has, therefore, been banned.

Bicycle ergometers that do not depend on rotational speed are predominantly used today. These are usually equipped with a computer-controlled eddy-current brake, and only the output to be attained is predefined; if the pedalling frequency is increased, the resistance decreases proportionally. The braking action is constantly compared with the rotational speed, the force expended, and the predefined stress. Deviations are corrected electronically by increasing or decreasing the braking force. The accuracy is specific to the measuring system and depends on the consistency and the control rate. In sound systems, deviations between 1% and 3% in the stress set are observed; the standard allows up to 5% deviations.

### Reduced Exercise ECG Leads

As with the other ECG leads, there are many ergometry lead programs. There are two main requirements for the reduced ECG leads during the exercise ECG [167]:

- Minimal susceptibility to faults due to superposition of muscle potentials and movement artefacts
- Qualitative and quantitative registration of ST-segment deviations

The limb leads can be applied respectively to the right and left sides of the shoulder blade and in the lateral regions of the right and left iliac wings. These show the least superposition from muscle potentials. The chest leads are exciting because ischaemic ST depressions and repolarization arrhythmias of the anterior wall appear most pronounced and occur most frequently in these leads. C2, C4, and C5 or C6 are the most popular electrode sites for chest leads.

Elevation or depression of the ST segment in the ECG under stress allows diagnostic conclusions to be drawn regarding coronary heart conditions, so this is a significant focus of measurements. Modern electrocardiographs, which usually provide an ergometry program, automatically measure and document the ST segment and amplitude. A distinction must be drawn between continuous and discontinuous ST measurement programs: in the case of continuous measurement, each QRS complex recorded is measured and analyzed directly. An average beat is generated continuously for each channel from several beats that exhibit good correlation. In contrast, in the case of discontinuous ST measurement, the average beat is generated from either values taken at timed intervals or just from a start and end complex [168, 169]. To obtain the average beat, the start and end points of the QRS complex are first determined. The ST amplitude and slope are measured at point J + x interval, which is determined as a heart rate function. The isoelectric line is established between the P wave and the start of the QRS complex.

### Exercise Test

Since the diagnostic issues and the composition of the patient clientele are assessed in very different ways, a uniform, standardized exercise tolerance test is not always possible. The guidelines compiled by the International Commission for the Standardization of Ergometry Application (ICSPE) have led to a largely standardized procedure in routine investigation and sports medicine.

- Stress Intensity
  In ergometry, there are two types of stress intensity in principle: maximal and submaximal stress. In case of maximal stress, the exertion increases until the test subject's physical output limit is reached. In case of submaximal stress, exertion is continued until medically relevant problems occur or their correlation with the exertion can be ascertained. The submaximal stress level depends on the medical problem and may be reached long before maximal stress is reached [170].
- Pulse Working Capacity
  Derived from the rules for assessing performance and the rules for stress limits, the PWC method allows the comparison of outputs standardized to the pulse rate. The PWC value assesses the performance in the submaximal range when the maximum rate has not been reached. The selected rate is added as an index [171]. The nominal values for the PWC are not dependent on age; they are calculated based on weight and gender. These values can be found in the PWC tables.
- Types of Exercise Tolerance Testing

- The general requirements for an evaluable exercise tolerance test can be summarized as follows: it should be capable of precise metering, physically measurable, and reproducible at any time. Many types of exercise do not satisfy these requirements, but they are mentioned below for the sake of completeness:
  - Forward bends and squats
  - Climbing stairs
  - Hand crank ergometer
  - Isometric stress (hand-grip)
  - Master's step test
  - Kaltenbach and Klepzigs step-climbing test
  - Treadmill ergometer
  - Bicycle ergometer
- Standardized Investigation Programs
- Several individual and standardized exercise tolerance testing programs have been employed since the early days of ergometry investigation. These are listed below:
  - Hollman's standard test method
  - The WHO's standard program
  - Knipping's vita maxima
  - Kirchhoff's square wave test

However, ergometry has increasingly evolved into a standardized method based on the internationally recognized regulations of the ICSPE. This has the advantage that results of investigations from different institutes and those obtained by different testing personnel can be compared and assessed according to the same standards. Therefore, all testing personnel must adhere to these regulations.

### *2.4.11 Clinical Applications*

As it illustrates the electrical excitation processes occurring in the heart, the ECG provides information about the origin and rhythm of excitation, the heart position and rate, pulse propagation, as well as repolarization and repolarization arrhythmias, which in turn can be caused by anatomical, mechanical, metabolic, or circulatory problems. However, the ECG has no direct informative value regarding the contraction and pumping capacity of the heart. The medical significance of the ECG is undisputed, although its capabilities should not be overestimated [172].

In cardiological investigations, the ECG is essential; in routine internal investigations, it is a valuable, and possibly even crucial, investigative tool. Caution is advised regarding the informative value of the ECG in determining the etiology and pathogenesis of cardiac disease, as well as the indications for and success of therapeutic measures. The ECG does not necessarily reflect the anatomical damage and functional faults of the myocardium. It is essential to note that the ECG's informative value depends on the knowledge and experience of the individual providing the assessment [173]. Inexperienced users will tend to interpret the ECG too broadly, while experienced users will provide a more reserved assessment and, where possible, avoid oversimplification and generalizations. It must be noted that, particularly with computerized evaluation programs, an individual's assessment is essential. Whereas incidents during noninvasive ECG recording are a complete novelty, serious arrhythmias can occur during intracardiac ECG registration [174, 175].

ST-segment variation during the exercise ECG is of the utmost importance for detecting temporary myocardial ischaemia. In addition, coronary heart conditions can be established unambiguously. Coronary angiography has contributed to improving the interpretation of the exercise ECG. However, there is a fundamental difference between the two: coronary angiography detects the morphological changes in the coronary arteries, whereas the exercise ECG detects the functional effects. An indication for an exercise ECG can be given for diagnostic, therapeutic, or prognostic reasons [176–178]:

- Investigation of a coronary heart condition
- Investigation of the blood pressure where there is suspicion of exercise-induced hypertension
- Investigation of the stress tolerance
- Assessment of cardiac arrhythmias
- Assessment of progress and therapeutic success of medication and exercise therapy, and heart surgery
- Assessment and classification of the degree of severity of stress-induced coronary insufficiency

### 2.4.12 Regulatory Considerations

Electrocardiographs are power-operated technical medical devices, with associated provisions, regulations, and standards that are applied to protect patients and operating personnel. ECG devices that measure intracardially, or are provided for that purpose, are subject to Annex 1 of the German Medical Devices Operator Ordinance. The protection classes that apply to ECG equipment are primarily protection class 1 and protection class 2. VDE 0750 allows devices to be equipped with a protection class switch, making the operation in either protection class possible. In order to maintain functional and operational safety, the equipment must be subjected to technical safety checks and tests at regular intervals [48, 179].

Most faults that occur during ergometry can be attributed to the patient. A large proportion of these faults is compensated for by modern equipment technology. Nevertheless, the test subject can be made aware that the necessary pedalling work can be carried out without excessive upper body movements. Incidents are extremely rare in the case of ergometry when performed correctly, and routine investigations are today predominantly carried out by well-briefed medical assistants [180]. The only ergometric investigations that the doctor must supervise over the entire duration of the exercise tolerance test are those in which, due to the general condition of the test subject, complications cannot be ruled out. A nurse or medical assistant must be present at the same time in order to assist or to provide immediate assistance if necessary. An emergency supply of equipment, medication, and a functioning defibrillator must be available at all times.

Exercise tolerance tests carry some risks. In order to minimize risks, safety measures should be taken before and after the exercise tolerance test. Information from the resting ECG, including anamnesis, should be analyzed. The patient should be examined and informed. It is important to tell the patient to report any subjective complaints during the exercise tolerance test, and to continue to monitor the test subject following the exercise tolerance test; a monitoring ECG should be re-recorded, and the blood pressure should be measured [181, 182]. The criteria for aborting ergometry are:

- Increasing retrosternal severe pain
- Horizontal or descending ST depression
- Cumulative monomorphic or polytopic ventricular extrasystoles
- Ventricular salvos
- Isolated extrasystoles that fall in the T wave of the previous cardiac action
- Atrial fibrillation or flutter
- Serious conduction defects
- Depolarization defects
- Systolic blood pressure >250 mmHg, diastolic blood pressure >130 mmHg, and drop in blood pressure
- Noticeable breathing difficulty
- Signs of the beginning of left ventricular insufficiency
- ECG signs of a fresh myocardial infarction.

### 2.4.13 Future Perspectives

The future of electrocardiography is the continued intersection of digital technology, artificial intelligence (AI), and mobile health technology. Of most promise is integrating AI-based algorithms with the potential to enhance ECG interpretation by detecting subtle patterns that sometimes elude human clinicians. Such systems can potentially identify early arrhythmia, myocardial infarction, and even structural heart disease more rapidly and accurately [128]. In addition, AI-assisted ECG interpretation can decrease diagnostic variability, improve screening in low-resource settings, and support clinicians in high-volume practices.

Another significant advancement is the development of wearable and portable ECG technologies. Small, battery-powered wireless monitors—from pocket-sized ECG recorders to smartwatch-based systems—are transforming cardiac monitoring and introducing continuous or on-demand ECG assessment into community practice, extending beyond traditional clinics [140]. They are especially advantageous for long-term monitoring of intermittent arrhythmias and for use in remote or rural populations where specialist availability is limited. These devices and cloud-based technology enable real-time data transmission, physician alerts, and teleconsultation capabilities [141].

In the future, the ECG will play an increasingly central role in preventive and personalized medicine. Innovations such as implantable loop recorders with several years of battery life, intelligent electrodes incorporating adaptive filtering, and ECG-spirometers hybrids are expanding the diagnostic potential of traditional electrocardiography [161]. As data interoperability improves and AI systems receive regulatory clearances, ECG equipment will be increasingly integrated into vast health data networks, enabling continuous patient monitoring and improved clinical outcomes. Ongoing integration of mobility, intelligence, and accessibility ensures that ECG technology will be at the forefront of cardiovascular diagnosis for years.

## 2.5 Blood Pressure Monitors

Blood pressure measurements have been part of the basic clinical examination since the earliest days of modern medicine. The origin of blood pressure is the heart's pumping action, and its value depends on the relationship between cardiac output and peripheral resistance. Therefore, blood pressure is considered as one of the most important physiological variables with which to assess cardiovascular hemodynamics [183]. Venous blood pressure is determined by vascular tone, blood volume, cardiac output, and the force of contraction of the chambers of the right side of the heart. Since venous blood pressure must be obtained invasively, blood pressure most commonly refers to arterial blood pressure, which is the pressure exerted on the arterial walls when blood flows through the arteries [184]. The highest value of pressure, which occurs when the heart contracts and ejects blood to the arteries, is called the systolic pressure (SP). The diastolic pressure (DP) represents the lowest value between the ejections of blood from the heart. Pulse pressure (PP) is the difference between SP and DP, i.e., PP = SP − DP. The period from the end of one heart contraction to the end of the next is called the cardiac cycle. Mean pressure (MP) is the average pressure during a cardiac cycle. Mathematically, MP can be decided by integrating the blood pressure over time [185]. When only SP and DP are available, MP is often estimated by an empirical formula:

$$\mathrm{MP} = \mathrm{DP} + \mathrm{PP} / 3$$

Note that this formula can be very inaccurate in some extreme situations. Although SP and DP are most often measured in the clinical setting, MP is particularly important in some situations because it is the driving force of peripheral perfusion. SP and DP can vary significantly throughout the arterial system, whereas MP is almost uniform in normal situations.

Blood pressure values vary significantly over 24 h according to an individual's activity. Three factors, namely, the diameter of the arteries, the cardiac output, and the state or quantity of blood, are mainly responsible for the blood pressure level. When the tone in the muscular arterial walls increases, causing them to narrow or become less compliant, the pressure rises above normal levels. Unfortunately, increased blood pressure does not ensure proper tissue perfusion. In certain instances, such as in cases of shock, blood pressure may appear appropriate even when peripheral tissue perfusion has nearly ceased [186]. Nevertheless, observing or monitoring blood pressure allows dynamic tracking of pathology and physiology affecting the cardiovascular system. This system, in turn, has profound effects on the other body organs.

### 2.5.1 *History*

Invasive arterial blood pressure monitoring has been the gold standard for blood pressure measurement in the critically ill for a long time, especially when noninvasive conventional methods like auscultation or oscillometry are not feasible. Its development was prompted by the need for continuous, beat-to-beat blood pressure monitoring in high-risk clinical environments like intensive care, anesthesia, and neonatal care [187]. Over time, the technique has evolved from cumbersome, manually calibrated devices to exact catheter-based systems with real-time pressure monitoring and access for blood gas sampling.

Previously, arterial catheterization was performed using reusable equipment and required high technical expertise. However, the greater availability of disposable sensor kits and minimally invasive techniques for insertion, like percutaneous catheter placement using guide wires, has expanded the use of this technology beyond specialist centers. Advances in catheter material, sterility precautions, and ultrasonic vessel location have all contributed to safer and more streamlined procedures, with advantages for both patient outcomes and operator convenience.

Since 2020, the emphasis has been on optimizing the accuracy, reliability, and reproducibility of these systems in dynamic clinical environments. Researchers have emphasized the necessity to control influences like air bubbles, tubing compliance, and zeroing techniques to minimize hydrostatic and kinetic errors. Through continued technological advancement, silicon microchip-based sensors and fast-flush test protocols ensure that direct arterial pressure monitoring remains an essential tool in modern hemodynamic management.

### 2.5.2 *Technical Characteristics*

The basis of any physiological measurement is the biological signal, which is first sensed, transduced, or converted from one form of energy to another. The signal is then conditioned, processed, and amplified. Subsequently, it is displayed, recorded, or transmitted (in some ambulatory monitoring situations). Blood pressure sensors

**Table 2.12** Estimated uncertainties of reproducibility

| | Auscultation | Oscillometry | Umbilical arterial catheter |
|---|---|---|---|
| Neonate | | | |
| Systolic pressure (mmHg) | N/A | 3.3 | 2.2 |
| Diastolic pressure (mmHg) | N/A | 3.4 | 1.8 |
| Adult | | | |
| Systolic pressure (mmHg) | 2.8 | 3.2 | N/A |
| Diastolic pressure (mmHg) | 2.2 | 3.5 | N/A |

often detect mechanical signals, such as blood pressure waves, to convert them into electric signals for further processing or transmission [186]. They operate on various principles, including resistance, inductance, and capacitance. A sensor should have good sensitivity, linearity, and stability for accurate and reliable measurements.

Each blood pressure assay technique has an issue of reproducibility of measurements given approximately similar conditions. Reproducibility quantifies the internal uncertainty of an individual method and instrument, whereas accuracy quantifies the external uncertainty when compared with a reference. When measuring blood pressure, it is essential to remember that even with standard methods, a certain amount of non-repeatable random error is inherent. Consequently, taking the average of repeated measurements or multiple readings is always recommended before making any serious recommendation or management decision (Table 2.12).

**Hardware**

A large variety of vascular catheters exists. Catheter materials have undergone testing to ensure that they have a minimal tendency to form blood clots on their surface. The catheter chosen may be inserted percutaneously over a hollow stylet into the blood vessel. Guide wires can facilitate longer or larger-diameter catheters into vessels, after the guide wires have been placed through a smaller catheter or needle. Less often, entry to a vessel requires a "cutdown," a direct exposure of the vessel after a skin incision. Ultrasonic devices may assist in locating the vessels not readily apparent at the skin surface.

Although pressure sensors can be located at the catheter tip, this presents a problem for calibration if left in place and a clot forms near the tip of the catheter, damping the pressure signal. Instead, most catheters connect to an external pressure sensor via fluid-filled low-compliance tubing. The signal from the sensor then transforms into a display or recording. The sensor may take one of several forms, from a variable resistance diaphragm to a silicon microchip [187]. A basic system can consist of an intravascular catheter connected to a rigid fluid-filled catheter and tubing that communicates the pressure to an elastic diaphragm, the deflection of which is detected electrically. There is a direct relationship between the diaphragm deflection and the voltage. The higher the voltage, the greater the pressure. Continuous low-rate infusion of heparinized saline is carried out to keep the catheter patent or free from coagulation [16]. The advent of disposable sensor kits has dramatically simplified the clinical use of intravascular monitoring. With the cost continually being lowered with the development of the semiconductor industry, disposable sensors become more and more cost-effective.

Although direct recording is considered the most accurate method, its accuracy may be limited by variations in the kinetic energy of the fluid in the catheter or the dynamic frequency response of the measurement system. The hydraulic link between the patient and the sensor is the primary source of potential errors and hazards for the monitoring. Damping and degrading the system's natural frequency, caused by trapped air bubbles, small catheters, various narrow connections, compliant and too long tubing, and too many components connected, are the two characteristic problems with a pressure sensor system. Extreme care should be exercised to eliminate all air bubbles from the fluid and provide an adequate dynamic response. The sensor should be zeroed at the heart level to eliminate hydrostatic error. A fast flush test is easy to use to inspect the dynamic response of the catheter, tubing, and sensor system. It can also help direct adjustments for the system to minimize dynamic artifacts.

**Software**

Recent advances in blood pressure monitoring software have focused on enhancing accuracy, ease of use, and compatibility with modern healthcare systems. In particular, devices like Oranta-AO have added arterial oscillography and machine learning to enable more comprehensive cardiovascular assessment and disease risk estimation, enhancing the clinical application of blood pressure monitors [188]. Similarly, software-based calibration-free monitors such as Lifelight offer contactless and scalable blood pressure and heart rate monitoring with mobile phones, improving access with acceptable clinical accuracy [189]. Efforts have also been made to integrate real-time monitoring into Internet of Things (IoT) platforms to enable remote monitoring and data logging on cloud platforms [190]. In addition, recent mobile applications now support gesture and OCR-based input from older devices, offering new modes of digitizing readings and facilitating remote monitoring [39]. These developments signify a trend toward intelligent, networked, and user-centric blood pressure monitors.

### *2.5.3 Types of Devices*

**Indirect Blood Pressure Measurement**

Indirect measurement is often called noninvasive measurement because the body is not entered in the process. The upper arm, containing the brachial artery, is the most common site for indirect measurement because of its closeness to the heart and convenience. However, many other sites may have been used, such as the forearm or radial artery, finger, etc. Distal sites, such as the wrist, although convenient to use, may yield significantly higher systolic pressures than brachial or central sites due to impedance mismatch and reflective waves [48, 191]. An occlusive cuff is usually placed over the upper arm and is inflated to a pressure greater than the systolic blood pressure. The cuff is then gradually deflated, while a detector system simultaneously employed determines the point at which the blood flow is restored to the limb. The detector system does not need to be a sophisticated electronic device. It may be as simple as manually palpating the radial pulse. The most commonly used indirect methods are auscultation and oscillometry, each is described below.

### Auscultatory Method

The auscultatory method most commonly employs a mercury column, an occlusive cuff, and a stethoscope. The stethoscope is placed over the blood vessel for auscultation of the Korotkoff sounds, which defines both SP and DP. The Korotkoff sounds are mainly generated by the pulse wave propagating through the brachial artery. The Korotkoff sounds consist of five distinct phases. The onset of Phase I Korotkoff sounds (first appearance of clear, repetitive, tapping sounds) signifies SP, and the onset of Phase V Korotkoff sounds (sounds disappear completely) often defines DP. Observers may differ significantly in their interpretation of the Korotkoff sounds. Simple mechanical error can occur in the form of air leaks or obstruction in the cuff, coupling tubing, or Bourdon gage. Mercury can leak from a column gage system. In spite of the errors inherent in such simple systems, more mechanically complex systems have come into use. The impetus for the development of more elaborate detectors has stemmed from the advantages of reproducibility across observers and the convenience of automated operation. Examples of this improved instrumentation include sensors utilizing plethysmographic principles, pulse-wave velocity sensors, and both audible and ultrasonic microphones. The readings by auscultation do not always correspond to those of intra-arterial pressure. The differences are more pronounced in certain special occasions such as obesity, pregnancy, arteriosclerosis, shock, etc. Experience with the auscultation method has also shown that determining DP is often more difficult and less reliable than determining SP [192]. However, the situation is different for the oscillometric method where oscillations caused by the pressure pulse amplitude are interpreted for SP and DP according to empirical rules.

### Oscillometric Method

In recent years, electronic pressure and pulse monitors based on oscillometry have become popular for their simplicity of use and reliability. The principle of blood pressure measurement using the oscillometric technique is dependent on the transmission of intra-arterial pulsation to the occluding cuff surrounding the limb. An approach using this technique could begin with a cuff around the upper arm and rapidly inflate it to about 30 mmHg above the systolic blood pressure, thereby occluding blood flow in the brachial artery. A sensor measures the pressure in the cuff. The pressure is then gradually decreased, often in steps, such as 5–8 mmHg. The oscillometric signal is detected and processed at each step of pressure. The cuff pressure can also be deflated linearly in a similar fashion as the conventional auscultatory method [48].

Arterial pressure oscillations are superimposed on the cuff pressure when the blood vessel is no longer fully occluded. Separation of the superimposed oscillations from the cuff pressure is accomplished by filters that extract the corresponding signals. Signal sampling is carried out at a rate determined by the pulse or heart rate. The oscillation amplitudes are most often used with an empirical algorithm to estimate SP and DP. Unlike the Korotkoff sounds, the pressure oscillations are detectable throughout the whole measurement, even at cuff pressures higher than SP or lower than DP. Since many oscillometric devices use empirically fixed algorithms, variance of measurement can be large across a wide range of blood pressures [193]. Significantly, however, MP is determined by the lowest cuff pressure of maximum oscillations and has been strongly supported by many clinical validations.

### Self-Measurement

The growing number of publications on the topic in recent years indicates a significant increase in interest in self-measurement of blood pressure. There is also evidence that the management of patients with high blood pressure can be improved if clinic measurements are supplemented by home or ambulatory monitoring. Research has shown that blood pressure readings taken in the clinic can be elevated, by as much as 75 mmHg in SP and 40 mmHg in DP, when taken by a physician. The tendency for blood pressure to increase in specific individuals in the presence of a physician due to stress response is generally known as “white-coat” hypertension [194].

When reasonably priced and easy to use, oscillometric devices became widely available in the early 1970s, public interest in self-measuring blood pressure increased, making it possible for patients to be more involved in the detection and management of hypertension. Health care costs may also be reduced by home monitoring. Indeed, a recent study found that costs were almost 30% lower for patients who measured their blood pressure than for those who did not. Measurements taken at a patient’s home are more highly correlated to 24-h blood pressure levels than clinic readings are. It has also been shown that most patients can monitor their blood pressure and may be more relaxed and assured, particularly when experiencing symptoms.

### Ambulatory Monitoring

There is significant value in ambulatory monitoring of blood pressure. Over a 24-h period, blood pressure is subject to numerous situational and periodic fluctuations. The pressure readings exhibit a pronounced diurnal rhythm in an individual, with a decrease of 10–20 mmHg during sleep and a prompt increase upon waking and walking in the morning. Readings tend to be higher during working hours and lower at home and they depend on the pattern of activity. After a bout of vigorous exercise or strenuous work, blood pressure may be reduced for several hours. The readings may be raised if the patient is talking during the measurement period. Smoking a cigarette and drinking coffee, especially when combined, may both increase blood pressure. When assessing the efficacy of antihypertensive drugs, ambulatory blood pressure monitoring can provide considerable information and validation of the drug treatment [152].

Although the technique of noninvasive ambulatory blood pressure monitoring was first described over three decades ago, it has only recently gained acceptance as a clinically useful procedure for evaluating patients with abnormal blood pressure regulation. It gives the best evaluation for patients who have white-coat hypertension. Technical advances in microelectronics and computer technology have led to the introduction of ambulatory monitors with improved accuracy and reliability, small size, quiet operation, and reasonable low price.

They can take and store several hundred readings over 24 h while patients may not be compromised with their everyday activities, thus becoming usable for clinical diagnosis. Theoretically, ambulatory monitoring can provide information about the level and variability of blood pressure experienced during day-to-day activities, covering the full range. It is now recognized to be a very useful procedure in clinical practice since blood pressure varies significantly during the course of 24 h, especially useful in detecting white-coat hypertension.

However, many studies have found that the accuracy of monitoring using current ambulatory monitors is acceptable only when patients are at rest, not during physical activity or under truly ambulatory conditions. In the latter situations, the report of error codes during operation is much higher [195].

### Cuff Size

Both the length and width of an occluding cuff are important for accurate and reliable measurement of blood pressure by indirect methods. A too-short or too-narrow cuff results in false high blood pressure readings. Several studies have shown that a cuff of inappropriate size about the patient's arm circumference can cause considerable error in blood pressure measurement [196]. The cuff should also fit around the arm firmly and comfortably. Some manufacturers have designed cuffs with a fastener spaced so that a cuff of appropriate width only fits an arm of appropriate diameter. With this design, the cuff will not stay on the arm during inflation unless it fits accordingly.

### Direct Blood Pressure Measurement

Direct measurement is also called invasive measurement because bodily entry is made. For direct arterial blood pressure measurement an artery is cannulated. The equipment and procedure require proper setup, calibration, operation, and maintenance [197]. Such a system yields blood pressures dependent upon the location of the catheter tip in the vascular system. It is particularly useful for continuously determining pressure changes at any instant in dynamic circumstances. When massive blood loss is anticipated, powerful cardiovascular medications are suddenly administered, or a patient is induced to general anesthesia, continuous monitoring of blood pressures becomes vital.

The most commonly used sites for continuous observations are the brachial and radial arteries. The femoral or other sites may be used as points of entry to sample pressures at different locations inside the arterial tree, or even the left ventricle of the heart. Entry through the venous side of the circulation allows checks of pressures in the central veins close to the heart, the right atrium, the right ventricle, and the pulmonary artery. A catheter with a balloon tip carried by blood flow into smaller branches of the pulmonary artery can occlude flow in the artery from the right ventricle so that the tip of the catheter reads the pressure of the left atrium, just downstream [198]. These procedures are very complex and there is always concern of risk of hazard as opposed to benefit. Invasive access to a systemic artery involves considerable handling of a patient. The longer a catheter stays in a vessel, the more likely an associated thrombus will form. In spite of well studied potential problems, direct blood pressure measurement is generally accepted as the gold standard of arterial pressure recording and presents the only satisfactory alternative when conventional cuff techniques are not successful. This also confers the benefit of continuous access to the artery for monitoring gas tension and blood sampling for biochemical tests. It also has the advantage of assessing cyclic variations and beat-to-beat changes of pressure continuously, and permits assessment of short-term variations.

## 2.5.4 Clinical Applications

Since the introduction of Dinamap™, an automated blood pressure monitor based on the oscillometric principle, many variants of oscillometric algorithms have been developed. However, the fixed or variable fractions of the maximum oscillations are still the fundamental algorithms of oscillometry. Typically, mean blood pressure was determined by the lowest cuff pressure with the most significant average oscillation. Systolic and diastolic blood pressure were determined by the cuff pressure, with the amplitude of oscillation being a fixed fraction of the maximum [199]. Performance of the algorithms may be improved by introducing a greater level of complexity or variables into the considerations. The Dinamap™ 1846SX (Critikon, Tampa, FL) oscillometric device offered two measurement modes. The normal mode uses two matching pulse amplitudes at each cuff pressure step to establish an oscillometric envelope or curve. Therefore, measurement time is heart rate dependent. The second mode, which the manufacturer refers to as "stat mode," is capable of faster determination by disabling the dual pulse-matching algorithm designed for artifact rejection. The stat mode does not appear to compromise accuracy in anesthetized patients, in which rapid blood pressure measurement is often more desirable, particularly during induction and management of anesthesia [200].

Protocol Systems developed another variant of the oscillometric algorithm. In addition to using pulse amplitude for primary artifact rejection, it further calculates the impulse value, the principal area of the pulse waveform, in constructing an oscillometric curve. This curve is smoothed by employing a Kalman filter that provides an expected mean and acceptable upper and lower bounds of prediction for the principal area of the subsequent pulse waveform. Smoothing of the oscillometric curve is accomplished by using the difference between the predicted and calculated area data of the pulse waveform for each cuff pressure step. Blood pressures are derived from the final smoothed oscillometric curve [201]. In a recent study, oscillometric algorithms utilizing an artificial neural network have been shown to yield more accurate estimates of reference blood pressures compared to the standard oscillometric algorithm. The subtle features and nonlinear relationships of the oscillometric envelope have been modeled using neural network training and processing. Empiricism of the oscillometric fixed fraction criteria is overcome, and measurement variances are significantly reduced.

Due to its low risk and cost, noninvasive continuous blood pressure monitoring represents another need in critical care monitoring to supplement invasive arterial catheterization. A significant development in this field is the arterial counterpulsation principle, proposed by Penaz and further developed by two major groups of people. Finapres™, a continuous finger arterial blood pressure monitor, was engineered and developed by Ohmeda, Denver, CO [199]. Many clinical evaluation reports of these devices have been published since then.

Recently, several other continuous blood pressure monitors have been made commercially available. Examples of these are Cortronic APM770, which monitors pulsation of the brachial artery with a slightly pressurized arm cuff and calibrates it to a continuous pressure waveform; Sentinel ARTRAC 7000, which monitors pulse transit time and correlates that to pressure change; Colin CBM-3000 and JENTOW (Colin Electronics, Komaki, Japan) and Nellcor NCAT N-500 (Nellcor, Hayward, CA), which are tonometric devices monitoring the radial artery pulse waveform by a matrix pressure sensor. All of these monitors require a frequent calibration reference [202]. Except for a few favorable reports with the tonometric method and devices, many reports so far are unfavorable. Nevertheless, noninvasive continuous monitoring represents an important and growing biomedical sensor and instrumentation research and development. Continuous monitors, which maintain cuff pressure, must periodically relieve pressure to prevent the risk of venous congestion, edema, swelling, and tissue damage.

### 2.5.5 Regulatory Considerations

The AHA recommendations provide a systematic step-by-step procedure for measuring blood pressure, including equipment, observer, subject, and technique. They extend considerations of blood pressure recording in special populations such as infants and children, the elderly, pregnant and obese subjects, etc. They also provide recommendations for self-measurement or home measurement of blood pressure and ambulatory blood pressure measurement [203].

The Association for the Advancement of Medical Instrumentation (AAMI) and American National Standards Institute (ANSI) published and revised a national standard for evaluating electronic or automated sphygmomanometers. This standard establishes labeling requirements, safety and performance requirements, and reference test methods for electronic or automated sphygmomanometers used to indirectly measure blood pressure. Specific requirements for ambulatory blood pressure monitors were also included [204]. Recently, AAMI/ANSI amended this SP10 standard to include neonatal devices. Some of the specific requirements, procedures, and limits were modified to fit neonatal applications, such as the maximum cuff pressure, ranges of age and weight, reference standards for validation, minimum sample size of data, etc. The overall system efficacy for both neonatal and adult devices requires that for systolic and diastolic pressures treated separately, the mean difference between the paired measurements of the test system and the reference standard shall be 5 mmHg or less, with a standard deviation of 8 mmHg or less. For manual or nonautomated indirect blood pressure measuring devices, the ANSI/AAMI SP9 standard applies.

The British Hypertension Society (BHS) also published and revised a protocol for assessing the accuracy and reliability of blood pressure measurement using automatic and semiautomatic devices. Many automatic and semiautomatic devices, including ambulatory devices, have been evaluated according to the BHS protocol. Such evaluation provided a quality-control mechanism for manufacturers and an objective customer comparison [102, 205]. However, many more devices are available on the market that have not been evaluated accordingly. Unlike the AAMI SP10 standard, in which indirect or direct blood pressure may be used as a reference standard, the BHS protocol relies exclusively on references to sphygmomanometer blood pressure measurement. It does not recommend comparison with intra-arterial blood pressure values. This could make accurate validation of ambulatory devices difficult because sphygmomanometer measurements are inaccurate during exercise and under ambulatory conditions.

The annual publication of the Medical Device Register is a comprehensive reference work that provides a wealth of detailed information on U.S. and international medical devices, medical device companies, OEM suppliers, and the key personnel in the industry [206, 207]. Blood pressure devices are listed in the sphygmomanometer directory. Price information on specific models for some providers has also been published. For example, A&D Engineering, Inc. listed prices from $51.95 (model UA701) to $179.95 (model UA-751) for a whole line of sphygmomanometers in the 1997 Medical Device Register. Since technology and the market can change rapidly, models, features, specifications, and prices may change accordingly. More specific and updated information may be available by contacting the manufacturers or distributors directly.

Many listed blood pressure devices have multiple evaluation studies; only a few study results are presented here. Given reference standards for comparison, although direct and indirect methods yield similar measurements, they are rarely identical because the direct method measures pressure, and the indirect method is more indicative of flow. Egmond et al. evaluated the accuracy and reproducibility of 30 home blood pressure devices compared to a direct brachial arterial standard. They found that the average offsets of all tested devices amounted to—11.7 mmHg for systolic and 1.6 mmHg for diastolic blood pressure, which were close to those of the mercury sphygmomanometer (−14.2 mmHg for systolic and −0.1 mmHg for diastolic pressure), indicating a significant difference between the two assessment standards. When selecting a blood pressure device for a specific application, the evaluation using the reference of a common practice in the intended population or environment may be more informative, since that reference has been the everyday basis for decision making in blood pressure diagnosis and treatment.

Different evaluation results for the same brand product can also be due to different versions of a model used for validation, where a later version may have performance improvement over the earlier one. Another source of discrepancies can come from utilizing different study protocols or only partially following the same protocols. It is recommended that the original clinical evaluation report be carefully examined to determine the desired efficacy that may meet the users' requirements. If the devices were FDA-approved for marketing in the U.S., one may request a copy of their clinical validation report directly from the manufacturer.

### 2.5.6 Future Perspectives

Hypertension is one of the most common and important risk factors for health in industrialized countries. It is the leading cause of death in the U.S. It is treatable by a variety of effective medications. It can cause serious damage to the heart and arteries, leading to cardiac infarction, stroke, or renal failure. Significant sudden changes in blood pressure may also precede a major physiological catastrophe such as cardiac arrest. There is now almost universal acceptance that basic physiological parameters such as blood pressure should constantly be monitored in the clinical setting.

There has been increasing interest in automatic blood pressure monitoring devices in recent years, and some clinicians are now advising patients to record their blood pressure at home over up to 3 months before starting antihypertensive medication. Self-monitoring of blood pressure has become very common with the development of microchip technology and oscillometric monitors. The patients no longer have to learn to listen for Korotkoff sounds [208]. This has also removed bias and observer errors, allowing more accurate measurement than conventional techniques using a stethoscope and a mercury sphygmomanometer.

Special populations have unique blood pressure assessment requirements. Newborns require miniaturized equipment. A blood pressure reading in a newborn may stimulate a series of movements, causing motion artifacts. The very obese may find it hard to fit correctly with a cuff at the upper arm if it is too conical rather than cylindrical. In pregnancy, auscultatory and oscillometric methods may correspond poorly with central pressures, although they are helpful in following trends. Even the proper Korotkoff sound (IV or V) to designate as diastolic pressure is uncertain.

Observing blood pressure has limitations. It may suggest what is happening with blood volume, but sometimes does not reveal that blood volume has become inadequate until circulatory collapse has occurred. Venous and left atrial pressures often clarify blood volume problems, but with uncertain results. Similarly, a satisfactory blood pressure does not always indicate adequate tissue perfusion. Some medications that increase blood pressure can do so at the expense of general perfusion. Since blood pressure is measured at specific sites in the arterial tree, if circulation has become nonhomogeneous, such as in arteriosclerosis, the region distal to the arteriosclerosis can be compromised without warning from blood pressure readings sampled at another site. Even mean blood pressure, so useful otherwise, can fail in these circumstances.

Despite inherent problems, observing blood pressure through old and new technologies retains more than enough usefulness to remain an essential aspect of patient care. The promise of improved technology to solve problems such as motion artifacts, noninvasive continuous monitoring, long-distance telemetry, rapid analysis of accumulated or concurrent data, and assessment of new inaccessible blood flow regions represents continued challenges for future biomedical research and development.

Recently, exciting research has revealed that comparing pressures taken at the arm and the ankle results in a handy but straightforward index for assessment of lower extremity vascular disease, with implications for general cardiovascular risk factors [209]. The possibility of obtaining noninvasive blood pressure readings from arteries in the forehead by stick-on oscillometric patches has also been proven. At least in anesthetized patients, the forehead noninvasive blood pressure corresponded reasonably well with central arterial pressures. Finger blood pressure monitors have found some applications in continuous ambulatory and sleep blood pressure assessments. A technology capable of continuously monitoring brachial or even central blood pressure continues to be a clinical demand and a future challenge.

## 2.6 Patient Monitors

Patient monitoring measures the patient's vital signs and organ functions by a dedicated device with automatic detection and alarming of abnormal or life-threatening conditions (e.g., violation of the selected parameter limits and arrhythmia events).

The physiological parameters are acquired continuously, at automatic intervals or else in individual measurements, analyzed, displayed as waveforms and/or numerical values, stored in trends, and, if required, printed out or, for example, forwarded to patient data management systems. After an introduction to the fields of use for patient monitoring systems, the types of monitors and displays are described, followed by sections on handling aspects such as controls, user guidance, and operating philosophy. This Chapter covers the important features of handling alarms and events, followed by a discussion of trend display, automated calculations, and an overview of monitor networks.

Traditionally, the monitoring function which is primarily used at the bedside or in the operating theater is carried out over a relatively short period (short-term monitoring, e.g., during an operation) or a relatively long period (long-term monitoring, e.g., in intensive care units), and is intended to reliably draw the medical staff's attention to physiologically unstable conditions as early as possible. This requires reliable and reproducible detection and display of measurements and includes both self-monitoring of the unit and monitoring of the effectiveness of life-supporting systems to which the patient is connected [49].

The conventional electronic measuring and monitoring unit or monitor has become a multifunctional, software-controlled system with extensive data collection and storage capabilities, which is used for diagnosis and, in combination with other clinical observations and assessments, both for therapeutic decision-making and for monitoring the effects of the therapy. In standards, the general term for such systems is Programmable Electrical Medical System (PEMS). For users, the ease of operation of the monitor and its accessories is a top priority, including their versatility and the reliability of all measurements and alarms. There should be as few false alarms as possible, and above all, a life-threatening situation should never remain undetected. Modern monitors are expected to be scalable, meaning they can be adapted to meet specific requirements at any time by adding or removing extra modules or software options [210]. By means of updates and upgrades, they must be forward-looking, keeping pace with new developments, and capable of extending, for example, with new measuring techniques. Modern monitors feature a highly intuitive operating philosophy and communicate with each other and with central monitoring stations via network connections. Communication with other units and networks in the hospital is one of their advanced system properties (Fig. 2.26).

## *2.6.1 History*

Developing central stations and integrated arrhythmia systems based on standard microcomputer-based server hardware and software platforms has led to wide-scale distribution in the clinical environment. These systems possess database and analysis functions previously reserved for larger systems.

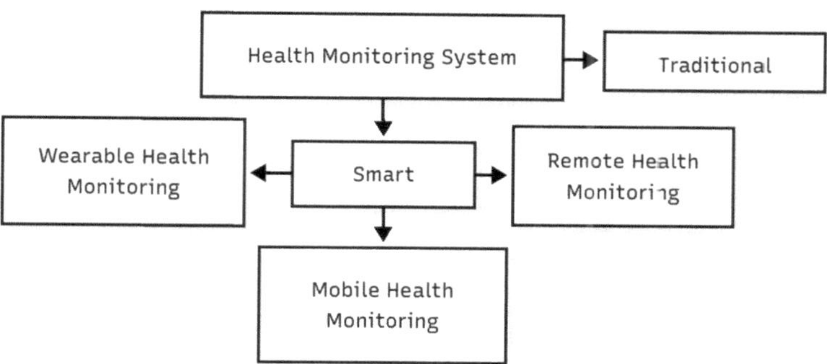


**Fig. 2.26** Classification of patient monitoring systems

In recent years, the bedside monitor has become a focal point for data entry and presentation. Most bedside monitoring systems sold today can also acquire and display data from clinical laboratories, bedside laboratory devices such as blood chemistry machines, and other devices such as ventilators. Unfortunately, each monitor has its proprietary communications protocol and data acquisition scheme. As a result, the user community faces bedside monitors that function like "mini" patient-data-management systems. Furthermore, the desire to capture and manage all clinical data for patients in a critical care setting (not just patient monitoring data) has resulted in the development of specialized ICU information systems [211]. It is common for hospitals to acquire computer-based bedside monitors, which must be interfaced with an ICU information system, which may be interfaced with a hospital's clinical information system. Several large, capable, and reputable manufacturers have supplied over 350 computer-based ICU information systems worldwide. Three of the major companies involved in the development of such computer-based charting and monitoring systems are Philips Medical Systems with its CareVue system, GE Medical Systems formerly Marquette Electronics with its Centricity Clinical Information system, and Eclipsys (formerly EMTEK) with its Continuum 2000 computerized charting application.

## 2.6.2 Technical Characteristics

Using microcomputers in bedside monitors has revolutionized the acquisition, display, and processing of physiological data. Virtually no bedside monitors or ventilators marketed today do not use at least one microcomputer. Physiological signals such as the ECG are derived from sensors that convert biological signals (such as pressure, flow, or mechanical movement) into electrical signals. Modern computerized monitors digitize these signals as close to the patient as possible (Fig. 2.27).

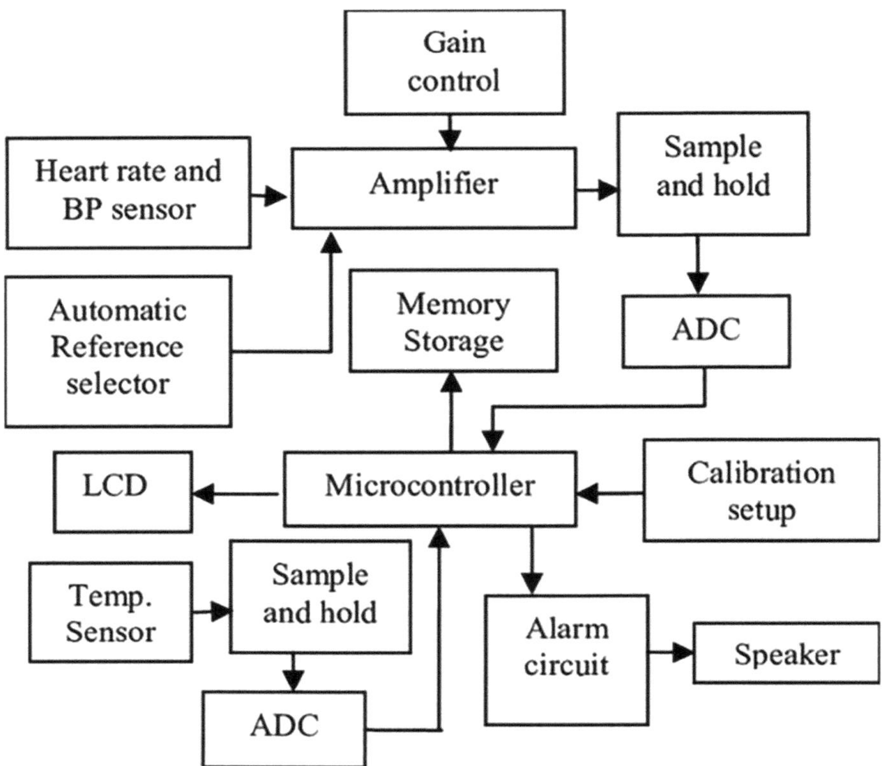


**Fig. 2.27** Block diagram of a modern bedside monitor

Transducers acquire physiological signals from the patient. These transducers convert the appropriate physiological signal into an electrical signal that is then amplified and conditioned (usually an analog filter of some sort) and then presented to an Analog to Digital converter (ADC). The ADC sends the data to a microprocessor-based signal processor, which extracts heart rate and blood pressure features. After processing, the physiological signals are displayed on a display device and usually sent to a centralized ICU display system and frequently to an electronic patient record [212].

Some biological signals, such as the currents trailing the heart, are already in electrical form and are recorded as the ECG. The ECG voltage signal derived from the electrodes at the body surface is small, only a few millivolts in amplitude. The patient is electrically isolated from the bedside monitor, and the analog ECG signal is amplified to a level sufficient for conversion to digital data using an analog-to-digital converter (ADC). Digital data can then be processed, and the results displayed.

Sampling rate is an important factor that affects the correspondence between an analog signal and that signal's digital representation. At a rate of 500 measurements per second, the digitized representation of the ECG looks like an analog recording of the ECG. All the features of the ECG, including the shape of the P wave (atrial depolarization), the amplitude of the QRS complex (ventricular depolarization), and the shape of the T wave (ventricular recovery), are reproduced faithfully. When the sampling rate is decreased to 100 measurements per second, however, the amplitude and shape of the QRS complex begin to be distorted [130, 213]. When only 50 observations per second are recorded, the QRS complex is grossly distorted, and the other features are distorted. At a recording rate of only 25 measurements per second, gross signal distortion occurs, and even estimating heart rate by measuring intervals from R to R is problematic (Fig. 2.28).

## Hardware

Patient monitoring devices in intensive care units (ICUs) have undergone a significant transformation in recent years, featuring modular designs and scalable components that meet diverse clinical needs. Microprocessor-based systems and high-performance transducers are utilized in current systems, offering greater flexibility, enhanced data accuracy, and seamless integration with electronic medical records (EMRs). These systems typically comprise compact-sized modular monitors that can switch dynamically between transport and bedside modes without disrupting the data acquisition process, demonstrating the "pick-and-go" concept [214]. Advances in digital signal acquisition with microcomputers have also enhanced hardware responsiveness and accuracy, particularly for vital sign acquisition in ECG, respiration, and hemodynamics monitoring [215].

One of the new trends in hardware design is the incorporation of wireless technology and sensor miniaturization. ICU monitors are currently equipped with Wi-Fi-based telemetry systems that remove the need for traditional cabling and enhance patient mobility, particularly for step-down and ambulatory care units [216]. These changes alleviate age-old complaints about kludgy cables and

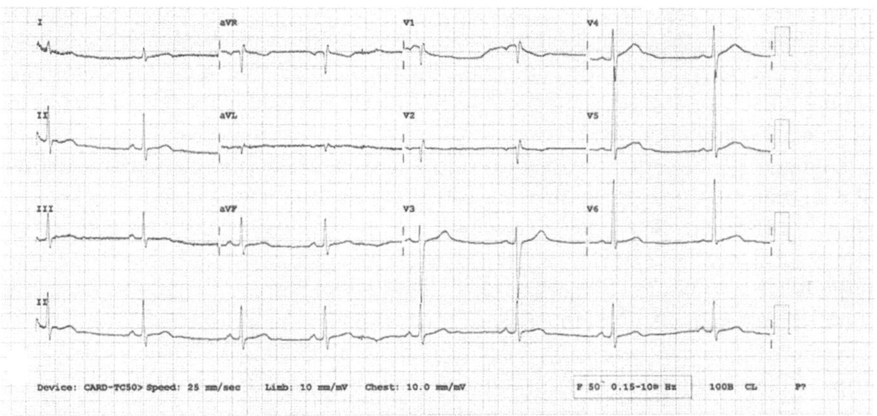


**Fig. 2.28** Electrocardiogram (https://upload.wikimedia.org/wikipedia/commons/d/df/12_lead_ECG.jpg)

relentless false-positive alarms by streamlining the monitoring hardware interface. Emerging designs also feature multi-lead ECG acquisition with real-time noise reduction and electrode status, helping clinicians detect and correct poor signal quality due to skin–electrode impedance.

Patient monitors are also being designed to incorporate predictive analytics solutions for improvement through early detection. For example, ICU monitoring now supports plug-in add-ons or dockable components that capture and analyze high-rate waveform data in real-time, including arrhythmia type classification and detection of ventilator-associated events. Such systems support redundancy and aggressive failover to ensure continuous operation, even in the event of patient transport or system failure [217]. As hospitals become increasingly digital, the modularity and upgradeability of patient monitoring devices make them essential instruments in scalable, efficient ICU management.

### Software

Today, bedside monitors contain multiple microcomputers, offering significantly more computing power and memory than the systems used by the pioneers of computer monitoring. Bedside monitors with built-in microcomputers have the following advantages over their analog predecessors [218].

The digital computer's ability to store patient waveform information, such as the ECG, permits sophisticated pattern recognition and physiological signal feature extraction. Modern microcomputer-based bedside monitors use multiple ECG channels and pattern recognition schemes to identify abnormal waveform patterns and classify ECG arrhythmias. Signal quality from multiple ECG leads can now be monitored and interference noise minimized. For example, the computer can watch for degradation of the ECG skin–electrode contact resistance. If the contact is poor, the monitor can alert the nurse to change the specified problematic electrode.

Physiological signals can be acquired more efficiently by converting them to digital form early in the processing cycle. The waveform processing (e.g., calibration and filtering) can then be done in the microcomputer. The same process simplifies the nurse's task of setting up and operating the bedside monitor by eliminating the manual calibration step.

Digitized physiological waveform signals are easier and more reliable, and digital data transmission is inherently noise-free. As a result, newer monitoring systems allow healthcare professionals to review a patient's waveform displays and derived parameters, such as heart rate and blood pressure, at the bedside, at a central station in the ICU, or at home via modem on a laptop computer. Figure 2.29 is a close-up of the signals and values from a typical bedside patient monitor.

Selected data can be retained easily if they are digitized. For example, ECG strips of interesting physiological sequences, such as periods of arrhythmias, can be stored in the bedside monitor for later review. Today's monitors typically store all of the waveform data from multiple leads of ECG and blood pressure transducers for at least 24 hours and sometimes for even longer. Measured variables, such as heart

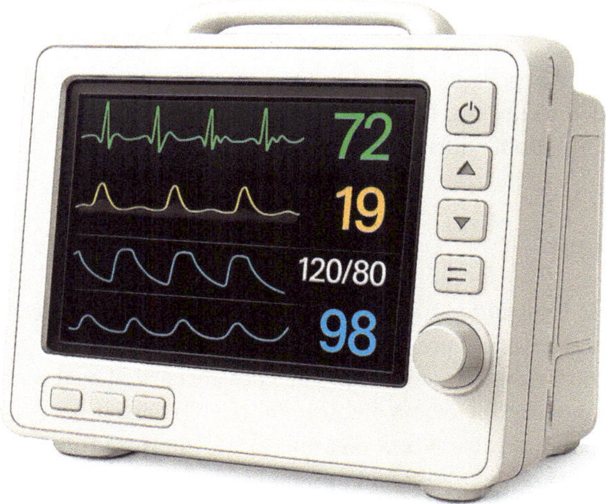


**Fig. 2.29** A bedside monitor display

rate and blood pressure, can be graphed over prolonged periods to aid in the detection of life-threatening trends.

Alarms from bedside monitors are now much “smarter” and raise fewer false alarms. In the past, analog alarm systems used only high–low threshold limits and were susceptible to signal artifacts. Now, computer-based bedside monitors can often distinguish between artifacts and real alarm situations by using the information derived from one signal to verify that of another and can confidently alert physicians and nurses to real alarms. For example, heart rate can be derived from the ECG or the arterial blood pressure. The system sounds an alarm if both signals indicate dangerous tachycardia (fast heart rate). If the two signals do not agree, the monitor can notify the health-care professional about a potential instrumentation or medical problem [219]. The procedure is not unlike that performed by a human verifying possible problems by using redundant information from simpler bedside monitor alarms. Despite these advancements in bedside monitors, false alarms are still very prevalent. Systems can be upgraded easily. Only the software programs in read-only memory (ROM) must be changed; older analog systems require hardware replacement.

## *2.6.3 Types of Devices*

### Stand-Alone Monitors

A stand-alone monitor does not communicate with other monitors or a central station and is often used only for selective measurement or short-term monitoring of a few patient parameters.

#### Transport Monitors

This type of monitor is portable and as light as possible. It has an integrated display and can be fastened to the bed or to the transport bed. It is used in battery-operated devices to monitor patients during transport.

#### Telemetry Monitors

These are portable transmitters (often without a display) for wireless monitoring of patients in a defined coverage area of an antenna system installed in the clinical environment. Unlike the transport monitor, such devices are carried by the ambulant patient. They are used to monitor the electrocardiogram (ECG) and, if necessary, the oxygen saturation and (noninvasively) blood pressure at a central station. Modern telemetry devices no longer utilize the traditional ultrahigh-frequency (UHF) and very high-frequency (VHF) bands, which require proprietary antenna and receiver systems. Instead, they employ a Wi-Fi radio network called WLAN (wireless local area network), utilizing certified, generally available components that comply with industry standards.

#### Compact Monitors

Such devices have an integrated display and a fixed and limited number of measurement parameters. Semi-Modular (compact) monitors can be expanded by a module for additional measurements. A recorder can be integrated. Integration in networks is usually possible nowadays. When equipped with accumulators, there is no strict distinction between use as a transport monitor and use as a transport monitor. When integrated in a WLAN, the monitor can work in the same radio network as a WLAN telemetry unit [220]. If the monitor is further miniaturized, it will undoubtedly become impossible to draw such strict boundaries between a telemetry device and a monitor.

#### Modular Monitors

The performance of these monitors is freely scalable by exchanging or adding modules (plugin units or external extensions) for the detection of further parameters and also using software options (e.g., for advanced arrhythmia monitoring). It can be adapted in each case to the specific requirements. These monitors, which have an integrated or separate screen, can often only be used in a stationary position at the patient's bedside or in the operating theater (OT) and are generally combined with monitor systems in a network.

A modular monitor suitable for transport throughout the hospital, combined with a logically associated medical-grade panel personal computer (PC). The monitor is docked at the bedside on a so-called docking station, which provides secure mechanical mounting and contains all the connections to the power supply, network, and, if required, to external devices and other display units. Simply by turning a lever, the mechanical connection and all electrical connections are disconnected, and the monitor is used as a transport monitor, without any interruption in monitoring (pick-and-go principle). On return from transport, the monitor is put on the docking station, and the lever is returned to its locking position, thereby re-establishing all previously disconnected connections. There is no need for any cables and/or modules between the bed monitor and transport monitor to be reconnected, and seamless patient monitoring is ensured, without any restrictions on the parameters [214, 220]. The dedicated bedside panel PC is first used for advanced monitoring to present the abundance of monitor information intelligibly and in large sizes in various screen layouts. Secondly, it acts as an information technology (IT) portal for doctors and nurses. It provides access to all electronically available information in the hospital about their patients [images, e.g., X-ray, magnetic resonance tomography (MRT), and ultrasound, test results, medical histories, and preexisting conditions] and to databases (red list, care guidelines). Thereby, essential information for decision-making on further therapy is available where it is needed—at the bedside, the point of care—without a time-consuming search. Thirdly, the PC can simultaneously be used for paperless documentation by running a patient data management system.

This system further develops the information monitor mentioned above and the pick-and-go principle. A convenient and light but mighty monitor with a touch-screen records all the vital signs and stays with the patient at all times (including during transport). At the bedside, it can be inserted into the automatically locking docking station with one hand and thereby connected to the information monitor, which is used for comprehensive operation. The information monitor acts simultaneously as an IT portal for all possible web-based or Citrix applications in the hospital. The standardized hardware provides a user interface that has the same design, not only for monitoring but also, for example, for respiratory therapy and anesthetic equipment. The aim is to always provide the user with the same operating philosophy in an integrated system, and as a result of this standardization to minimize both the cost of training and the sources of operator errors throughout all the wards and departments, from accident and emergency (A&E) units to the OT, and from the recovery room to intensive care units [48, 214]. The system is scalable according to the various requirements in the different wards and departments, facilitates intelligent data transfer, and ensures effective transport without any loss of time.

### 2.6.4 Clinical Applications

Patient monitoring systems are mainly used in general and specialized operating theaters (OT) (especially cardiac, vascular, and neurosurgical) [221]:

- Induction and postanesthetic rooms, recovery rooms, and observation wards
- General and special intensive care units (ICU), including neonatal (NICU) and coronary (CCU) care units as well as stroke units, accident and emergency

(A&E) units, procedure rooms, outpatient clinics, emergency services, and patient transport.

Furthermore, monitors are regularly used in wards and units that take patients from intensive care units at a very early stage (step-down units). There are at least five categories of patients who need physiological monitoring:

1. Patients with unstable physiological regulatory systems; for example, a patient whose respiratory system is suppressed by a drug overdose or anesthesia
2. Patients with a suspected life-threatening condition; for example, a patient who has findings indicating an acute myocardial infarction (heart attack)
3. Patients at high risk of developing a life-threatening condition; for example, patients immediately after open-heart surgery or a premature infant whose heart and lungs are not fully developed
4. Patients in a critical physiological state, for example, patients with multiple trauma or septic shock.
5. Mother and baby during the labor and delivery process.

Care of the critically ill patient requires prompt and accurate decisions so that life-protecting and life-saving therapy can be appropriately applied. Because of these requirements, ICUs have become widely established in hospitals. Such units use computers almost universally for the following purposes:

- To acquire physiological data frequently or continuously, such as blood pressure readings.
- To communicate information from data-producing systems to remote locations (e.g., laboratory and radiology departments).
- To store, organize, and report data.
- To integrate and correlate data from multiple sources.
- To provide clinical alerts and advisories based on multiple sources of data.
- To function as a decision-making tool that health professionals may use in planning the care of critically ill patients.
- To measure the severity of illness for patient classification purposes.
- To analyze the outcomes of ICU care in terms of clinical effectiveness and cost-effectiveness.

One of the goals of bedside patient monitoring is to detect life-threatening events promptly so that they can be treated before they cause irreversible organ damage or death. Care of critically ill patients requires considerable skill and prompt, accurate treatment decisions. Healthcare professionals collect numerous data through frequent observations and testing, and more data are recorded by continuous monitoring equipment. Physicians prescribe complicated therapy for such patients [47, 222]. As a result, enormous amounts of clinical data accumulate. Professionals can miss important events and trends if the accumulated data is not presented in a compact, well-organized form. In addition, the problems of managing these patients have been made even more challenging by economic pressures to reduce the cost of diagnostic and therapeutic interventions.

Continuity of care is essential for critically ill patients. Teams of physicians, nurses, and therapists generally serve such patients. Data is often transferred from one individual to another (e.g., the laboratory technician calls a unit clerk who reports the information to a nurse who, in turn, passes it on to the physician who makes a decision). Each step in this transmission process is subject to delay and error. The medical record is the principal instrument for ensuring the continuity of care for patients [223] (Figs. 2.30 and 2.31).

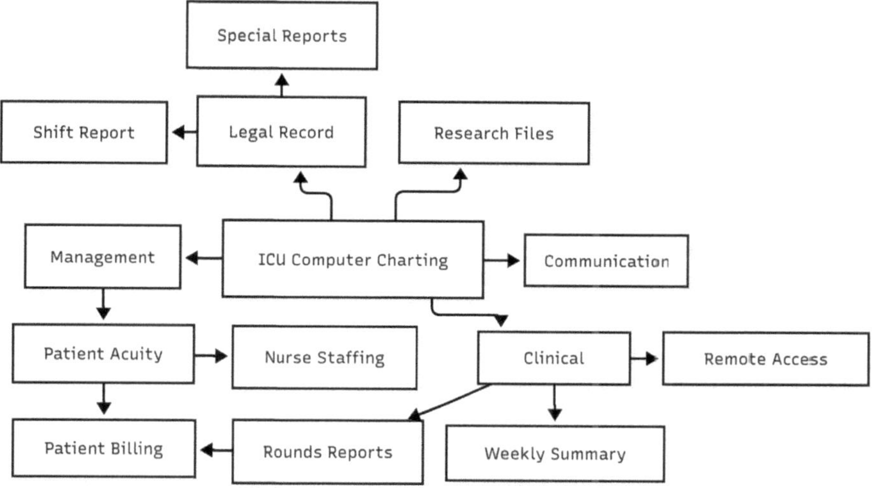


**Fig. 2.30** The six major areas healthcare professionals interact with computer-based ICU charting to make patient care more effective and efficient

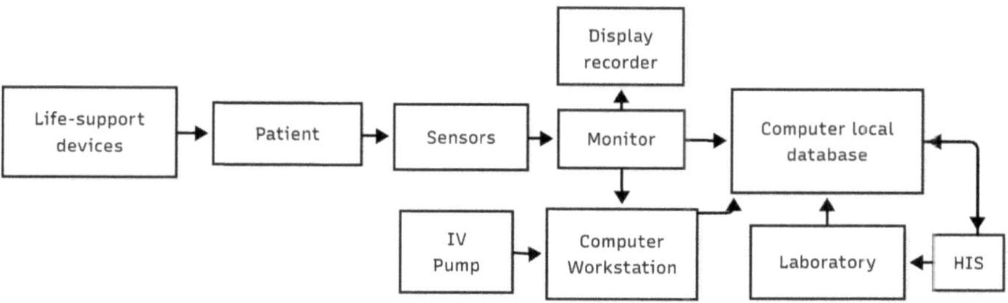


**Fig. 2.31** Block diagram of a distributed-database ICU system with networking

### 2.6.5 Regulatory Considerations

Existing regulatory policies for patient monitoring systems have prioritized post-market surveillance (PMS) and conformity assessment, particularly under the EU Medical Device Regulation [224]. Traditional conformity assessments do not account for real-world conditions, so new methods have emerged. There is a harmonized approach to patient monitor conformity assessment, including metrological performance, visual integrity, and safety features assessment during routine use [79]. The approach enhances compliance monitoring and device traceability per the updated MDR requirements.

Furthermore, some used this model on infant incubators to prove its generalizability to other high-risk medical devices. Their study corroborates the necessity of structured conformity testing that ensures long-term performance reliability and minimizes risks associated with equipment deterioration. Supporting studies have also called for harmonizing PMS strategies and regulatory alignment with international standards to enhance transparency and global device safety [79].

Such initiatives align with broader regulatory reforms towards proactive, evidence-based regulation. For instance, artificial intelligence (AI) in PMS designs has been proposed to maximize signal detection and risk management [225], enabling regulators to enhance the detection and response to new safety concerns in real time.

### 2.6.6 Future Perspectives

In the coming times, the conformity assessment model will serve as an entry point for digitalization in medical device regulation. The method enables automated performance testing and structured documentation to integrate AI in clinical device management [79]. AI-driven systems can revolutionize monitoring through real-time alerts, predictive maintenance, and enhanced anomaly detection analytics, ultimately resulting in improved patient outcomes and operational effectiveness [226].

Further, next-generation systems will incorporate these standardized conformity solutions with hospital-wide information systems to provide intelligent, networked infrastructure among ICUs and operating rooms. The models' scalability allows them to be adapted to various categories of devices, e.g., infusion pumps and mechanical ventilators [79]. The tools also offer device-specific monitoring and centralized, institution-level performance analytics.

In short, as healthcare becomes increasingly digitally mature, AI-driven conformity assessment will be at the center of it. These innovations will drive continuous quality assurance, reduce adverse events, and ensure critical patient monitoring systems are safe, effective, and fully compliant with evolving clinical and regulatory requirements [175].

## 2.7 Mechanical Ventilators

To supply the body with oxygen, the volume of the lungs increases during inhalation. When breathing in, the pressure in the lungs drops, and in this way atmospheric air is sucked into the lungs. The reverse applies when breathing out: thoracic and respiratory muscles return to their idle state, reducing lung volume. The resulting intrapulmonary increase in pressure causes the expiratory gas, which contains carbon dioxide, to be expired. In an idle state, this procedure is repeated approximately 10–20 times per minute in an adult. For a body weight of 75 kg, the volume moved with each breath varies between 350 and 850 mL. Considering additional physical activities, which can result in a significant increase in respiration, it is more than possible that our respiratory musculature shifts a total volume of 10,000–15,000 L of air over a day. These figures underline the fundamental importance of our respiratory system for the entire organism [227]. Suppose the interplay of the organs and muscles involved in respiration is interrupted. In that case, ventilators can completely take over breathing or share the breathing work if the patient is breathing too shallowly. Many reasons may require a ventilator, but in principle, it can be allocated to five different issues.

Use of a ventilator can also be required due to undesired respiratory depression caused by strong pain relievers or the use of muscle relaxants. The examples listed make it clear that patients can depend on breathing gas supplied to them via specialized gas dosage equipment for various reasons. A differentiation must be made here between a patient who is still breathing spontaneously and only needs to be offered an increased concentration of oxygen from a ventilation therapy device and a patient who is no longer able to perform the necessary breathing work and must be ventilated by a ventilator [228]. Regardless of the breathing disruption, a long-term ventilator performs a life-saving function in all cases. Against this background, the ventilator must fulfill three different tasks [48]:

- Oxygenation of the patient: Provide and supply oxygen and air.
- Partial or total assumption of respiratory work: Generate and dose defined gas flow and respiratory pressure.
- Monitoring of the device and patient: Generate alarms and visualize changes.

Ventilation therapy primarily aims to support or replace the patient's breathing, thus guaranteeing efficient gas exchange. For this reason, the ventilator user must ensure that the selected device configuration supplies the patient with adequate oxygen and that the ventilation sufficiently reduces the amount of carbon dioxide in the body. Efficient control is achieved through arterial blood-gas analysis. With a long-term respiratory device, the therapist is provided with a tool that enables them to simultaneously train and strengthen the patient's respiratory musculature, allowing the patient to gradually become accustomed to breathing independently. This weaning process can last hours, days, or even weeks. One reason for this wide range is the different duration of ventilation, during which atrophy of the respiratory musculature can occur. Furthermore, the duration of the weaning phase is influenced by the clinical picture of the patient, the recovery process, and the overall clinical situation (Fig. 2.32).

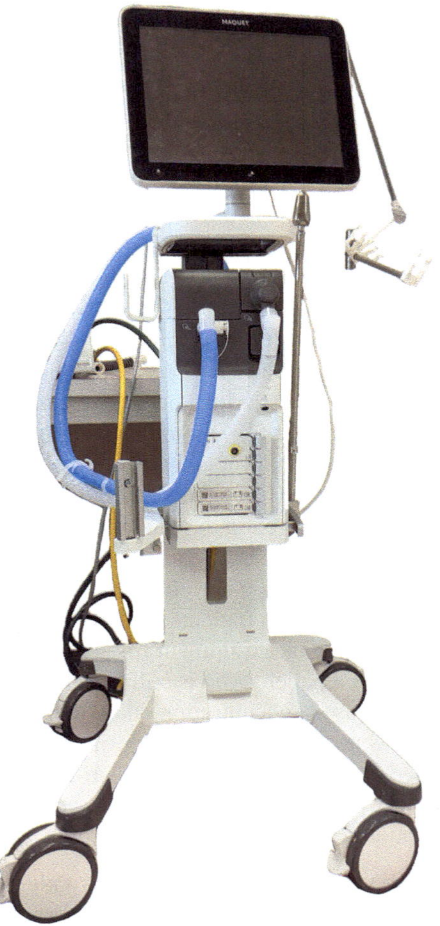

**Fig. 2.32** Intensive care ventilator (https://upload.wikimedia.org/wikipedia/commons/3/31/Servo_I_Ventilator.jpg)

## 2.7.1 History

Long-term mechanical ventilation (LTMV) has been shaped by technology and growing recognition of its usefulness in managing chronic respiratory failure. Initially developed for acute care, mechanical ventilation was later adapted for long-term use following the polio epidemics. Eventually, it became the norm for the management of conditions like neuromuscular diseases, chronic obstructive pulmonary disease (COPD), and obesity hypoventilation syndrome. Over time, ventilation was relocated from the hospital to the home setting, giving patients a higher quality of life and economic advantage.

Since the 1980s, countries like Switzerland have seen an abrupt rise in the use of LTMV, which reflects expanding clinical assurance in invasive and non-invasive methods. Its spread of use was maintained through clinical evidence demonstrating increased survival and symptom relief in a wide range of conditions [229]. Concurrent with the extended applications, a similar development in engineering has made it possible to create compact, portable, and sophisticated ventilators suitable for home and ambulatory use, especially relevant for pediatric and geriatric populations [230].

The most recent LTMV history is characterized by integration with digital technology, such as remote monitoring and smart alarms. This development is a step in the broader direction towards telemedicine and personalized care, with modern devices capable of delivering real-time feedback and data exchange to clinicians outside the hospital setting. The increased application of LTMV is a clinical necessity and a sign of growing social needs for home healthcare alternatives that focus on autonomy, safety, and efficiency.

## *2.7.2 Technical Characteristics*

If the patient's respiratory activity is insufficient, some form of external substitution or complementary intervention is required to transport the breathing gas to the lungs. Artificial respiration can be achieved by the delivery of defined gas flows and by the creation of positive pressure. There is a significant difference from spontaneous breathing: When the patient breathes spontaneously, the intrapulmonary pressure stays roughly at the baseline of atmospheric pressure. In contrast, the breathing gas is supplied to the lungs with positive pressure during artificial respiration. A hose or breathing circuit interfaces the ventilator and the patient. It is generally designed as a dual-hose circuit for clinical intensive care ventilators [231, 232]. In principle, the patient can be connected with the ventilation system via a face mask or a tube inserted into the trachea. The user will decide which method to use based on the respective circumstances, such as the expected ventilation period, and take the appropriate medical measures to prepare the patient. Different system components are required for the technical implementation of a long-term ventilator.

### **Hardware**

#### Power Supply

Ventilators require electric power, oxygen, and compressed air to operate correctly. The devices are usually supplied via an external power source and the hospital's central gas supply. In functional areas without a central gas supply or during transportation of patients within the hospital, it is necessary to ensure the device's functioning by other means. Potential solutions include using separate compressors, compressed gas cylinder packs, and accumulators. Increasingly, ventilators that are not dependent on compressed air, which provide ventilation by filtering and using ambient air, are also being used. Only an oxygen source and a power supply are needed to operate such ventilators [233].

### Gas Mixer

The gas mixer allows the user to vary the oxygen concentration of the inspiratory gas between 21% and 100% by volume. While ventilators often used to be supplied by external mechanical gas mixers, technological developments have resulted in an electronically controlled gas mixer integrated in the ventilator becoming standard. Gas mixers usually have a dual function: they ensure that the breathing gas to be supplied is prepared and delivered in the required quantity and at the correct rate. Often, the threshold ranges pose the most significant challenges to these metering systems [234]. If, for example, a volume of 20 mL with an oxygen concentration of 30% by volume is required for ventilation, 17.7 mL of gas must be delivered via the compressed air valve and 2.3 mL via the oxygen valve.

### Pressure Generator

The pressure or flow generator is responsible for delivering the mixed gas prepared by the gas mixer according to the ventilation parameters set in the operating unit. At the simplest level, the gas flow or pressure can be created manually using a manual ventilation bag. Technically comparable methods are to be found in older ventilators and anesthesia workstations. These devices generate the inspiratory gas flow using mechanically moving parts, such as bellows or piston pumps. On the other hand, modern intensive ventilators feature combined gas mixture and metering devices that provide the required gas quantities directly from the gas supply systems [116]. From a technical point of view, these components can be designed as a flow or a pressure generator. A flow generator is a controlled valve whose output provides a defined gas flow; the output pressure is not specified. A pressure generator, on the other hand, behaves similarly to a compressor, whose output provides a defined pressure with an unspecified gas flow. Pressure generators are often used to drive ventilators that are not dependent on compressed air and use suctioned ambient air for patient ventilation.

### Breathing System

The breathing system forms the interface between the patient and the ventilator. Clinical long-term ventilators are usually connected with the patient via an inspiratory and an expiratory hose. The expiratory valve is closed during the inspiratory phase. The gas flow delivered through the inspiratory port passes through a breathing gas humidifier before entering the patient's lungs, adapting it to the climatic conditions in the patient's lungs. After the inspiratory phase, the patient exhales when the expiratory valve is opened. Thus, the expiratory gas passes through the ventilator again, but is not reused for the following inspiration as with an anesthesia workstation [235]. Based on this characteristic, the breathing systems of long-term ventilators are also referred to as non-rebreathing circuits.

For completeness, it should be mentioned that ventilators with one-tube circuits are used in individual clinical function areas. These circuits are also non-rebreathing; however, in this case, the expiratory valve is not positioned on the side of the device but near the patient. The improved handling provided by the single hose is thus in conflict with an expiratory valve arranged in the field of vision of the patient. Ventilators with single-hose circuits have become the standard in emergency and intermediate care based on individual product requirements. In intensive care units, on the other hand, ventilators with two hose circuits are more common due to the required expiratory volume monitoring.

#### Gas Humidifier

Breathing gas humidifiers are used to warm and humidify the inspiratory gas. Since the dry and relatively cool supply gas would dry out the patient's airways, it is vital to humidify and warm the breathing gas to avoid the risk of causing irreversible damage to the ciliated epithelium. Active or passive breathing gas humidifiers are available for this purpose. Active breathing gas humidifiers are located in the inspiratory limb and use electrical energy to heat a water bath. When the cold, dry gas passes over the water surface, it absorbs water molecules and is thus warmed and humidified. Passive breathing gas humidifiers, termed heat and moisture exchangers (HMEs), are placed close to the patient, between the tube and the Y-piece. These products are designed to buffer a significant fraction of the moisture and heat expelled by the patient. This retained moisture is then used to condition the inspired gas passing through the HME during the next inspiration [236]. Using an HME with an active breathing gas humidifier in a single breathing circuit is not permitted, as it would significantly impair the resistance of the HME. HMEs are also unofficially referred to as filters, which is a misnomer as they have nothing in common with each other, unless they also fulfill a hygienic function.

#### Expiratory Valve

Besides the above-mentioned switchover function, the expiratory valve is responsible for two additional important tasks. A positive end-expiratory pressure (PEEP) is created in the lungs if the valve is not entirely opened during expiration. This PEEP pressure is therapeutically important because it increases the gas exchange surface of the lungs. An adequate PEEP can also prevent the collapse of individual alveolar areas. The expiratory valve can also fulfill another function, providing that the ventilator controls the valve during the inspiratory phase [237]. In this case, the expiratory valve can compensate for undesired pressure rises in the breathing system caused, for example, by the patient coughing.

Operating and Display Unit

The operating and display unit interfaces with the ventilator and the user. These units are often touchscreens designed to display pressure and flow curves and multiple menus for setting different ventilation modes, adjusting alarm limits, or measured value overviews, etc. The parameter settings entered in the operating unit control the other device components and therefore significantly influence the ventilation pattern applied to the patient.

Alarm System

The monitoring and alarm system ensures that the ventilation parameters set in the operating and display unit are applied. It also issues audible and visual alarms to alert staff to critical changes in the patient's condition or technical malfunctions. The following are measured: the inspiratory oxygen concentration, ventilation pressure, and ventilation volume. In addition, using an active breathing gas humidifier makes inspiratory breathing gas temperature measurement with an alarm system obligatory.

Patient Monitoring

Patient monitoring is used to monitor the patient's vital functions. This includes, for example, an electrocardiogram, blood pressure, oxygen saturation, and the measurement of the carbon dioxide concentration in the breathing gas. Although patient monitors sometimes display ventilation data, these devices are to be seen as an independent display unit with an alarm facility. This makes patient monitoring a significant component of the intensive care workstation, but not part of the ventilator.

**Software**

Inverse Ratio Ventilation

Usually, the inspiratory period is shorter than the expiratory phase. However, the inspiratory time may need to be increased at the expense of the expiratory phase when treating diseases with severe oxygenation disorders. The term inverse ratio ventilation (IRV) merely states that ventilation takes place with an inverse inspiration-to-expiration ratio; in other words, the inspiratory time is longer than the expiratory time. The designation IRV alone does not provide information on whether the ventilation is volume or pressure controlled [238].

### Sigh

By observing one's spontaneous breathing, you will notice that breathing is not always even. Occasionally, we inhale more air than usual, i.e., we sigh. Initially, the sigh function was introduced in ventilation to reproduce the typical variations in volume that occur during spontaneous breathing, thereby breaking up the monotonous and unphysiological ventilation pattern of controlled ventilation. The sigh function, also called intermittent PEEP, is accomplished by temporarily increasing the PEEP pressure to a higher value. In the Evita ventilator, the PEEP pressure is increased, for example, every 3 min for two breathing cycles [239]. The term sigh results from the deep drawn inspiration whose discharge creates a noticeable flow murmur similar to a spontaneous sigh. The use of a sigh could not become established as initially conceived. However, the sigh function has become an important therapeutic tool for reopening collapsed alveoli (recruitment).

### AutoFlow

The AutoFlow function is an optional addition that is available in all volume-controlled ventilation modes on Drager ventilators (except ILV). The ventilation mode is set using the parameters that are valid for the respective mode. When AutoFlow is activated, the ventilator replaces the constant flow typical of volume-controlled ventilation modes with the decelerating flow pattern known from pressure-controlled ventilation modes. This combines the benefits of pressure-controlled ventilation with the strengths of volume-controlled ventilation. The modified volume-controlled ventilation can be characterized as follows [240]:

- AutoFlow ensures that the user-defined tidal volume is applied at the lowest possible ventilation.
- AutoFlow automatically adjusts the ventilation pressure to pulmonary compliance changes, eliminating the need to correct the inspiratory pressure in pressure-controlled ventilation manually.
- AutoFlow tolerates spontaneous breathing activities by the patient at any time, thus adding the benefits of a free breathing system listed under PC-BIPAP to volume-controlled ventilation.
- AutoFlow eliminates the peak pressure usually occurring during volume-controlled ventilation, which might cause partial overinflation of individual lung areas.
- AutoFlow takes over the responsibility for setting the „Flow "controllers. The reduction of parameters makes it easier to set volume-controlled ventilation.

The sequence of inspiration, expiration, and control characteristics is as follows: The chronological sequence of inspiration and expiration remains unaffected by the AutoFlow function and corresponds to the behavior of the respective ventilation mode. After activation of AutoFlow, the ventilator applies the next mandatory ventilation stroke with a minimum constant flow. The ventilation pressure measured at the end of this inspiration is used as the inspiratory pressure in the following inspiratory phase. The flow is then delivered with a decelerating flow profile. After the switchover to expiration, the ventilator compares the applied tidal volume with the user-defined set value. The inspiratory pressure of the following mandatory phase is slightly increased or decreased to offset the differences. The adjustment mechanism is limited to a fluctuation margin from breath to breath [241]. The pressure increase is stopped when the inspiratory pressure approaches the upper airway pressure alarm limit of up to 5 mbar. If this pressure is insufficient to apply the set tidal volume completely, the device generates an inconsistent alarm volume. Although spontaneous breathing activities can lead to fluctuations in the expiratory volume, AutoFlow ensures that a constant tidal volume is applied on average over time. AutoFlow is always possible and useful, provided there are no special pulmonary restrictions and the patient is receiving volume-controlled ventilation anyway. Irrespective of the current ventilation situation, the upper airway pressure alarm limit is fundamental because of the above-mentioned dual function [242, 243].

## *2.7.3 Types of Devices*

Ventilators differ according to their gas flow behavior. Devices that provide ventilation by generating a continuous gas flow are used, as well as demand flow devices that only provide a gas flow during the inspiratory phase.

### Flow Systems

Continuous Flow Systems

A continuous flow of oxygen and compressed air is supplied from the pressurized gas sources via metering valves. This gas flow is guided via an inspiratory hose to the patient and from there via an expiratory hose to an expiratory valve. Thus, a spontaneously breathing patient can always cover their air requirements from the gas flow. If the patient needs to be ventilated, the expiratory valve is closed for a defined period. This leads to a pressure rise in the breathing system, and the gas flow is supplied to the patient's lungs. An adjustable pressure control valve limits the inspiratory ventilation pressure. With the switchover to expiration, the expiratory valve is opened, and the pressure in the breathing system returns to the ambient or the PEEP pressure. The breathing gas exits the lungs through the decrease in pressure, is mixed with the constant flow, and flows through the expiratory valve. In practice, continuous flow systems are preferably used in neonatal respiration and in respiration therapy [244]. Respiration therapy, or continuous positive airway pressure (CPAP) devices, can only generate a constant, positive pressure. The use of a respiration therapy device is thus reserved for spontaneously breathing patients, who are, for example, dependent on an increased oxygen concentration (Fig. 2.33).

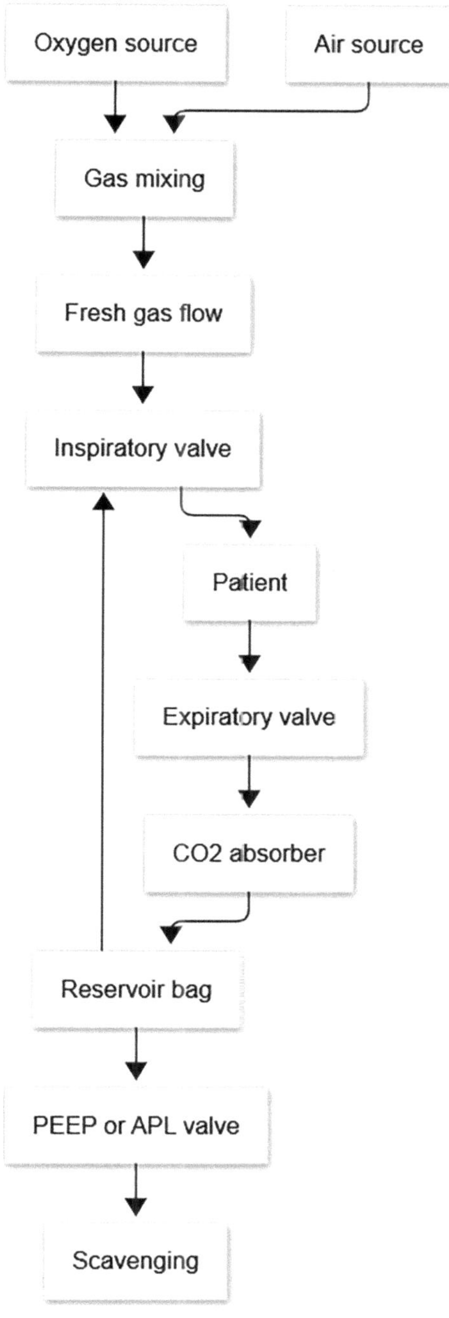


**Fig. 2.33** Continuous flow system

### Demand Flow Systems

In contrast to the above-mentioned continuous flow systems, demand flow systems only supply a gas flow during the inspiratory phase. In the case of controlled ventilation, the gas flow is generally synchronized by the user-defined time pattern. This can be defined with controllers, for example, for the inspiratory and expiratory time according to the operating philosophy of the device. Demand flow systems respond to spontaneous breathing activities by implementing a trigger criterion. Demand flow systems reduce gas consumption considerably and are used in inhalers to promote the patient's breathing depth and/or apply aerosols synchronized with inspiration.

### Combined Flow Systems

Some ventilators use combined flow systems for technical reasons or due to special operational requirements. These deliver a low constant or base flow on the order of some liters per minute compared with the patient's gas requirement. When inspiration is triggered, these systems increase the gas flow to meet the respective requirement [69]. Combined flow systems are used, for example, in ventilators that need to cover the entire spectrum of patients, from premature babies to adults (Fig. 2.34).

## Ventilation Control

### Start of Inspiration

After the expiratory time has elapsed, the start of an inspiratory phase is mandatory in controlled ventilation modes. In ventilation modes during which the ventilator merely supports the patient's breathing work, the ventilator must recognize the patient's breathing activities and provide an adequate gas flow. The ventilator trigger acts as a detector for the spontaneous breathing efforts. This is a device function with a user-adjustable threshold. Although the patient's spontaneous breathing activity is reflected in pressure and flow changes in the breathing system, both signals could be used in current ventilators because the tendency for artifacts is low. In this case, the ventilator responds to the patient's flow signal, and the trigger threshold can be adjusted in units of 1/min.

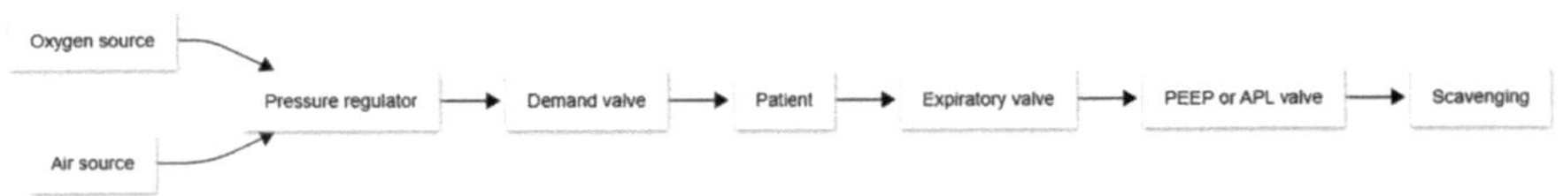


**Fig. 2.34** Demand flow system

Switchover Behavior

The long-term ventilator control influences the ventilator's switchover behavior from inspiration to expiration or vice versa. In this regard, a distinction can be made between four different types of control [245]:

- Time-cycled mode
  User-adjustable time parameters define the duration of the inspiratory and expiratory phases and, thus, also the switchover time. This control type often implements controlled (mandatory) ventilation modes, as it enables patient ventilation with a defined ventilation ratio.
- Pressure-cycled mode
  In pressure-cycled modes, the switchover from inspiration to expiration occurs when an adjustable ventilation pressure has been reached. Inspiration occurs after a time phase has elapsed, by patient activity, and on reaching a trigger criterion. The pressure-cycled mode is mainly used with impermissibly high pressure rises connected to an audible alarm as a safety element.
- Volume-cycled mode
  In this case, the switchover from inspiration to expiration occurs after the delivery of a ventilation volume to be defined by the user. As with the pressure-cycled mode, the next inspiration takes place after a time phase has elapsed or by a patient's activity. The volume-cycled mode is sporadically used in supporting ventilation modes. Moreover, in the US and American-influenced markets, it is also used in mandatory ventilation modes.
- Flow-cycled mode
  This control is primarily used for supporting ventilation modes and initiates the expiratory phase when the gas flow decreases to a defined value. In flo-cycled modes, inspiration is mainly initiated by a patient's activity and on reaching a trigger criterion.

### Ventilation Procedures

Ventilators can only follow two different behavior patterns despite the endless ventilation modes. These are controlled and supported ventilation methods. The main difference between these techniques is as follows: During controlled ventilation, the behavior of the ventilator is defined by the user-configured ventilation parameters. In supported ventilation modes, on the other hand, the ventilator follows the patient's breathing activities and only provides support by increasing the pressure in the breathing system [16]. Variations of these two ventilation methods are spontaneous breathing without support pressure and mixed ventilation modes with alternating mandatory and supporting phases (Table 2.13).

**Table 2.13** Forms of respiration and mechanical ventilation

| | Spontaneous breathing | Supported spontaneous breathing | Controlled ventilation | Mixed ventilation |
|---|---|---|---|---|
| Respiratory muscles | Sufficient | Weak | Intact or paralyzed | Weak |
| Breathing control system | Intact | Intact | Not available | Restricted or unstable |

## Controlled Ventilation (Total Respiratory Substitution)

The ventilation modes in this category are characterized by the fact that the patients do not breathe spontaneously and that the ventilator performs the total work of breathing. The different modes can be divided into volume-controlled modes and pressure-controlled modes. Volume-controlled modes are characterized by a user-defined volume ventilating the patient. In volume-controlled modes, the airway pressure is a resulting parameter and provides information on lung expansibility and airway resistance. In contrast, the user specifies an inspiratory ventilation pressure in pressure-controlled modes [108]. Conversely, in these modes, it is not the ventilation pressure but the tidal volume that provides information on the condition of the patient's lungs. In some cases, ventilation modes are manufacturer-specific, but naming also varies in international linguistic usage. To enhance usability, particular operating philosophies or a prefix to the ventilation mode have been implemented by the manufacturers.

### Volume-Controlled Ventilation

This mode is suitable, for example, for patients with healthy lungs but without spontaneous breathing. It is important to note that in this mode, the device does not respond to the patient's spontaneous breathing activities. The chronological sequence of inspiration and expiration is as follows: At the beginning of inspiration, the ventilator closes the expiratory valve and delivers the inspiratory flow according to the flow setting. This leads to an increase in pressure in the breathing system and the lungs. Suppose the inspiratory flow setting is so high that the set tidal volume is reached before the inspiratory time Tinsp elapses. In that case, the inspiratory valve closes, and the delivery or breathing gas stops. Due to pressure compensation between the breathing system and the patient's lungs, the ventilation pressure decreases from the peak pressure Ppeak to the plateau pressure Pplat.
The expiratory valve remains closed until the inspiratory time Tinsp has elapsed. This inspiratory pause can be recognized as a plateau pressure phase, Pplat, in the pressure curve. The expiratory valve opens when the inspiratory time Tinsp has elapsed. Therefore, the pressure in the breathing system falls to the PEEP pressure level generated by the expiratory valve. The expired gas leaves the lungs and is

transported via the expiratory branch of the ventilator into the atmosphere. The next inspiration follows after the expiratory phase, whose length is determined by the respiratory rate setting, has elapsed. To avoid pressure peaks, the maximum inspiratory working pressure of the ventilator can be limited via the Pmax controller. If provided by the device, pressure limitation is available in all volume-controlled ventilation modes. The term pressure-limited ventilation used in this context does not, therefore, provide any information on the ventilation mode that is currently being applied. The abbreviation PAW used in the graphic stands for airway pressure.

The user should remember that the sudden resumption of spontaneous breathing in this ventilation mode can lead to serious dyssynchrony between the patient and the ventilator. In such an event, the patient would fight against the mandatory ventilation pattern with spontaneous breathing. Activating the trigger function can compensate for this deficiency to an extent. However, in this operating mode, the device will respond to every inhalation effort by the patient by applying the set ventilation stroke. The increase of the respiratory rate and the minute volume leads to a decrease in the arterial carbon dioxide concentration. The breathing drive is thus reduced and may lead to respiratory standstill. Volume-controlled ventilation or intermittent positive pressure ventilation is becoming less important, as the VC-SIMV ventilation mode provides an identical ventilation and features a weaning mode [246].

#### Independent Lung Ventilation

Independent lung ventilation (ILV) is the independent ventilation of each lung using a special double-lumen tube whose ends are each connected to a separate ventilator. Evita ventilators, for example, can be electrically connected using a special connection cable to chronologically synchronize the actions of both ventilators. One of the ventilators assumes the master function, determining the breathing rhythm. Depending on the selected presetting, the second ventilator, also called the slave, performs ventilation in parallel, delayed, or inversely to the master's actions. ILV is only available as volume-controlled ventilation.

#### Pressure-Controlled Ventilation

During classic pressure-controlled ventilation, user-defined pressure alteration intervals are used for patient ventilation. Pressure-controlled ventilation dominates in neonatology intensive care units and is extremely important for treating adults with pulmonary damage, but it is not reserved only for this group. There are significant differences between the conventional pressure-controlled ventilation (PCV) and pressure control-biphasic positive airway pressure/pressure control continuous mandatory ventilation regarding spontaneous breathing characteristics [247]. While the patient's activities in PCV can create undesired pressure rises and lead to corresponding alarms, the PC-BIPAP and PC-CMV ventilation modes give patients the complete freedom to inhale or exhale at any time.

The chronological sequence of inspiration and expiration is as follows: At the beginning of inspiration, the ventilator closes the expiratory valve and delivers an initial flow, which causes a rise in pressure in the breathing system. Although the user-defined inspiratory pressure Pinsp is built up very rapidly in the breathing system, the time required until the prevalent pressure in the breathing system can be built up in the lungs is much longer because of the resistance of the tube and the expansion of the lungs. The continuously decreasing pressure difference between the pressure in the breathing system and the pressure in the lungs in this phase is reflected in a decelerating gas flow delivery. The ventilator stops the gas flow delivery after achieving a total pressure balance. The expiratory valve opens when the inspiratory time has elapsed. Therefore, the pressure in the breathing system falls to the PEEP pressure level generated by the expiratory valve. The expired gas leaves the lungs and is transported via the expiratory branch of the ventilator to the atmosphere. The next inspiration follows after the expiratory phase, whose length is determined by the respiratory rate setting, has elapsed. The ramp controller can adjust the time when the ventilator changes the pressure from PEEP pressure to the inspiratory pressure level.

In pressure-controlled ventilation, the trigger function can also be activated to synchronize the rise of pressure with the patient's spontaneous breathing efforts. The PC-CMV mode then changes to pressure control-assist control (PC-AC). The result is that the ventilator responds to every inspiration effort by the patient with a mandatory inspiration phase. The PC-AC mode is called BIPAP Assist on some ventilators but behaves as described above.

### Supported Spontaneous Breathing

In principle, the modes belonging to this group have several similarities, including, for example, that the spontaneously breathing patient triggers the start of inspiration and that the ventilator responds by producing a positive pressure in the breathing system. For this reason, spontaneous breathing supported by pressure is often referred to as pressure-supported spontaneous breathing. Internationally, the abbreviations for pressure support (PS) and assisted spontaneous breathing (ASB) differ, but generally, users are familiar with both names. The switchover from inspiration to expiration occurs when mode-specific criteria, such as flow or volume target values, are met. Spontaneous breathing suits patients with weakened respiratory muscles and an intact respiratory drive [248].

#### Conventional Pressure Support

The chronological sequence of inspiration and expiration is as follows: As soon as an inhalation effort triggers the ventilator, the ventilator delivers a gas flow and generates the inspiratory pressure defined by the adjuster. The ramp controller can influence the speed at which the ventilator achieves the set pressure support level. A rapid rise in time results in a high initial flow and reduces the patient's breathing effort. The switchover to expiration occurs when the pressure support level has been reached and after the inspiratory gas flow has decreased to a defined inspiratory flow. Although in this method, the patient is always provided with the same pressure support irrespective of the intensity of his breathing efforts, spontaneous breathing volumes can vary depending on patient activity.

#### Proportional Pressure Support

The proportional pressure support (PPS) and proportional assist ventilation (PAV) modes are further developments of the pressure support mode described in the last section. While in conventional pressure support, the ventilator provides the support pressure itself when the patient no longer actively breathes, in PPS (PAV) mode, the ventilator supports the patient in proportion to the work of breathing performed by the patient. This also results in the markedly high variability of tidal volumes, which follow the natural course of spontaneous breathing. The main idea and objective of proportional pressure support is that the ventilator should only take over that part of the breathing work that the patient cannot perform himself. Since the work of breathing is determined by the airway resistance and the elastic recoil force of the lungs, PPS can be individually adjusted to the patient's respective disease using two different adjustment parameters [249]. This differentiation is necessary because a patient with increased airway resistance has to cope with a fundamentally different problem than a patient with pathologically changed elasticity.

In the first case, the gas flow is impaired, whereas in the second case, the volume of spontaneous breathing is insufficient. A different pressure curve profile is therefore allocated to the controllers. When the resistive work of breathing increases, support is provided using a flow-proportional pressure characteristic. If, on the other hand, the disease is characterized by a marked elastic work of breathing, the pressure curve is proportional to the tidal volume. The pressure support, which is effective for the patient, results from the overlap of the two curve functions. Support that has been calculated too generously can result in the patient receiving a greater volume than intended because of the reinforcing characteristics of the system. For this reason, the pressure and tidal volume alarm limits are significant here.

#### Variable Pressure Support

Observing one's own breathing activities reveals that breathing volumes are not constant but vary within a certain range. Variable pressure support is available in the spontaneous breathing mode SPN-CPAP, which tries to mimic the physiologic course of respiration. For this purpose, the level of pressure support changes from breath to breath. Variations in pressure result from the settings and the Press. Preliminary findings indicate that this mode might have beneficial effects on oxygenation.

Volume Support

This method also varies the level of pressure support. However, the main objective and circumstances differ from the modes described above. Activating volume support ensures that the patient receives the user-preselected tidal volume. The tidal volume will be delivered even if the lung compliance changes or spontaneous efforts decrease [250].

### Spontaneous Breathing (Without Respiratory Support)

The patient receives neither pressure support nor mandatory ventilation strokes in these modes. The modes allocated to this group are not ventilation but spontaneous breathing modes (SB). Spontaneous-continuous positive airway pressure facilitates spontaneous breathing at a specific pressure level, which the user can set by adjusting the PEEP controller. If the patient inhales, causing the pressure in the breathing system to fall slightly, additional gas is immediately delivered to ensure the pressure level remains constant. This method requires that the patient's spontaneous breathing and breathing drive are sufficiently stable, and the patient can be responsible for the respiratory rate and the tidal volume. The task of the ventilator is limited to providing the required breathing gas, creating the PEEP pressure, and monitoring the patient's physical condition, which requires the breathing activities to be closely monitored. This also means it is possible [251]:

- To prevent the collapse of individual alveolar areas
- To increase the gas exchange surface of the lungs by a positive airway pressure and
- To provide the patient with an increased oxygen concentration.
- To increase efficiency, CPAP can be combined with a support method. This turns a purely spontaneous breathing mode into a supported spontaneous breathing mode.

### Mixed Ventilation

As already described, different ventilation modes allow adaptation of ventilators to meet individual patient requirements. In a figurative sense, the different ventilation modes also represent the patient's transition from controlled ventilation to spontaneous breathing. Reducing respiratory or ventilatory support should be started as early as possible to allow the patient to breathe independently. Not only is this in the patient's interest, it is also important from an economic point of view. The ventilation modes belonging to mixed ventilation combine elements from controlled ventilation and support spontaneous breathing. The mandatory phases take place in either pressure- or volume-controlled form, as already known from controlled ventilation, and ensure a certain minimum ventilation. The user will determine the weaning strategy based on the type of controlled ventilation and gradually reduce the breathing work performed by the ventilator [252]. In practice, this reduction is achieved by reducing the mandatory frequency or by reducing the inspiratory pressure. The ventilation modes in this category are especially suitable for patients whose breathing drive is unstable and whose respiratory muscles are weak. These modes also require that the user pay close attention to the fact that the ventilator settings correspond to the physical working capacity of the patient.

#### Volume-Controlled Mixed Ventilation

The volume control-synchronized intermittent mandatory ventilation, with or without pressure support mode, ensures a defined, constant, mandatory, volume-controlled ventilation irrespective of any spontaneous breathing activities by the patient. VC-SIMV can therefore replace the VC-CMV mode and is already being used in the controlled ventilation phase. In VC-SIMV mode, the ventilator ensures that mandatory ventilation is as comfortable as possible for the patient. For this reason, in VC-SIMV mode, the ventilator can vary the time between the mandatory ventilation strokes while maintaining the number of ventilation strokes per minute. As with VC-CMV, the mandatory minute volume results from the respiratory rate and the set tidal volume [253]. The patient is supplied with additional breathing gas at the start of spontaneous breathing, so the total minute volume consists of mandatory and spontaneous minute volumes.

The chronological sequence of mandatory and supported phases is as follows: In VC-SIMV mode, a trigger window is present before the mandatory ventilation stroke. If the patient inhales during this phase, the ventilator will start the ventilation stroke, which was about due anyway. The time difference between the regular default cycle time and the actual cycle time is added to the next spontaneous breathing phase, not to exceed the user-defined number of ventilation strokes per minute. The ventilator supports spontaneous breathing with pressure support from the end of a mandatory phase until the trigger window is activated again. This produces alternating mandatory phases in which the ventilator delivers a set ventilation pattern and supported phases in which the patient is allowed maximum freedom [254]. Although, in principle, there is nothing wrong with this method, unfortunately, overlaps frequently occur between mandatory and spontaneous activities in clinical practice. This results in unpleasant dyssynchronous alarms and increased alarms for the medical staff because the ventilator does not respond to the patient's requirements in the mandatory phase. Therefore, this type of situation is equally undesirable for the patient and medical staff and should thus be avoided by all means, also in view of the weaning duration. In this context, ventilation modes or additional functions, which also tolerate spontaneous breathing during the mandatory phase, can provide a remedy.

If the patient is not breathing spontaneously, the volume control-mandatory minute volume ventilation mode behaves in the same way as a volume-controlled ventilation mode and, under these conditions, is not different from the previously described VC-SIMV mode. The only crucial difference between the two modes is that the mandatory ventilation part in VC-MMV can vary depending on the spontaneous breathing activities. Controlled ventilation stroke is not applied if the patient breathes a large volume independently. Thus, VCMMV provides the patient unlimited freedom from pure controlled ventilation to total spontaneous breathing [255]. For example, the mode has proven itself during postoperative ventilation, but it is not a substitute for individual breathing training. As in other volume-controlled ventilation modes, overlapping unpleasant spontaneous and mandatory phases can occur during VC-MMV. The implementation of an additional function, if available, may improve tolerance of these interferences, like in VC-SIMV.

The chronological sequence of mandatory and supported phases is as follows: The mandatory minute volume is determined by setting the respiratory rate and tidal volume controller. Controlled ventilation takes place according to the known pattern. At the start of spontaneous breathing, the ventilator continuously calculates and forecasts the volume the patient will reach in a minute. If the calculation is positive, the ventilator automatically stops mandatory ventilation.

If the calculation is negative, the ventilator delivers a corresponding number of synchronized mandatory strokes to reach the user-defined minute volume. In apnea, ventilation occurs according to the predefined adjustment parameters. Pressure support can be used to support spontaneous breathing. Furthermore, adequate adjustment of the spontaneous breathing rate alarm limit RRspon is significant in VC-MMV to detect abnormally fast respiration.

#### Pressure-Controlled Mixed Ventilation

PC-BIPAP is equally suitable for patients with pulmonary function disorders and those with healthy lungs. The PC-BIPAP ventilation mode is a time-cycled, pressure-controlled form of ventilation that allows the patient to inhale or exhale at any time. Therefore, PC-BIPAP is often compared to the time-controlled switchover between two SPN-CPAP levels. The mandatory and spontaneous activities do not alternate chronologically as in VC-SIMV, but take place simultaneously. This device behavior, also called a free breathing system, significantly improves patient comfort and facilitates the smooth transition from controlled ventilation to complete spontaneous breathing. The technical basis of the mode is the dynamic interplay of the inspiratory gas metering device and an active expiratory valve. In the case of a pressure loss, the gas delivery unit supplies the additional required gas flow. On the other hand, a sudden pressure rise is compensated by the limited controlled opening of the expiratory valve [256]. This special pressure-controlled ventilation offers different benefits to both the patient and the user.

- The ventilator always responds to the patient's requirements, eliminating the struggle against closed valves, ensuring patient ventilation is less stressful.
- The harmonized interaction between the device and the patient enables shallower sedation, which might reduce costs and increase the patient's breathing drive.

- An awake and responsive patient can be activated and motivated, positively influencing the healing process.
- Communication with the patient optimizes pain medication or ventilator settings.
- The patient's spontaneous breathing allows the reduction of mandatory ventilation and improves the pulmonary gas distribution and the gas exchange.
- Spontaneous breathing decreases intrathoracic pressure forces, relieves the heart, and positively affects the venous return flow to the heart.
- The patient contributing to the work of breathing as early as possible can reduce the ventilation period and thus the risk of infection.
- The free breathing system reduces the number of alarms triggered by dyssynchronization, making ventilation less stressful not only for the patient but also for medical staff.

These benefits are also available to users in volume-controlled ventilation when using the AutoFlow function.

The chronological sequence of mandatory and supported phases in PC-BIPAP is as follows: As with VC-SIMV, a trigger window is present before the mandatory ventilation stroke. If the patient inhales during this phase, the ventilator will already deliver the pressure change, which was about due anyway. The time difference between the regular default and actual cycle times is added to the next spontaneous breathing phase. This offset ensures that the user-defined respiratory rate remains constant. The ventilator supports spontaneous breathing with pressure support from the end of a mandatory phase unit, and the trigger window is activated again.

The pressure rise time defined by the user with the ramp setting influences both the supported and mandatory pressure rise. Thus, the patient always receives the breathing gas with a uniform flow characteristic, whose decelerating course is generally perceived to be significantly more pleasant than a constant flow. As a further feature, PC-BIPAP has an additional trigger window to synchronize the pressure change from inspiratory pressure to the PEEP level with spontaneous breathing. This may mean that the length of the inspiratory period can also vary to a certain extent. Like for the ventilation frequency, the intervals are also corrected and compensated accordingly by the inspiratory period adjustment in the following mandatory ventilation phase [257].

#### Pressure Control-Synchronized Intermittent Mandatory Ventilation

This ventilation mode behaves like the volume-controlled pressure control-synchronized intermittent mandatory ventilation (VC-SIMV) variant regarding the chronological switchover between mandatory and spontaneous ventilation phases. The only difference from volume-controlled VC-SIMV is that the mandatory ventilation strokes are pressure-controlled in this case. The free breathing system described under PC-BIPAP is not obligatory here or has limited availability depending on the manufacturer.

Pressure Control-Airway Pressure Release Ventilation (PC-APRV)

Although the main characteristics of PC-APRV are very similar to the PC-BIPAP ventilation mode, this mode is based on an entirely different ventilation philosophy. In contrast to all the other modes in which the mandatory inspiration produces a pulmonary pressure rise, the volume change in PC-APRV occurs by a brief pressure relief. This release phase enables an extremely short and incomplete expiration. To better understand this situation, it may be helpful to imagine a patient who breathes spontaneously at an increased pressure level. If spontaneous breathing subsequently deteriorates, increasing arterial carbon dioxide, it will be necessary to increase ventilation. Until recently, the pressure in the breathing system increased, thus the volume transported to the lungs. PC-APRV, on the other hand, utilizes the fact that the positive pressure already fills the patient's lungs and causes a brief expiration by reducing the pressure in the breathing system. The pressure relief phase in PC-APRV is extremely brief, typically 0.5 s. Since this time does not allow for a complete expiration in adult ventilation, only the lung compartments that can be quickly emptied and filled are ventilated in the release phase. The regions where the gas only reaches slowly due to increased airway resistance are hardly influenced by the brief pressure change [258]. However, often it is precisely these lung regions that can only be ventilated with difficulty using conventional ventilation and/or are susceptible to collapse. By stabilizing the pressure conditions in these critical parts of the lungs, PC-APRV can usually provide gentler ventilation and improved gas exchange. The PC-APRV adjustment parameters differ slightly from the usual designations and parameters due to the specific features of the ventilation mode. In PC-APRV, for example, the expiratory time Tlow can be set instead of the respiratory rate. This makes it easier for users to set the brief release phases. Accordingly, the inspiratory time is referred to as Thigh and the inspiratory pressure as phigh.

PC-APRV does not provide pressure support as it would conflict with the ventilation mode's philosophy. Otherwise, PC-APRV has the same spontaneous breathing characteristics as PC-BIPAP, i.e., the patient can inhale or exhale at any time. PC-APRV has been used successfully in treating patients with severe gas exchange disorders and is gaining importance, at least in this application. PC-APRV can, in principle, be used for patients with healthy lungs, but it is seldom observed due to the described deviations from physiological respiratory patterns.

### Noninvasive Ventilation

Noninvasive respiratory therapy is gaining in importance as a means of avoiding intubation or as a supporting respiration therapy after extubation, not to mention the tremendous drive to cut costs in the health-care sector. However, mask ventilation presents the user, patient, and ventilator with special challenges. These include, for example, the availability and acceptance of suitable face masks and the communication and cooperation between the user and the patient. There are also special technical challenges concerning the performance of the ventilator, since leaks and disconnections occur frequently during mask ventilation. Noninvasive ventilation is optional and should be available as an adjunct to all standard ventilation modes. Due to the wide range of manufacturer-specific features, only a few fundamental aspects of mask ventilation are considered here. The quality of mask ventilation is determined by whether the ventilation is prone to self-trigger due to leaks at the breathing mask. Depending on the ventilator, the user either automatically or manually adapts the trigger sensitivity [259]. In this context, it must be mentioned that not all ventilators provide volume-controlled ventilation in NIV. However, even if this feature is available, applied volumes might vary significantly based on device performance. In any case, high-performance leak compensation is essential in such applications. Leak compensation continuously compares the set tidal volume with the expiratory measured volume and increases the inspiratory gas delivery in the event of leaks. Last, monitoring and alarm limits must meet special demands during noninvasive ventilation. For example, if the position of the mask needs to be corrected, which involves temporarily removing and refitting the mask, it would usually result in a near-immediate disconnect alarm under normal conditions. Such an alarm can be avoided by an adjustable alarm delay time, usually only available in the NIV operating mode.

**Apnea Ventilation**

The ventilator and patient are responsible for the total minute volume during the weaning process. If apnea occurs in this phase because the patient cannot cope, the remaining mandatory volume applied may not be able to ensure sufficient ventilation anymore. For this reason, to avoid hypoventilation, the apnea alarm can be combined with the apnea ventilation in modes that allow or support spontaneous breathing. In this case, the ventilator ensures the defined controlled ventilation of the patient until the user can attend to the current patient situation [260]. In adult ventilation, apnea ventilation is generally implemented as volume-controlled ventilation, whereas pressure-controlled ventilation in neonatology.

## *2.7.4 Clinical Applications*

Mechanical ventilation is a cornerstone in treating acute and chronic respiratory failure. Its use in clinical practice spans a wide range of critical illnesses, including Acute Respiratory Distress Syndrome (ARDS), exacerbations of Chronic Obstructive Pulmonary Disease (COPD), and trauma-related respiratory compromise. Ventilation is initiated specifically to support gas exchange and reduce the work of breathing in patients who cannot maintain adequate ventilation by themselves [261]. Effective mechanical ventilation improves oxygenation, prevents respiratory muscle fatigue, and reduces the risk of death if applied appropriately.

Mechanical ventilation is also key in the management of difficult weaning and in preventing ventilator-induced lung injuries. Ventilator setting individualization based on patient-specific pathophysiological data has been emphasized to limit complications like barotrauma, volutrauma, and ventilator-induced diaphragm dysfunction [262, 263]. Furthermore, innovations in ventilation modes, such as pressure support and synchronized intermittent mandatory ventilation, are intended to promote greater synchrony between machine and patient to allow better patient comfort and recovery outcomes. Beyond the critical care units, mechanical ventilators are increasingly being utilized in long-term and home care, particularly for patients with neuromuscular diseases and chronic hypoventilation syndromes. The evolution of non-invasive ventilation has enabled early treatment of respiratory failure and, in many cases, the avoidance of intubation, most notably in COPD patients [233]. With advancing healthcare, integrating mechanical ventilation into varied care settings ensures enhanced quality of life and extended survival for those with complex respiratory needs.

Intubated patients have to perform considerably more work to breathe due to the artificial narrowing of their airways. This additional work of breathing results from the pressure difference arising along the tube, which the respiratory muscles must also counteract. The tube type (endotracheal tube or tracheal cannula), the tube diameter, and the gas flow delivered through the tube are major determining factors. To better understand the gas flow's importance and effect, try to breathe for several minutes through a straw while holding your nose closed. You will notice that considerably greater breathing efforts are required to create larger gas flows. Consequently, this means that the patient should be informed about the flow. Based on this idea, automatic tube compensation increases the pressure in the breathing system during inspiration by the pressure drop induced by the flow between the tube connector and tube tip. During expiration, compensation occurs by a brief reduction of the PEEP level. This gives the patient the impression that he is not intubated. However, the dynamic pressure changes in the breathing system lead to significant changes in the pressure-time curve. These curve progressions, which are initially unusual for the user, merely reflect the variations in pressure before the tube and do not thus correspond with the pulmonary pressure curve. More detailed information on the pressure at the tube tip can be provided by devices that calculate this pressure and display it as a separate pressure curve.

Tube compensation is available in all ventilation modes. It can be adjusted to the current ventilation situation by entering the tube type, diameter, and the desired compensation as a percentage. Since ATC greatly simplifies the patient's work of breathing, the user significantly reduces the pressure support, or even switches it off temporarily, before activating the ATC function. Tube compensation is, in principle, suitable for all intubated patients, but can be configured to be limited to the inspiratory phase, for example, for patients with obstructive respiratory diseases [264].

### 2.7.5 Regulatory Considerations

Although the ventilator automatically monitors many device functions, the user must manually set alarm limits for other measured values. The importance of patient monitoring has already been shown using the example of apnea ventilation [265, 266]. Despite this, many users often view alarms as an unpleasant side-effect of ventilation. A more positive picture emerges when you compare the adequate adjustment of the alarm limits to a protective fence surrounding the patient. As long as patient activities remain within the limits of the fenced-off area, there is no cause for worry or reason for alarm. However, when the patient tries to leave the protective zone created for him, the device will report this breakout attempt by generating a corresponding alarm. Inevitably, this raises the issue of the importance of the different alarm limits and how they should be set. The following can be stated [267, 268]:

- There are no unimportant alarm limits. It must be noted that the patient's situation may change at any time. Therefore, the alarm limits that do not currently appear relevant should also be adjusted according to the patient's needs.
- Alarm limits should always be set based on the current respective measured values to allow as much freedom as possible while prioritizing safety.
- All alarm limits must always be checked and adjusted to meet the patient's current needs whenever a ventilation mode is set or changed. These steps can avoid predictable alarms and unnecessary stress.
- There are no useless alarms. Each alarm is generated by a change in the patient's condition, a user's misjudgment, or a technical fault requiring the user's immediate attention.

The task of monitoring and alarm systems changes as the work of breathing is transferred to the patient during the weaning process. During controlled ventilation, the monitoring and alarm system is mainly used to monitor the device's functioning and effect on the patient. However, it also assumes responsibility for monitoring respiratory sufficiency in the weaning phase. The physiological fluctuations of the respiratory rate and the tidal volume require that the alarm limits, based on the current measured value, are set much more tightly in controlled ventilation than during mixed ventilation or (supported) spontaneous breathing [269].

Over the last 3 years, the regulatory focus on ventilators has strengthened, particularly for post-market surveillance (PMS). The European Medical Device Regulation (MDR) also requires more stringent, third-party conformity tests to ensure safety, reliability, and performance throughout a device's life cycle. Therefore, a new conformity assessment process was brought into play to close major regulatory loopholes in mechanical ventilator testing. This method strictly examines safety, visual integrity, gas volume, flow, and pressure delivery to ensure compliance with fundamental metrological and patient safety standards [79].

The technique validation in different healthcare institutions between 2018 and 2021 revealed significant improvements in device performance and risk reduction. By emphasizing traceability and measurement equivalence, such a disciplined approach fulfills MDR criteria for high-end PMS protocols and enables healthcare centers to identify potential divergences in the early stage [79]. Remote testing software and quality testing are even more important, especially where the ventilator function should be validated under varied clinical loads [270].

### 2.7.6 Future Perspectives

The new testing model is not just regulation-compliant but also paves the way for integration with emerging digital technologies. This encompasses potential applications of artificial intelligence (AI) to offer automated conformity checks, detect anomalies, and predict equipment failure before it affects patient treatment [79]. Such capabilities are growing in interest in bright ICU spaces, where ventilator data can be entered into central systems for real-time monitoring and risk alert.

The trend towards AI-assisted ventilator control is also gaining scholarly steam. For instance, one 2024 article proposed pairing deep Q-learning models with ventilator control to enhance decision-making during uncertainty, one aspect of a broader trend toward intelligent, adaptive respiratory support systems [271]. Ultimately, the trend is not simply compliance with existing regulations but an affirmative movement towards building solid, data-sourced ventilator infrastructure that supports next-generation healthcare standards.

## 2.8 Anesthesia Machines

Anesthesia is an essential component of modern healthcare, enabling patients to undergo surgeries and procedures without experiencing pain, anxiety, or distress [272]. The practice of anesthesia has evolved significantly since its inception in the nineteenth century. Today, it is a highly specialized field that integrates pharmacology, physiology, and technology to provide safe and effective care for patients undergoing medical interventions [273].

The role of anesthesia machines in this field cannot be overstated. These machines are integral to administering anesthesia agents safely and maintaining patient safety throughout a procedure. They deliver a controlled mixture of gases, manage patient ventilation, and continuously monitor vital signs during surgery [274].

Anesthesia machines are designed to ensure that patients receive a controlled and consistent supply of gases during surgery [275]. They are equipped with several components that regulate the flow of anesthetic gases, oxygen, and nitrous oxide, while also providing mechanical ventilation to support or fully control breathing when necessary.

These machines have sophisticated monitoring systems that measure vital signs such as oxygen, carbon dioxide, heart rate, and blood pressure. This constant monitoring helps anesthesiologists ensure that the patient remains stable throughout the procedure and that any deviations from the desired parameters are addressed immediately [272].

In addition to providing gas delivery and ventilation support, anesthesia machines reduce the risk of complications arising from improper gas mixtures, mechanical failure, or human error. By maintaining accurate control over the administration of anesthesia, these machines are critical in preventing adverse outcomes, such as hypoxia, hypercarbia, or anesthesia awareness.

### 2.8.1 History

The first recorded use of anesthesia was in the 1840s, when ether and nitrous oxide were discovered as anesthetic agents. Early anesthesia techniques were rudimentary, relying on manual delivery of gases and simple equipment to administer ether or nitrous oxide.

As surgical procedures became more complex and the need for greater precision in anesthesia delivery grew, technological advancements developed more sophisticated anesthesia machines. In the early twentieth century, devices that could automatically regulate the flow of gases and deliver controlled doses of anesthetic agents were introduced. Over the decades, further advancements in automation, safety features, and monitoring capabilities have shaped the modern anesthesia machines used in operating rooms today (Fig. 2.35).

### 2.8.2 Technical Characteristics

Anesthesia machines are complex systems designed to deliver a controlled mixture of gases, including oxygen and anesthetic agents, to the patient during surgical procedures. Understanding their working principles is crucial for ensuring safe and effective operation [48]. The process involves several key components that work

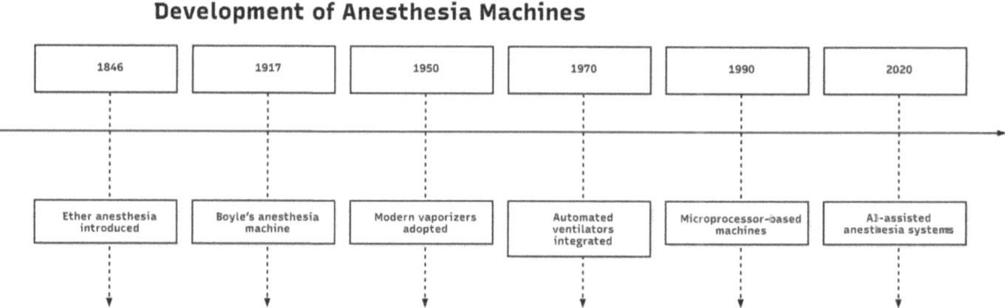


**Fig. 2.35** Timeline showing key milestones in the development of anesthesia machines

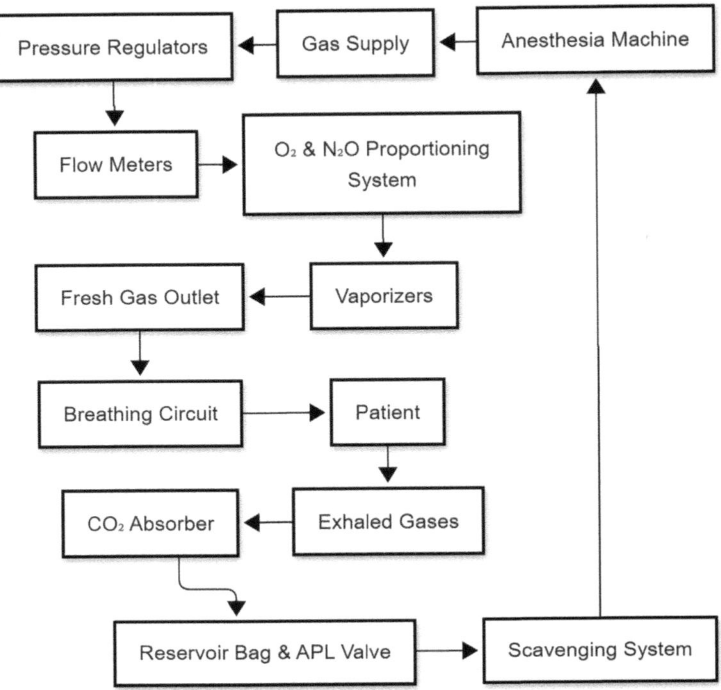


**Fig. 2.36** Block diagram of anesthesia machine

together to ensure the patient receives the appropriate gases, with precise control over flow rates, ventilation, and oxygenation (Fig. 2.36).

The gas flow system in an anesthesia machine is responsible for delivering a mixture of gases to the patient. This system includes components such as flowmeters, pressure regulators, and control valves, which allow the anesthesiologist to adjust the flow of gases. Flowmeters display the flow rate of each gas, such as oxygen or nitrous oxide, and control valves adjust the flow based on the clinical needs. These adjustments are crucial in ensuring that the proper gas mixture is delivered to the patient in the correct proportions [276].

In many anesthesia machines, the oxygen flow rate can be adjusted independently of other gases, which allows the clinician to tailor the oxygen concentration according to the patient's needs. This flexibility is significant during complex surgical procedures, where oxygen levels must be carefully regulated to avoid complications.

The breathing circuit is vital in delivering the anesthetic gases to the patient's lungs. In many cases, the system uses positive pressure ventilation to assist the patient in breathing during anesthesia. Positive pressure is applied to force air into the lungs, especially when the patient is under general anesthesia and cannot breathe independently [277]. The ventilation system includes a ventilator that can be set to deliver a specific volume of gas with each breath or a set pressure, depending on the mode selected by the anesthesiologist. The volume and rate of ventilation are tailored to the patient's specific requirements and adjusted based on the clinical scenario [278, 279].

The carbon dioxide removal system is an essential feature of the breathing circuit, which ensures the patient does not re-breathe carbon dioxide. As the patient exhales, carbon dioxide accumulates in the gas mixture, so it must be removed to prevent respiratory acidosis. A carbon dioxide absorber captures the exhaled $CO_2$, ensuring the gas delivered during the next breath is free from excess carbon dioxide. This allows for continuous, safe ventilation [280].

The vaporization system is vital in delivering anesthetic agents in their gaseous form. These agents, which include halothane, sevoflurane, or desflurane, are initially in liquid form, and the vaporizer heats the liquid anesthetic to produce a gas [281]. The anesthesiologist adjusts the vaporizer to control the concentration of the anesthetic agent in the gas mixture, with typical concentrations ranging from 1% to 4%. The vaporizer is calibrated to specific anesthetic agents, preventing mix-ups and ensuring that only the intended agent is used during surgery.

## Hardware

Anesthesia machines have several key components, each designed to fulfill a specific function in administering and monitoring anesthesia. The proper functioning of these components largely determines the anesthesia machine's effectiveness and safety.

The gas supply and delivery system forms the core function of an anesthesia machine. This system ensures the continuous and controlled supply of medical gases, such as oxygen ($O_2$), nitrous oxide ($N_2O$), and sometimes air, to the patient [282].

- Oxygen and Nitrous Oxide Supply [274]
  The primary gases used in anesthesia are oxygen, nitrous oxide, and occasionally air. Oxygen is crucial for maintaining the patient's respiratory needs, while nitrous oxide is a potent anesthetic agent used with other volatile anesthetics. These gases are delivered from either a gas cylinder (for portable or backup systems) or the hospital's pipeline system. Oxygen is typically supplied at higher pressures, requiring a regulator to reduce the pressure to a safe level for delivery to the patient.
- Pressure Regulators [273]
  Pressure regulators control the gas pressure from the cylinders or pipeline, reducing it to a safe, usable level for the anesthesia machine. The regulators ensure that gases are delivered to the machine at a stable pressure (usually around 50 psi) to maintain consistent flow.

- Pipeline and Cylinder Systems [275]
  Anesthesia machines can be supplied with gases from either pipeline systems installed in the hospital or from portable cylinders. Pipeline systems are connected directly to the machine and supply gases through specialized hoses. Cylinder systems are backup sources typically used when the pipeline supply fails. Cylinders are stored in specific areas; each gas type has a dedicated cylinder (e.g., oxygen cylinders, nitrous oxide cylinders) (Fig. 2.37).

## Vaporizers

The vaporizer is another critical component of the anesthesia machine. Its purpose is to convert liquid anesthetic agents, such as sevoflurane or isoflurane, into a vaporized form that the patient can safely inhale [272]. Vaporizers are designed to precisely control the temperature and gas flow to deliver the correct anesthetic agent concentration to the patient. The anesthesiologist can adjust the vaporizer settings to achieve a specific anesthetic concentration, typically expressed as a percentage of the total gas mixture. Vaporizers are also equipped with safety features to prevent overdosing or underdosing of anesthetic agents, and some machines include

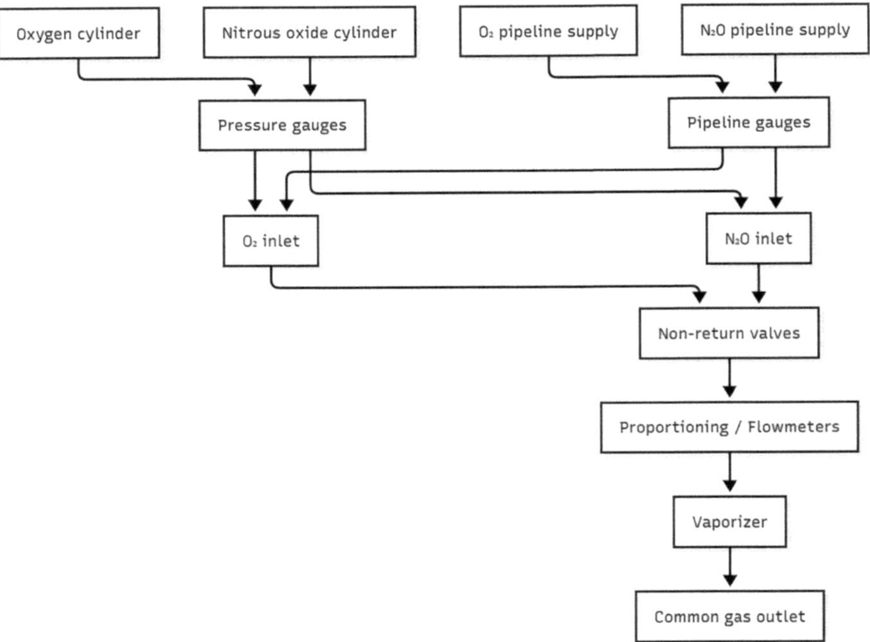


**Fig. 2.37** Diagram showing the gas supply system of an anesthesia machine

automatic compensation mechanisms to adjust for temperature or gas flow changes, ensuring a consistent output. Types of vaporizers [282]:

- Out-of-Circuit Vaporizers: These vaporizers are located outside the breathing circuit, and their output is mixed with the other gases before delivery to the patient. They are more common in modern anesthesia machines.
- In-Circuit Vaporizers: These vaporizers are built directly into the breathing circuit. They are less common but can be found in older machines or specialized devices.

Vaporizers need to be calibrated regularly to ensure their accuracy. Calibration involves verifying that the correct anesthetic gas concentration is delivered, usually through a gas analyzer. Regular maintenance is essential to avoid malfunction, such as leaks or incorrect concentration delivery (Fig. 2.38).

The breathing circuit connects the anesthesia machine to the patient's airway. It is designed to deliver the gas mixture to the patient and remove exhaled gases [274]. The breathing circuit typically includes a flowmeter, a Y-piece, hoses, and airway attachments such as endotracheal tubes or face masks. The system is designed to facilitate the flow of oxygen and anesthetic gases to the patient while also allowing for the removal of exhaled carbon dioxide. Components of the breathing circuit may also include a humidifier to moisten inspired gases, mainly when mechanical ventilation is used. Types of Circuits [275]:

- Mapleson Circuits: These are simpler, non-rebreathing circuits often used in anesthesia for patients with short, uncomplicated procedures.
- Circle System: This is a more complex, closed-circuit system that allows the patient to rebreathe some of their exhaled gases, with the carbon dioxide being removed by a carbon dioxide absorber. It is the most commonly used system in modern anesthesia machines for lengthy procedures.

Anesthesia machines have advanced monitoring systems that track patients' vital signs during surgery. These systems allow the clinician to observe real-time oxygen saturation, carbon dioxide levels, and other critical parameters. Pulse oximeters measure oxygen saturation, providing immediate feedback on the patient's oxygenation status, while capnographs measure exhaled carbon dioxide levels, helping to assess ventilation. Alarms are integrated into these systems to alert the anesthesiologist if any parameter falls outside acceptable limits, ensuring patient safety is always prioritized [282].

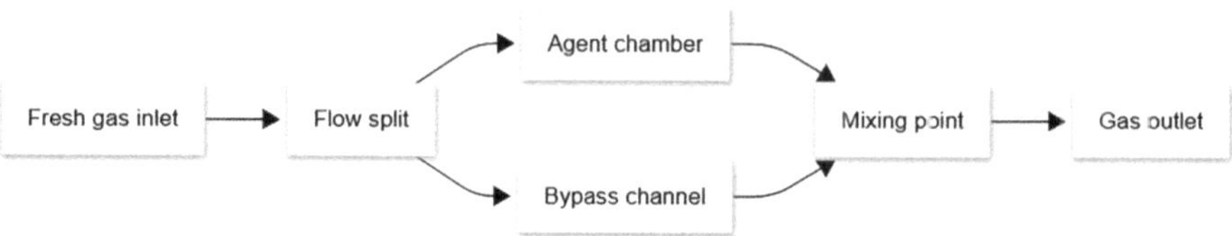


**Fig. 2.38** Schematic of an out-of-circuit vaporizer

- Key Monitoring Parameters:Oxygen Saturation ($SpO_2$): Monitored continuously to ensure the patient maintains adequate oxygen levels.
- End-tidal $CO_2$ ($EtCO_2$): This measure of the carbon dioxide level in the exhaled breath provides insights into the patient's ventilation status.
- Heart Rate and Blood Pressure: Vital for detecting changes in cardiovascular function.
- Temperature: Monitoring body temperature to prevent hypothermia or hyperthermia during surgery.

The monitoring system is integrated into the anesthesia machine's control panel, providing real-time feedback to the anesthesiologist. Advanced systems can alert the anesthesiologist of potential issues (e.g., low oxygen levels or abnormal heart rate) through alarms.

**Software**

Software components are a standard feature of modern anesthesia machines, providing precise control of gas flow, real-time monitoring, and automated safety. These software components communicate with sensors and actuators to regulate gas composition, monitor patient physiological parameters, and sound alarms for abnormalities such as low oxygen or disconnection of the circuit. As anesthesia machines evolved into complex workstations, the software is now an essential part not only of control but also of data and diagnostic integration [277].

The most recent software development has been about user-friendly user interfaces and the integration of clinical decision support. For example, machine learning algorithms are increasingly being utilized to automate anesthesia depth, ventilation settings, and alert prioritization [283]. These AI systems alleviate the burden on anesthesiologists and enable predictive analytics to identify potential complications before they escalate into a crisis. With remote updating and in-use performance assessment, software updates are also becoming more modular and efficient. Maintenance and regulatory requirements have vastly improved as a result. Modern anesthesia machines incorporate version control methods that verify software integrity before they can be activated, so it is less probable that system failure will happen due to mismatched or outdated software versions [232, 269].

Moreover, software systems enable the integration of anesthesia machines with hospital information systems (HIS). Anesthesia data can be captured and analyzed seamlessly, critical for post-operative reviews and quality assurance. Real-time data transfer to electronic health records (EHRs) is increasingly common, ensuring continuity of care and facilitating research in anesthesia outcomes [283]. Briefly, the role of software in anesthesia machines has developed from straightforward control towards comprehensive integration with intelligent monitoring, machine learning applications, and hospital IT systems. They are building the future of anesthesia delivery, improving patient safety, and maximizing workflow for clinicians.

### 2.8.3 Types of Devices

The ventilator in an anesthesia machine is a critical component, especially when the patient cannot breathe independently. Mechanical ventilation can be set to deliver a fixed volume of air (volume-controlled ventilation) or to maintain a set pressure within the lungs (pressure-controlled ventilation), depending on the patient's condition [272]. These settings are chosen based on the patient's lung compliance, surgical procedure, and overall health. Mechanical ventilation ensures that the patient receives adequate ventilation, even during lengthy surgeries when manual ventilation may not be sufficient [284].

1. Types of Ventilators Used in Anesthesia:
   - Pneumatic Ventilators: These are driven by compressed gases (usually oxygen or air) and provide ventilation to the patient based on the volume or pressure settings.
   - Electronic Ventilators: These are powered by electricity and offer more sophisticated control over ventilation parameters, such as tidal volume, respiratory rate, and inspiratory pressure.
2. Modes of Ventilation:
   - Volume-Controlled Ventilation (VCV): The machine delivers a preset volume of gas to the patient with each breath.
   - Pressure-Controlled Ventilation (PCV): The machine delivers gas until a preset pressure is reached, which is helpful in patients with compromised lung compliance.
   - Assist-Controlled Ventilation (ACV): This is a combination of both, in which the ventilator provides breaths when the patient is unable to initiate them.

The scavenging system is essential for removing waste anesthetic gases from the operating room to prevent exposure to healthcare workers and the environment. Anesthesia machines have waste gas collection systems that transport exhaled gases away from the patient and exhaust them safely into the atmosphere or a disposal system [274]. Without this system, anesthetic gases would accumulate in the operating room, leading to potential health risks for staff and the patient.

- Types of Scavenging Systems:Active Scavenging System: A vacuum actively draws waste gases away from the operating room.
- Passive Scavenging System: Relies on gravity and the natural flow of gases to carry waste anesthetic gases away.

### 2.8.4 Clinical Applications

Anesthesia machines play a crucial role in clinical practice by ensuring safe and efficient delivery of anesthetic medication and respiratory therapy during surgery and emergency procedures. Their integration into modern surgical procedures enables precise control of the depth of anesthesia, oxygenation, and ventilation, which are essential to minimize intraoperative risks and postoperative complications. Clinical application of such equipment has evolved with the incorporation of newer technologies like bispectral index (BIS) monitoring, which allows anesthesiologists to monitor the hypnotic state of patients and reduce the risk of awareness under anesthesia [285].

Machine learning and closed-loop systems are increasingly incorporated into anesthesia machines to support clinical decision-making, improve patient outcomes, and personalize anesthetic delivery. These technologies use real-time data to automatically adjust anesthetic dosing and ventilation, enhancing the safety and accuracy of care, particularly in high-risk environments like critical care units [286]. These systems also address issues of operations, such as reducing clinicians' workload and minimizing human error, which remains a leading cause of anesthesia-related accidents.

In the COVID-19 pandemic, operating room anesthetizing equipment was versatile and proved its worth beyond the operating room. When intensive care unit (ICU) ventilators were in short supply, anesthesia equipment was called upon to perform mechanical ventilation for critically ill patients. However, the evidence shows that these machines were not substituting in the long term for ICU ventilators, testifying to their usefulness and limitations in extreme situations [287, 288].

Their application in low-resource and austere environments has also grown. For instance, the Universal Anesthesia Machine (UAM) is explicitly designed to operate in environments where electricity and oxygen supply are not guaranteed. It has been successfully utilized in field hospitals and disaster relief camps to deliver safe anesthesia in restrictive conditions. Such adaptability enhances the usability of anesthesia machines globally and helps deliver safe surgical care to underserved regions.

### 2.8.5 Regulatory Considerations

Safety is paramount when using anesthesia machines, and these devices come equipped with various safety mechanisms designed to prevent errors, ensure consistent gas delivery, and protect both patients and clinicians.

One of the most critical safety features is the oxygen fail-safe system, which ensures that the anesthesia machine will not deliver a hypoxic mixture (a mixture with too little oxygen). If the oxygen supply to the machine is interrupted or falls below a certain pressure, the fail-safe mechanism kicks in. Depending on the system's design, it either stops the flow of gases altogether or reduces the flow of anesthetic gases. This ensures that the patient will not be exposed to an inadequate oxygen supply, which could lead to hypoxia [272].

In addition to the oxygen fail-safe, modern anesthesia machines have hypoxic guard systems. These systems prevent the machine from delivering a gas mixture with insufficient oxygen, even when nitrous oxide or other gases are added to the mix. For example, if the oxygen supply falls below a preset level, the system may automatically limit the flow of nitrous oxide to maintain an appropriate oxygen concentration. This is particularly important in ensuring that the patient's oxygen levels are always maintained within safe limits, regardless of the mixture of gases being delivered [48, 72].

The anesthesia machine is also designed with alarm systems that alert the anesthesiologist if any critical parameters deviate from their preset limits. These alarms are essential for ensuring patient safety and preventing dangerous situations. If, for example, the oxygen concentration falls too low or the pressure in the breathing circuit rises unexpectedly, the machine will immediately sound an alarm, prompting the clinician to take corrective action [289]. These alarm systems are integrated with the machine's gas flow and ventilation systems, ensuring that any malfunction or dangerous condition is quickly detected.

Furthermore, anesthesia machines are equipped with features to detect mechanical and electrical failures. If a system component, such as the ventilator or gas delivery system, fails, the machine will alert the clinician. Some machines also have battery backup systems, ensuring critical functions, such as ventilation and monitoring, continue even during a power failure. Additionally, pressure and flow monitoring systems are in place to detect any abnormal conditions in the gas delivery system, such as low oxygen pressure or excessive gas flow, and trigger alarms to ensure that the patient's safety is not compromised [290].

When working together, these safety features create a comprehensive system that minimizes the risk of harm to the patient. The combination of failsafes, alarm systems, and continuous monitoring ensures that anesthesia machines can provide safe and effective care during even the most complex and high-risk procedures [291].

In the context of the EU Medical Device Regulation (MDR), there is an increasing need for uniform conformity assessment procedures for moderate- to high-risk medical devices like anesthesia machines. The traditional post-market surveillance (PMS) procedures lack proper real-world testing tools. This method evaluates both the metrological and technical characteristics, focusing on the precision of measurements, reproducibility of gas delivery, and reliability of safety systems under clinical applications [79].

This method supports regulatory frameworks by offering objective parameters to assess device performance following market introduction. Its inclusion supports hospital MDR and ISO 80601-2-13 conformity by offering reproducible test environments and risk-based evaluations of anesthetic gas delivery systems. The use of PMS with this system further supports early fault detection and reduces user error, vital in the prevention of intraoperative adverse effects due to gas delivery malfunctions [292].

Applying such standardized test protocols makes it easier for regulators to audit compliance and arms healthcare facilities with evidence-based decision support. By providing a consistent assessment outcome, the strategy improves traceability, device certification renewal, and corrective action, which is an essential element of device lifecycle management and regulatory transparency [277].

### 2.8.6 Future Perspectives

The conformity assessment methodology also provides entry for incorporating smart technologies into anesthesia equipment. Its structured data collection lends itself to the easy incorporation of AI-informed solutions that can also predict machine malfunction or gas output deviation. This predictability is commensurate with the global movement toward digital healthcare infrastructure, where real-time monitoring of device condition and advanced scheduling of upkeep are possible [79].

In the future, integrating networked anesthesia workstations with conformity assessment modules may lead to entirely automated quality assurance systems. These systems can report anomalies independently, can be connected to hospital information systems, and can allow real-time regulatory reporting. AI-driven algorithms can further optimize alarm management by canceling false alarms and contextualizing data-driven prioritized alerting, improving clinical workflow and patient safety [277].

Finally, the broad application of this method could influence the design of the next generation of anesthesia devices. By including conformity verification at hardware and software levels, manufacturers can ensure ongoing conformity with safety standards. This maximizes operational efficiency and sets an international standard for regulatory harmonization of medical device monitoring and control [292].

## 2.9 Pacemakers and Defibrillators

Variable impulse generation or conduction can cause arrhythmias, impairing the coordination of the myocardial fibers, which is impaired, suspended, or even plunged into chaos (fibrillation). Ventricular fibrillation is uncoordinated myocardial fibrillation with no ejection from the ventricles, characterized on an electrocardiogram (ECG) by irregular and disorganized depolarizations with high frequency. Pulseless ventricular tachycardia is characterized by a regular and rapid sequence of broad QRS complexes, and, as with ventricular fibrillation, there is no ejection. Both types of rhythm are life-threatening conditions of the cardiovascular system and are thus indications for defibrillation [293]. Defibrillation is understood as meaning a brief, phasic pulse of energy which is intended to bring about simultaneous depolarization of all the myocardial fibers, which means that, after approximately 5 s of administering an electrical pulse, no ventricular fibrillation or ventricular tachycardia can be detected any longer in the ECG. This measure aims to terminate tachycardic ventricular and supraventricular arrhythmias so that, following a refractory period generally lasting between 200 and 500 ms, the sinus nodes once more assume the pacemaker function as the primary excitation center. Defibrillators are electrotherapeutic high-voltage devices used during resuscitation and to terminate tachycardic ventricular and supraventricular arrhythmias [294] (Fig. 2.39).

## 2.9.1 History

The following chronological events are of particular significance in ICD development. The first transthoracic defibrillation with direct current was carried out by Lown in 1962. The first model of an implantable automatic defibrillator (automated implantable cardioverter defibrillator) was presented by Mirowski as early as 1969 and was implanted in a human for the first time in 1980. This system detected ventricular flutter and fibrillation using the heart rate criteria and/or absence of isoelectric ECG portions. Detection of arrhythmias was done using myocardial screw-type electrodes. A programmable ICD system was used in clinical practice 1988, and a multi-programmable ICD system in 1989. The first dual-chamber ICD came onto the market in 1997, while an atrial defibrillator was implanted as early as 1996. ICD electrodes placed intra-arterially are a safe and effective method for terminating atrial fibrillation. The advantages of this are firstly the low energy output and secondly that the patient does not require short anesthesia [295, 296].

A combined atrioventricular defibrillator was first implanted in 1997. More sophisticated atrioventricular defibrillators have the advantage that, besides providing fully automated detection of atrial and ventricular signals, they also deliver electrical pulses to both ventricles in order to terminate arrhythmias that occur. So-called implantable CRT defibrillators for cardiac resynchronization therapy have been available since 2001. These devices deliver a shock to interrupt and therefore stop tachycardia. The right and left ventricles are also stimulated simultaneously to coordinate the cardiac beats (Fig. 2.40).

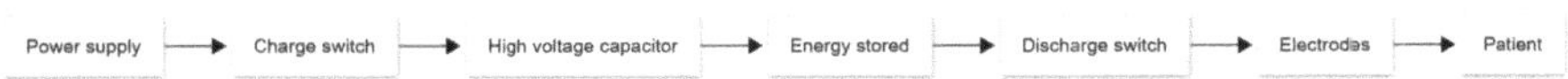


**Fig. 2.39** Diagram of defibrillator charge and discharge

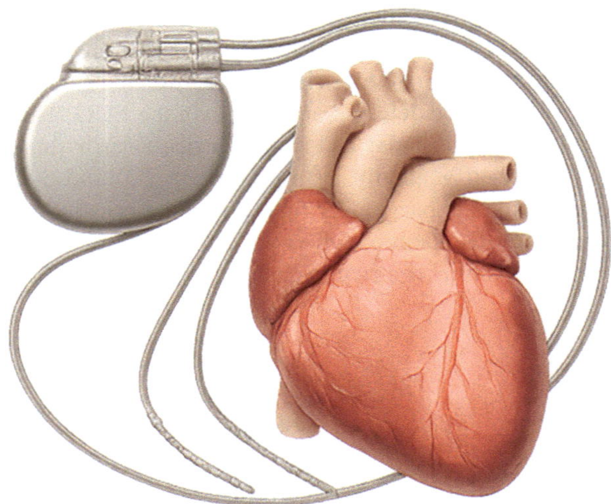

**Fig. 2.40** Implantable biventricular or CRT-ICD system

### *2.9.2 Technical Characteristics*

The portable defibrillator is a direct-current (DC) voltage system that is usually not dependent on mains electricity and that is essentially composed of the following system components [297]:

- The energy supply via mains connection or rechargeable batteries
- A capacitor as an energy store (capacity = n pulses at 360 J)
- A charging circuit for the capacitor (duration of charging, i.e., when the maximum energy is reached, is on average 10–8 s, considerably less in some manufacturers' models), and a discharge circuit which delivers the current pulse at different, preselectable energy levels.

The DC pulse stimulation ranges between 3 and 8 ms at a current of 10–27 A (internally) and 22–60 A (externally). Automatic safety discharge should occur when no shock is triggered, when the defibrillator shock is triggered, when a new energy level is preselected, and in the event of technical malfunction (Fig. 2.41). The energy (E) which can be stored in the capacitor can be determined from the capacity (C) and the available voltage (U) as

$$E = CU2/2(VA = W)$$

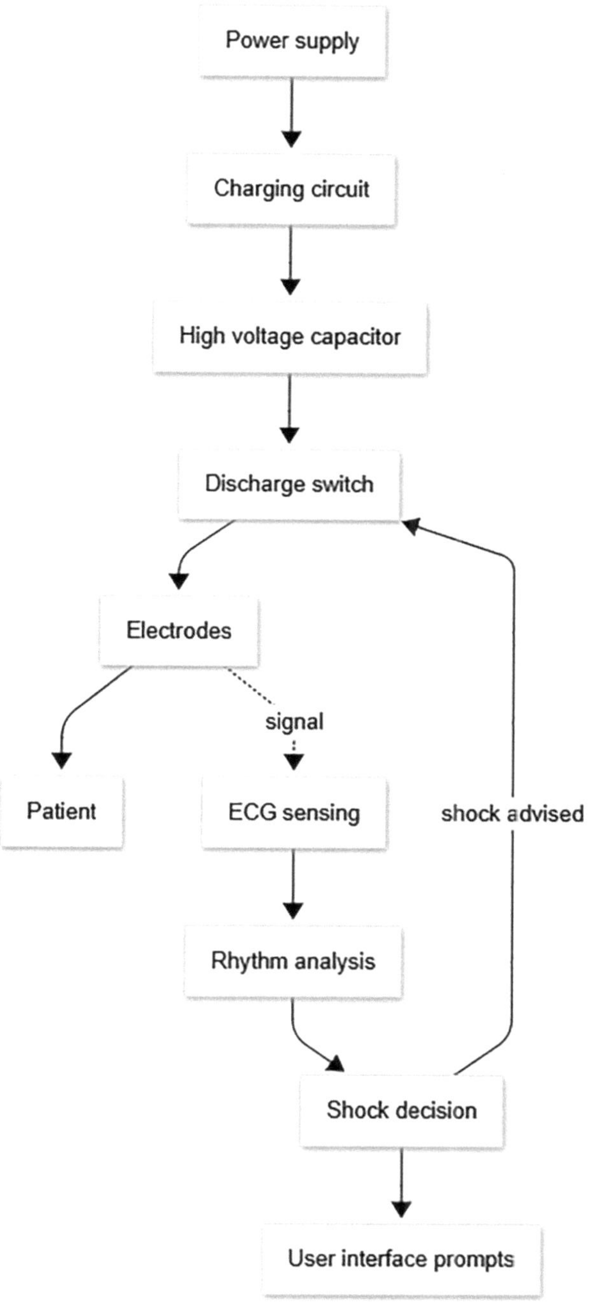


**Fig. 2.41** Block diagram of a semiautomated DC defibrillator

### Waveform of the Energy Shock

The terms waveform and curve technology refer to the time-based sequence of energy output. The shape of the wave dictates firstly how much energy is supplied to the patient and secondly over what period this energy is administered. The optimum amount of energy for the defibrillator pulse is the amount of energy that causes the least myocardial damage.

A distinction is made between mono-, bi-, and triphasic defibrillation shock configurations. Whereas, in the case of the monophasic waveform, the current only flows in one direction and the polarity does not change, with the biphasic waveform the current is delivered in one direction, interrupted, and continued in the opposite direction. Here, the polarity changes with every phase. The main forms of the biphasic discharge characteristic are the truncated exponential curve and the square pulse [298]. Today, particularly in the case of implantable and automatic external defibrillators, biphasic shock forms are preferably used, which differ as a result of varied adaptation to the thoracic impedance of the patient and are more effective on the first shock administered than monophasic shocks. Biphasic defibrillators are generally more effective and gentler on the heart than monophasic ones and have the advantage that the shock-induced dysfunction of the myocardial cells is less and that defibrillation success can be achieved with lower energy and voltage. The device-dependent amount of energy is 150–200 J for the first defibrillation and 200–360 J for all others, whereas it is always 360 J in the first monophasic defibrillation. In addition, biphasic pulse forms allow devices to be further miniaturized (Fig. 2.42).

Whereas the optimum energy flow in monophasic defibrillation is somewhere in the range from 30 to 40 A, with biphasic shock it is believed to be in the range from 15 to 20 A. Defibrillators whose administered shock corresponded to the real transthoracic flow would be preferable. Some of the biphasic defibrillators which are available on the market use very different manufacturer-specific pulse forms. There is currently no general consensus about the effectiveness and potential negative effects of the various pulse forms on offer. The operating modes are divided into

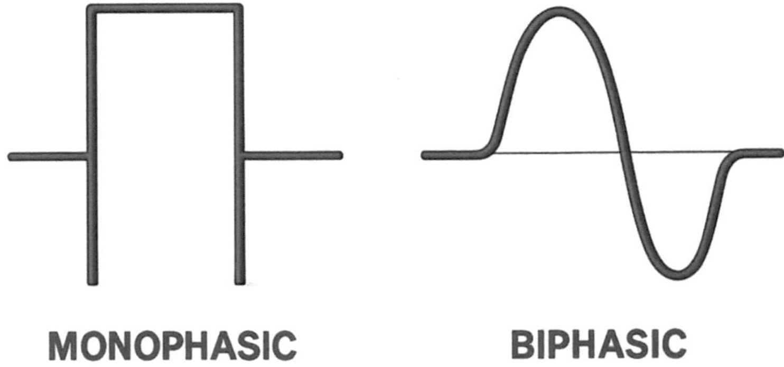


**Fig. 2.42** Monophasic and biphasic pulse forms

asynchronous and synchronous operation: whereas the heart's own pulses are taken into account in the synchronous operating mode. The latter operating mode should be reserved for strictly emergency defibrillators. Only the synchronized operating mode is suitable for cardioversion [299].

### Thoracic Impedance

Thoracic impedance is the resistance in the body which opposes the energy pulse or flow from the defibrillator. It ranges between 15 and 150 Ω; usually it is 70–80 Ω. The impedance should therefore be taken into consideration when the necessary energy is administered, as the patient's thoracic impedance is crucial to the amount of energy required. Because the impedance varies to a large degree in humans, dynamic adaptation of the waveform of the energy pulse is an important feature. In modern devices, the thoracic impedance is automatically measured and taken into account before defibrillation, meaning that energy can be delivered more accurately [300]. Larger electrodes incidentally reduce the impedance.

### Defibrillation/Cardioversion

This synchronization is carried out to prevent the pulse being delivered in the vulnerable phase (T wave) and to prevent the risk of ventricular fibrillation being triggered. In contrast, asynchronous cardioversion, which takes place independently of the R wave, is what is known as fibrillation. From a hemodynamic point of view, blood is no longer or is hardly pumped into the circulatory system during ventricular flutter and fibrillation, as the individual muscle fibers do not contract in a coordinated fashion. In the case of atrial flutter and fibrillation, approximately 20–30% less blood is ejected since the filling capacity of the ventricles is not optimized as a result of atrial contraction being stopped. Indications for electrical cardioversion are:

- Atrial flutter and fibrillation
- AV junctional reentrant tachycardia
- WPW (Wolff—Parkinson—White—Syndrome) and ventricular tachycardia

With ventricular fibrillation, defibrillation is the only therapy that can be used that has any prospect of success. Electrical cardioversion is contraindicated in digitalis overdose, hypokalemia, and atrial fibrillation (Fig. 2.43).

### Hardware

In addition to conventional manual defibrillators, there are semi-automated and automated systems (AEDs), which perform an automatic ECG analysis via attached electrodes and have an integrated display. Defibrillators without a monitor, display,

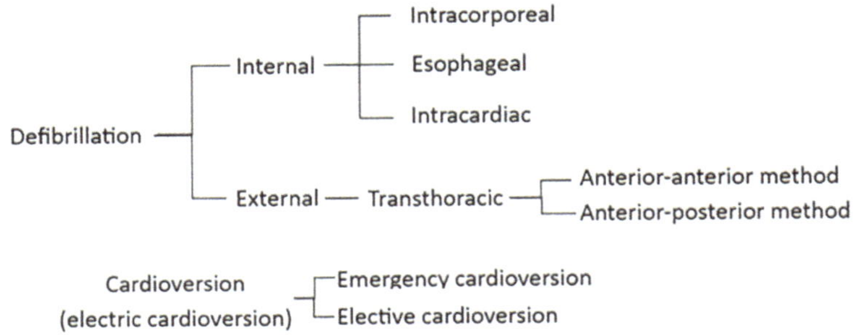


**Fig. 2.43** Method overview for defibrillation/cardioversion

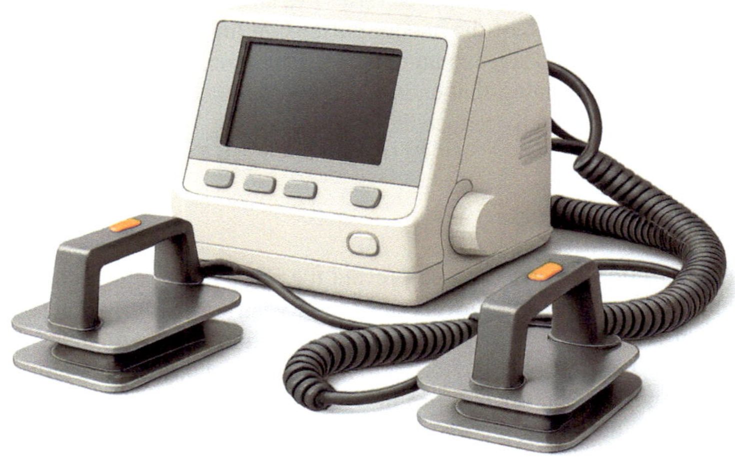

**Fig. 2.44** Semi-Automated defibrillator with paddles

or rhythm analysis are known as blind defibrillators. Modern defibrillators have a quick-look monitoring device in the paddles. When ventricular fibrillation is detected in a semiautomated device, the user is recommended to defibrillate [301, 302] (Fig. 2.44).

The expandable functionality, which is usually achieved using pluggable modules, makes the fundamental system properties possible in semi-automated defibrillators and modules: integrated external pacer, noninvasive blood pressure, $SpO_2$, capnography, arrhythmia detection, and a recording component for documentation. Within the scope of quality assurance for a defibrillation that has been performed, complete recording by the device is of particular interest, including ECG recording and 12-channel ECG reports as well as recording of all other relevant data for later evaluation and documentation. The possibility of remote data transmission, from the ambulance to the hospital's emergency department, will also play a relatively significant role in the future.

### System Technology

Miniaturized construction, more effective defibrillation due to low-energy pulses, and improved and updated software enable subpectoral implantation with transvenous electrode insertion under local anesthetic to be standard practice today. Conventional products have a volume <40 cm and a weight <80 g, with an average device lifespan of 4–6 years. Today, ICD technology provides fine-tuned, integrated systems [79]:

- Single-chamber ICD with the therapeutic possibility of antitachycardia stimulation, cardioversion, and defibrillation. The defibrillator electrode is placed in the right ventricle.
- Dual-chamber ICD with an additional atrial electrode or single-lead ventricular pacing with atrial tracking-ICD.
- Triple-chamber ICD with the additional possibility of cardiac resynchronization therapy. The electrode fixed in the right ventricle is supplemented by a further electrode that selectively stimulates the left ventricle.

Just as there is the international pacemaker code, there is also a code for ICDs. An ICD system consists of a generating unit and an electrode. The generating unit includes the housing, the battery, capacitors, a microprocessor, an amplifier, a magnetic switch, an audio transducer for signals, an antenna for telemetry, and an electrode connection head. The electrode consists of an isolated electrode body with a multilumen construction. The conductors for detection, stimulation, and defibrillation are arranged inside the electrode, isolated from one another. Depending on the ICD model, the therapy possibilities are:

1. Pacing
2. Antitachycardia pacing
3. Cardioversion
4. Defibrillation

Integrated ventricular demand rate-responsive pacing or dual chamber rate-responsive pacing pacemaker circuits are standard in modern ICD technology. The operational lifespan of dual-chamber systems is somewhat shorter than that of single-chamber systems. New shock forms, improved electrode systems, and optimized shock delivery are leading to a considerable reduction in the defibrillation threshold, which today is generally below 15 J. There is also the fact that short and constant charge times prevent the DFT from increasing. Biphasic or sequential defibrillator pulses are currently preferred in clinical use. Studies have confirmed that the pulse of energy required increases with the duration of ventricular fibrillation and with the increase in conduction fronts, and conversely, that the sooner the ventricular fibrillation is terminated after it arises, the lower the energy [303]. Comprehensive diagnostic program memories, which in the context of patient aftercare enable validation of the therapeutic intervention, are part of today's standard equipment. Some ICD devices provide the option of telemetry transmission of recorded intracardiac electrograms via an antenna in the head of the ICD implant.

The periodic or event-triggered reports are transmitted via mobile telephony to an Internet-based database using a mobile patient unit. The attending doctor can access the transmitter data online [304].

### Electrodes

If ICD implantation was still a complex surgical procedure at the beginning of the 1990s, then developing a transvenous electrode was a considerable simplification. Combining transvenous electrodes with subcutaneous defibrillation electrodes is a vital step forward.

The electrically active generating unit housing and/or proximal section of the defibrillation probe is used as the anode, while the electrode section in the proper ventricle functions as the cathode. A distinction is drawn between two configurations: the single-coil probe from the right ventricle to the ICD housing, and the dual-coil probe with a defibrillation surface between the right ventricle, the superior vena cava, and the ICD housing, which is the most favorable in terms of energy. If the electrode section in the right ventricle functions as an anode due to programming, this reversal in polarity likewise results in a reduced energy requirement during defibrillation. This measure is particularly suitable for patients with a very high defibrillation threshold. The signal detection function and anti-bradycardic stimulation are performed via the probe's tip, which is constructed in true bipolar or integrated bipolar fashion [305].

Correct application of the adhesive electrodes is necessary to achieve faultless ECG recording and ultimately to prevent equipment-related interpretation errors. Although more expensive, self-adhesive defibrillation electrodes (pads) are safe and effective and should be preferred over standard plate electrodes (paddles). Another advantage of adhesive electrodes from the operator's viewpoint is that it is possible to defibrillate from a safe distance without leaning over the patient. It is also quicker to administer the first energy pulse using self-adhesive electrodes than paddles. Whereas with paddles, contact gel is needed between the skin surface and the metal plate to reduce the skin impedance—and thus improve the electrical contact—and prevent burns, this is not necessary with adhesive electrodes [306]. Compared with electrode paste and gels, gel pads are favorable for safe operation because they avoid the risk of arcing or short circuiting and thus prevent ineffective defibrillation. The Association for the Advancement of Medical Instrumentation (AAMI) recommends a minimum electrode area of 150 cm2, since larger electrodes have a lower impedance or even lead to a decrease in the transmyocardial flow. The diameter of customary electrodes is 8–12 cm for adults and children with body weight >10 kg and 4.5 cm for children with body weight <10 kg.

Modern ICD electrode bodies have a multi-lumen construction; a few are coaxial. Silicone is predominantly used as the insulation for the external layer of the probe and offers a high level of biocompatibility and flexibility, but is very sensitive to mechanical stress. Other distinguishing features of transvenous probes are the number of defibrillation probes and coils. Active or passive fixing of ICD electrodes can be done using fixed screws or extensible screws and using anchors [307].

Atrial, epicardial, and coronary sinus electrodes are additional pacing/sensing electrodes. The CS electrode has an acceleration sensor at its distal end, which records and differentiates acceleration values in at least two different directions. A special shock probe is the array electrode, which is implanted subcutaneously. This electrode has up to three shock coils and is used additionally when there is an insufficient defibrillation threshold. The individual coils of the finger electrode are connected in parallel with the right-ventricular shock coil via a Y-connector. The single-lead VDD-ICD is an electrode system for a dual-chamber ICD. The atrial signals are recorded at this electrode, which is fixed in the apex of the right ventricle, using two electrode rings. This electrode thus replaces the otherwise additional atrial electrode. Bipolar and tripolar ECG leads in ICD systems enable reliable ischemia detection, which has considerable advantages over the conventional surface ECG, owing to the early detection of ischemias and their severity and duration.

#### Programming

Communication with an implanted device is realized using a specialized device called the programmer. It enables programming of parameters of electric stimuli, measurement of sensed signals of the heart's beat and electrical features of the system, and selection of all other parameters. Data transfer between the programmer and the device uses telemetric inductive coupling or a wireless radio signal. Programmers are computerized devices with their operating systems. They contain general service software and special applications for particular devices or groups. The user interface is a touch screen that includes buttons for sending data to the implanted device, diverting the therapy, or selecting the paper advance speed in a case of electrogram (EGM) or electrocardiogram (ECG) records. Furthermore, the built-in parts include an ECG monitor, an internal printer, a device for data disc input (diskettes, flash drive), slots for connecting an external printer, monitor, or keyboard, and inputs from electrophysiological monitoring systems. Cross-referenced entries are available on the system's main screen, enabling access to information on the set functions before input to application software, language selection, an easy-to-use diagnostic ECG monitor, a quick automatic device interrogation mode, and others. Regarding the ECG monitor, it is possible to change the speed of motion, to set an input amplifier or an input filter of the surface ECG, or to display electric stimulus spikes. Identification of the implanted device using a telemetric sensor positioned over the pacemaker and downloading data from it is designated reading or interrogation [308]. The interrogation is the first step of all sessions during follow-up. At the initial interrogation, the information on, for example, the parameter settings, patient data, diagnostic data, and battery status, is copied from the device memory. Parameter values might be changed by touching the pointer to the appropriate parameter window and by lifting the pointer off the screen. After executing changes to parameter values, the change will appear in the window until it is programmed into the device. After defining a new parameter, its interactions with the other parameters are evaluated immediately. If a new value breaks the limits of interaction within the application, an icon will appear that reports parameter failure. The failure is described in the interaction window, and a solution is proposed [309]. To continue programming changes, correcting the affected parameter first is necessary. Suppose it is necessary to permanently record the data interrogated at a follow-up. In that case, the programmer offers printed reports containing actual values of parameters, data on therapy history, information on the device's battery status, and programmed data about a patient (date of implantation, type of leads, indication for device implantation, etc.).

#### Software

To determine the optimum time to deliver the defibrillation pulse when fibrillation characteristics are present, computer-aided form analysis of ECG signals is a promising and innovative new development currently being researched. It involves evaluating the frequency and amplitude characteristics of the surface ECG using so-called fibrillation scoring algorithms. This algorithm is based on linear (e.g., Fourier analysis, wavelet theory) and nonlinear methods (such as an N(a) histogram, which can be used to investigate the degree of randomness in a signal). Further advantages of this technology may be that ineffective energy pulses are avoided, damage to the myocardium is thereby limited, and information is provided about the quality of the resuscitation performed [296, 310].

#### Algorithms

Internal ECG signal detection algorithms analyze the ECG's amplitude, frequency, and slew rate. Errors in interpreting tachycardic arrhythmias can lead to false ICD discharges and erroneous failure to detect ventricular arrhythmias. Different algorithms are used to detect and differentiate ventricular arrhythmias from supraventricular arrhythmias. The emerging cardiac rhythm frequencies are classified and assigned to up to six detection zones: a bradycardia zone, a sinus rhythm zone, a fibrillation zone, and one to three tachycardia zones.

ICD algorithms distinguish between supraventricular and ventricular tachycardias based on criteria such as frequency stability, QRS width criterion, sudden-onset rapid heartbeat, the relationship between atrial and ventricular signals, the site of acceleration and AV association, or distinguishes between different variants in the AV relationships using detection of a pattern over a period between two RR intervals. Detection criteria can be programmed in the sensing system responsible for detection and re-detection. Furthermore, it is also possible to include atrial events in the detection algorithms. The mode switch algorithms induce an automatic change of operating mode from the DDDR to the dual chamber demand rate-responsive pacing mode to ensure that, after high atrial frequencies have been detected, the triggered mode for ventricular stimulation is actuated in aid of inhibited operation [311]. To increase the sensitivity and specificity of the detection of ventricular tachycardias in ICD therapy, in addition to the electrical criteria, it is also a good idea to consider information about the hemodynamic situation, such as the contractility of the left ventricle.

### 2.9.3 *Types of Devices*

Defibrillators can be divided into manual defibrillators, semi-automated and automated external defibrillators (AEDs), fully automated defibrillators, and defibrillator implants. The criterion for distinguishing between semi- and fully automated defibrillators is that, with the semi-automatic defibrillator, the user is shown to trigger a defibrillator recommendation and the administration of the pulse, whereas this is done automatically with a fully automated defibrillator. The electrodes used are so-called paddles, adhesive electrodes, or internal paddles [312] (Fig. 2.45).

#### Automated External Defibrillator

AED systems—predominantly using two-phase curve technology—only deliver a defibrillation pulse if a life-threatening cardiac arrhythmia is present, which is recognized as such by the device. The user is also guided using a control menu. Modern systems additionally offer a voice-controlled user interface. The American Heart Association (AHA) takes the view that up to a third of all deaths resulting from sudden cardiac death could be prevented by widespread AED use. The use of AED systems is classified as an integral part of basic resuscitation measures [302, 313].

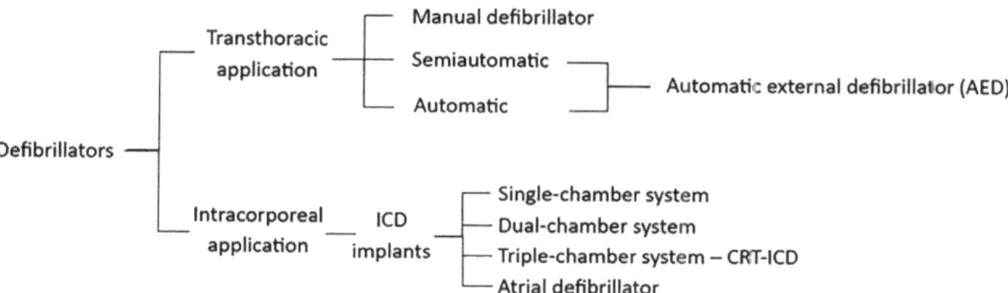


**Fig. 2.45** Overview of types of defibrillator devices

## Implantable Cardioverter-Defibrillators

Implantable cardioverter-defibrillators (ICDs) are primarily used for reliable detection and treatment of life-threatening cardiac arrhythmias (ventricular tachycardia and fibrillation), which originate in the ventricles and which cannot be treated with medication. The American and European Societies of Cardiology also recommend ICD implantation in patients who have survived sudden cardiac death, which did not occur as a result of myocardial infarction, and also for primary prophylaxis in patients with restricted cardiac pumping function. When necessary, ICD systems can also administer pacemaker pulses in bradycardic phases. ICD systems can also stimulate antitachycardia, cardioversion, and defibrillation [314] (Fig. 2.46).

## Pacemaker

A pacemaker is a small device placed in the chest or abdomen to help control abnormal heart rhythms. This device uses electrical pulses to prompt the heart to beat. Pacemakers are used to treat arrhythmias. Arrhythmias are problems with the rate or rhythm of the heartbeat. During an arrhythmia, the heart can beat too fast, slow, or irregularly [315]. Pacemakers use low-energy electrical pulses to overcome this faulty electrical signaling. Pacemakers can:

- Speed up a slow heart rhythm.
- Help control an abnormal or fast heart rhythm.
- Make sure the ventricles contract normally if the atria are quivering instead of beating with a regular rhythm (a condition called atrial fibrillation).

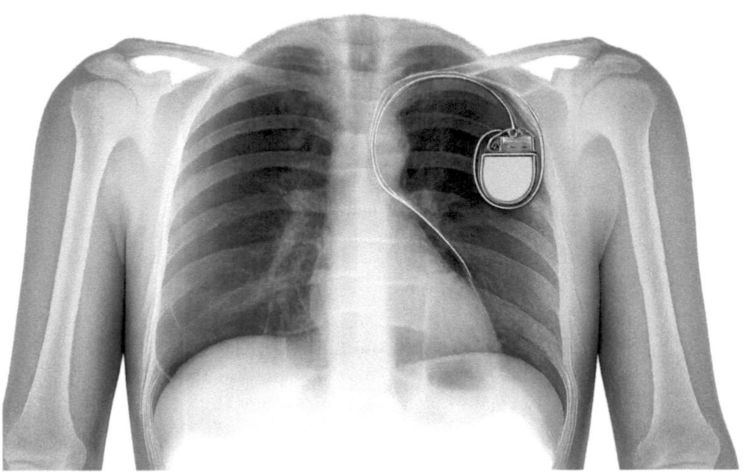

**Fig. 2.46** Chest X-ray with implanted ICD system

- Coordinate electrical signaling between the upper and lower chambers of the heart.
- Coordinate electrical signaling between the ventricles. Pacemakers that do this are called cardiac resynchronization therapy (CRT) devices, and they are used to treat heart failure.
- Prevent dangerous arrhythmias caused by a disorder called long QT syndrome.

Pacemakers can also monitor and record your heart's electrical activity and rhythm. Newer pacemakers can monitor your blood temperature, breathing rate, and other factors. They can also adjust your heart rate to changes in your activity. Pacemakers can be temporary or permanent. Temporary pacemakers are used to treat short-term heart problems, such as a slow heartbeat that's caused by a heart attack, heart surgery, or an overdose of medicine [316].

Temporary pacemakers are also used during emergencies. They might be used until your doctor can implant a permanent pacemaker or a temporary condition disappears. If you have a temporary pacemaker, you will stay in a hospital as long as the device is in place. Permanent pacemakers control long-term heart rhythm problems [317] (Fig. 2.47).

Cardiac pacing principles are based on creating an electrical field between the electrodes and the surrounding myocardium using an electric stimulus. To create an action potential and its subsequent spontaneous propagation, it is necessary to ensure that a difference in potential between the extracellular and intracellular domains of the ectoplasm falls to the value of the threshold potential, from about −80 to about −60 mV. The intracellular domain is charged relatively negatively. The extracellular domain, however, is positively charged. The electrode fixed to the endocardium is compared with practically all cells in the extracellular domain. The closest surroundings of the electrode are at the same potential as the electrode. So, under an electric stimulus, the extracellular domain is polarized in compliance with the stimulus [299]. The purpose is to induce an action potential on the membranes

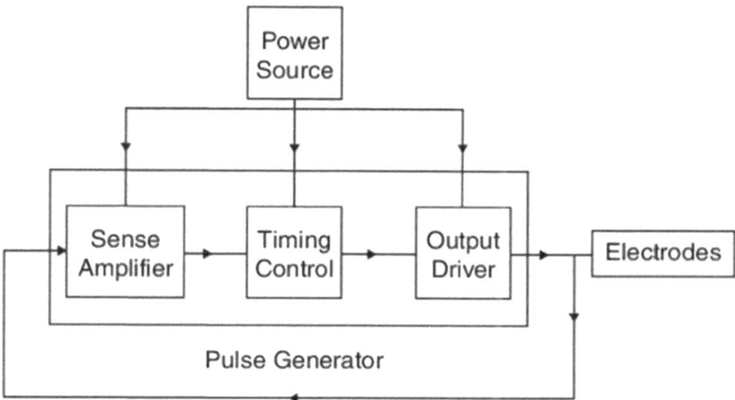


**Fig. 2.47** Simple block diagram of a pacemaker

by changing the electric potential to above the membrane potential value. Because the intracellular domain is charged relatively negatively, a decrease in membrane potential can be achieved by decreasing the potential of the extracellular domain using a negative pulse. A positive electric stimulus can also be used for pacing. However, the amplitude must be higher. The action potential created in the cellules depolarized directly by the electrode is propagated by biophysical mechanisms to the surrounding cellules and depolarized. The highest current density from the electrodes is at the edge between the electrode and the tissue [318]. It decreases as the distance from the electrode increases. A pacing threshold is a minimal value of a certain physical quantity at which a consistent cardiac depolarization has been safely created and propagated. The pacing threshold can be expressed in amplitude, pulse width, or energy according to the direct proportion E » U2*t. Cardiac pacing uses rectangular electric stimuli with programmable amplitude and width. Excitability of the heart muscle can be expressed by parameters of a cardiac electric stimulus that can activate cardiac depolarization, and the so-called Hoorweg-Weiss curve (strength–duration curve) that expresses a relation between current amplitude and pulse width of the pacing threshold is used for this. The curve has the shape of a hyperbola, and two characteristic values are defined on it:

- Rheobase—a minimal pacing threshold current for the theoretically infinite width of the pulse.
- Chronaxy—a pulse width at which the pacing threshold equals twice the rheobase.

In practice, within the rheobase definition, the infinite width of the pulse is substituted by a definite one, for example, 2.0 ms. A doubled value of the voltage threshold or a tripled value of the pacing threshold width is considered a safe reserve of an electric stimulus output. The issue of the pacing threshold is much more complicated and complex. The pacing threshold is influenced by, for example, the type and material of the lead used, the distance between the electrodes, and the state of the tissue. The pacing threshold also changes within the time after a lead implantation. However, a considerable increase has not been observed yet, thanks to the use of steroids. Within a daily cycle, the pacing threshold is higher during sleep; it falls during waking and decreases even more distinctly during physical exertion. The pacing threshold is also influenced by pharmaceuticals: it rises especially after the use of β-blockers and class I antiarrhythmics but falls after corticosteroid use. Occasionally, a brisk and inexplicable rise of the pacing threshold of some patients can be observed. This is designated as an exit block [319].

## 2.9.4 Clinical Applications

Synchronized defibrillation is called electrical cardioversion, i.e., the pulse of energy is triggered by the R wave in the ECG. Externally, transthoracic defibrillation is performed using electrodes and pulses of energy from 2 to 360 J. As a guide value dependent on the body weight, a pulse strength of 3 J/kg is recommended for adults and 2 J/kg for children. In terms of electrode application, a distinction is made between the anterior-anterior method and the anterior-posterior method. In contrast, the anterior-posterior method, which is primarily used in emergencies, involves placing both electrodes on the thorax; in this method, a large-area electrode is placed on the back. The anterior-posterior method is preferred for electrotherapy in the case of arrhythmias, since the most significant proportion of the administered pulse of energy flows directly through the myocardium [296, 310]. For internal, or intracorporeal, defibrillation, sterile internal paddles are used. In the case of an open thorax, these paddles cover the exposed heart, meaning the electrodes must be in contact with the myocardium over its entire area. For internal defibrillation, the energy pulse is a maximum of 50 J.

An esophageal pulse electrode (cylindrical electrode at the end of the catheter) is placed at the level of the left atrium. The counter electrode is attached to the thorax. An additional electrode to the cylindrical electrode enables bipolar stimulation and recording of an esophageal ECG signal, which synchronizes the energy pulse [320]. Intracardiac is likewise carried out using a catheter. One electrode lies at the apex of the right ventricle, while the second electrode is placed in the superior vena cava.

ICD implantations have increased significantly in numbers. The following reasons are vital to this development:

- A simplified implantation technique reduces the rates of mortality resulting from surgery.
- Very low morbidity.
- High level of patient acceptance.
- ICD therapy has considerable advantages over medicinal therapy for the prevention of sudden cardiac death, within the scope of secondary prophylaxis, for example, following hemodynamic ventricular tachycardia.
- For idiopathic ventricular fibrillation, there is currently no alternative to ICD therapy.
- A further indication is primary prophylaxis for high-risk patients with no symptoms.
- The costs of ICD therapy have decreased considerably as a result of a reduction in product prices alongside increasing product life.

#### Technical Safety Aspects

- Avoid direct contact with the electrodes, conductive contact with the patients or others.
- There should be no moisture on the patient's skin, and the patient should also be positioned such that he is electrically isolated.
- Only perform cardioversion if the ECG is free from artifacts and if reliable ECG monitoring is possible. Too much electrode contact paste on the paddles can cause an electrical bridge to form.

- All additional devices connected to the patient must be defibrillation-proof; otherwise, they must be disconnected from the patient during cardioversion/ defibrillation.
- Caution should be exercised with patients with energized implants: the implant's functioning may be restricted or suspended, and it may be damaged or even become unusable.

In principle, all commercially available defibrillators are operated similarly and are suitable for internal and external defibrillation. As a rule, a visual and/or acoustic signal is generated when the defibrillator is operational, i.e., when the capacitor is charged. The electrodes, which are provided with gel, are placed firmly on the thorax and pressed on, and the preselected energy dose is triggered. This is usually done directly via a trigger on the handles. According to the 2005 ERC Guidelines, the practice of performing defibrillation three times within a minute using mono- and biphasic defibrillators is now obsolete. This application model has been replaced by delivery of a single shock at full energy; i.e., with a monophasic shock, 360 J is recommended for delivery of the shock. At least 150–200 J is advised for all discharge characteristics for the first biphasic shock. Following each shock, cardiopulmonary resuscitation should be performed for 2 min before administering the next shock. If further shocks are necessary, with monophasic defibrillators, the energy level is, in contrast, successively increased [302].

The energy pulse delivered and its amplitude, the form and polarity of the shock, the electrode size and position, and the homogeneity of the current density on the cardiac muscle (myocardium) are all crucial for efficient defibrillation or cardioversion. Cardioversion and defibrillation can result in the following serious and minor complications:

- Induced ventricular fibrillation, e.g., as a result of incorrect triggering, which can ultimately lead to asystole (cardiac arrest).
- Post Defibrillation arrhythmias such as ventricular and supraventricular extrasystoles and ventricular flutter.
- Arterial embolism.
- Burns and skin irritation, for example, due to insufficient electrode contact paste being used on the electrode surface.

### 2.9.5 Regulatory Considerations

- Defibrillators belong to class IIb of the German Medical Devices Act (MPG, Medizinprodukte Gesetz).
- Defibrillators must only be used in an explosion-proof atmosphere.
- Devices that are not defibrillator-proof must be disconnected from the patient.
- Equipment should be labeled according to DIN-IEC 601 as defibrillator proof.
- Maximum energy 360 J.
- Trigger buttons are only on both paddles (connected in series).

- Protective circuits ensure a reduced power setting when the defibrillator is switched off and ensure energy recovery no later than 1 min after defibrillator charging.
- Because of their unforeseeable and frequently changing use, defibrillators should always be connected to mains electricity at their device base locations so that they are operational and ready for use on an ad hoc basis.

### Complications

The spectrum of ICD complications ranges from harmless complications, such as skin irritations and minor burns on the areas where the electrodes have been applied, to serious complications, such as the emergence of extrasystoles following defibrillation, ventricular tachycardia, ventricular fibrillation or the occurrence of asystole following electric cardioversion in the case of sick sinus syndrome. ICD-specific complications can be caused, on the one hand, by the generating unit:

- Pressure-related necrosis
- Risk of infection
- Technical errors and malfunctions as a result, for example, of strong external magnetic fields or battery depletion
- Perforation of the generating unit, and on the other hand, by the electrodes:
  - Electrode dislocation can cause stimulation of muscles
  - Inadequate administration of shocks as a result of the detection of muscle potential or external sources of interference
  - Fractures in the electrodes, defects in the insulation, or a rise in the sensitivity threshold can cause electrode malfunction.

One malfunction in the detection function is undersensing or oversensing. In the case of undersensing, life-threatening arrhythmias are not detected or are detected too late, whereas with oversensing, the shocks administered are inadequate.

### Function Checking

In the early days of ICD device technology, it was still necessary for technical reasons to test the functioning of an ICD patient's implant every 2 months, but this check is now carried out independently by the device itself. Function checking of the system every 3–6 months is sufficient. If there is an indication of incorrect detection, a chest X-ray is generally performed to identify insulation defects in the probe. Due to the advancements in battery technology, the shelf life of single-chamber systems is expected to be 9 years, dual-chamber systems 7 years, and triple-chamber systems 5 years. Therefore, the device's lifespan will be considerably longer than previous ICD systems. Replacement of the generating unit is also only necessary at a later point in time. Stored data, such as treatment episodes, electrograms, battery state, and electrode resistance, can be queried via telemetry [39]. For function checking, various device parameters are measured intraoperatively during pacemaker and ICD implantations and, if necessary, adjusted.

Pacemaker and defibrillator conformity testing is underway to address the necessary evolution of these devices due to their life-or-death nature. The aim is to balance weaknesses in standardized test procedures for such devices by introducing systematic performance validation following installation. A new conformity assessment method, compatible with the International Organization of Legal Metrology (OIML) system, supports the independent testing of defibrillators and ensures their continuous compliance with clinical safety standards. Tested in many healthcare facilities, the method gives a reproducible and systematic testing process that enhances device traceability and minimizes risks of device malfunction.

The new strategy allows regulators and healthcare providers to shift from reactive to proactive safety management. It includes compliance testing as a regular part of hospital procedures, providing real-time feedback that enhances the reliability of pacemakers and defibrillators. As regulatory agencies move towards more evidence-based regulation, standardized conformity assessments by product type will be essential to safeguard patient outcomes.

### 2.9.6 Future Perspectives

In the coming years, standardization of conformity assessment is among the key measures for making medical device management digital. With all this digital interconnection, future systems will be able to utilize AI-based diagnostics to forecast anomalies, heighten the sensitivity of healthcare delivery, and limit unwanted occurrences [175, 321]. This might even enable globally uniform standards for device testing, especially needed for devices implemented in emergency care like defibrillators. Lastly, this advancement in conformity assessment lays the ground for more customized and adaptive medical device regulation, keeping safety measures up to date with technological advancements. As intelligent health technologies become increasingly embedded in healthcare settings, this will become a model for the regulation of next-generation cardiac devices [232].

## 2.10 Incubators

Each year, 15 million babies are born preterm, and their survival chances vary dramatically around the world. In order to prevent the death of infants, the baby incubator was invented. An incubator is a clear plastic box. For a premature baby, this box is the next best thing to being inside its mother's belly. An incubator creates an artificial environment for infants who are too small or sick and cannot maintain their

bodies warm enough for survival. Incubators also help to protect an infant from noise, light, and germs that may cause illness and infections.
The care of newborns had traditionally been regarded as the province of mothers. The incubator set into motion a three-way contest between mothers, obstetricians, and pediatricians regarding who should care for the premature infant. The first physicians who attempted to treat premature babies following the invention of the incubator in 1880 found gaining the mother's confidence and cooperation to be at least as challenging as applying the new technology. Further complications in their efforts were the fact that doctors themselves were divided. Both obstetricians and pediatricians at the turn of the century claimed that their specialty was better situated to deal with the problems of prematurity. In the nineteenth century, medical writers grouped all tiny babies into "premature and weak infants". Such babies were suffering from a lack of energy or vitality, and those dying from respiratory distress were diagnosed as having congenital atelectasis secondary to feeble breathing. Like other newborns, the premature infants were almost always born at home, and mothers were accustomed to providing considerable medical care for their infants. Many died in the first days of life from hypothermia, infection, or weight loss. The high overall mortality of infancy hid the mortality of these infants. In the late nineteenth century, 15–20% of all infants in American cities never lived to see their first birthday.

### *2.10.1 History*

The first significant challenge between doctor and mother was the invention of a medical technology directed towards premature infants: the incubator. In 1880, the French obstetrician Stephane Tarnier was inspired to install a device for infant care when he visited the chicken incubator display in Paris [322].

Tarnier's first incubator housed several infants warmed over a hot-water reservoir attached to an external heating source. He quickly simplified the apparatus to a single infant model heated by hot-water bottles, which were replaced manually by the nurse every 3 h. Ventilation relied on simple convection, with air entering at the base and circulating upward around the infant. Tarnier faced numerous criticisms, but one aspect that often went overlooked was his most significant contribution: convincing his colleagues that incubators made a difference. So he decided to compare premature infant mortality before and after the device's introduction in a large case series that eventually comprised 500 infants.

The results appeared impressive since the mortality of infants fell from 66% to 38%. Because of that, the Paris municipal board rushed to set up incubators in all of its maternity hospitals. Pierre Constant Budin was included in the new generation of obstetricians, and he had finalized the project of hospitalizing premature infants apart from their mothers. Budin died unexpectedly from infuenza in 1907, and because of that, obstetric leadership in the infant welfare movement passed on to Pinard, who continued to focus on maternity leave while retaining a secondary role for incubator care. In Nice, Alexandre Lion, a physician, developed a much more sophisticated incubator than that of Tarnier in the 1890s. A large metal apparatus equipped with a thermostat and an independent forced ventilation system, but the problem was that none of its features came cheaply, limiting its appeal to charity or government-supported hospitals. Lion created so-called "incubator charities" and his high point of career was the opening of the child hatchery (1896), an elaborate incubator baby show that became the surprise sensation of the Berlin Exposition. Thanks to the efforts of one of Lion's associates, the physician showman Martin Couney, incubator shows came to the United States. The shows were the first celebrations of technology and its future promise in rescuing the lives of premature infants [322, 323].

In 1870, German pediatrician Dr. Martin Couney invented the modern baby incubator. Dr. Couney's daughter was born premature and lived to adulthood under her father's care. After inventing the baby incubator, Dr. Couney faced skepticism from other medical professionals who did not believe his methods would work. Banks were unwilling to finance the production of his incubators, believing that no hospital would want the devices. Couney set out to prove them all wrong.

The incubators Couney used were the latest models, imported directly from Europe. Each incubator was more than 1.5 m tall, made of steel and glass, and stood on legs. A water boiler outside supplied hot water to a pipe underneath a bed. The bed was made of fine mesh on which the baby slept, while a thermostat regulated the temperature. Another pipe carried fresh air from outside the building into the incubator, passing through absorbent wool suspended in antiseptic or medicated water, then through dry wool to filter out impurities. On top, a chimney-like device with a revolving fan blew the exhausted air upwards and out of the incubators.

Caring for premature babies was expensive. 1903 costs about $15 a day ($405 or £277 today). But Couney did not charge the parents a penny for their medical care. They came in such numbers that Couney easily covered his operating costs, paid his staff a good wage, and had enough left to begin planning more exhibits. These made Couney a wealthy man [324, 325].

Joseph B. DeLee was an obstetrician who opened an incubator station at the Chicago Lying-in Hospital in 1900. He intubated and inflated the lungs of premature infants and created his thermostats for his incubator. He had also set up a transport service whereby a portable incubator could be dispensed with a doctor and nurse to pick up premature newborns amid the Chicago winter. DeLee's station lasted only 10 years because of economic issues. A 1919 review article noted that "the use of the incubator is becoming increasingly unpopular, and the United States Children's Bureau advised mothers in 1920 that 'incubators are not now generally used even in hospital cases." The explanation for the stalemate involves two factors: increasing differentiation of obstetrics and pediatrics characterizing the period, and the traditional preponderance of home birth was diminishing during World War I [326].

In 1914, Hess developed his own version of the incubator, an electrical "heated bed" reminiscent of Crede's design that surrounded the infant in a hot water jacket. His success in raising financial support to move beyond single incubators to an organized incubator station was more important than the fact that he developed his own incubator. While many of Hess's contemporaries had rejected incubators, he realized they were useful. He expanded the function of the incubator itself into an oxygen chamber and developed an automobile-based transport system. Moreover, Hess worked with his head nurse, Evelyn Lundeen, to develop a staff of trained nurses following specific protocols. One physician recalled head nurse Lundeen as "an autocrat who knew more about the care of the premature than the doctors did", which makes sense because the nurse had replaced the mother. Premature infants were now born mainly in the hospital, and their care was provided by specialized nurses supervised by pediatricians rather than obstetricians. Mothers gained access to far more powerful technologies to assist their infants.

## 2.10.2 *Technical Characteristics*

### Hardware

Baby incubators are biomedical devices whose performance must be maximum because of the type of patient they are suited for. A neonatal incubator is a rigid box in which infants needing medical care are placed. The most important feature of the incubator is its controlled environment. The term controlled environment means maintaining all environmental parameters, such as humidity, oxygen level, temperature, and air flow, at a constant level [327, 328]. Basic parts of every incubator are (Fig. 2.48):

1. Heater
2. Fan
3. Temperature control
4. Humidifier
5. Oxygen supply
6. Alarms and safety features
7. Access ports for nursing care

In a typical infant incubator, the baby lies on a mattress in a closed, transparent cabinet where the entire environment is completely controlled. The cabinet has portholes so that nurses can access the baby if any help is needed. The compartment containing control mechanisms is located under the cabinet. Different models of incubators have additional equipment suited for specific purposes [329] (Fig. 2.49).

The principle of action of the entire incubator depends on the fan action and its function in humidifying the air and controlling the incubator's temperature [330].

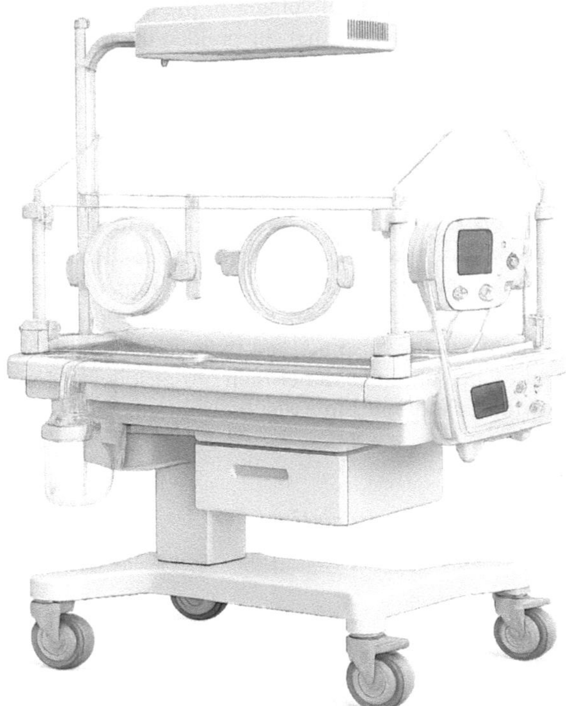

Fig. 2.48 An overview of an infant incubator

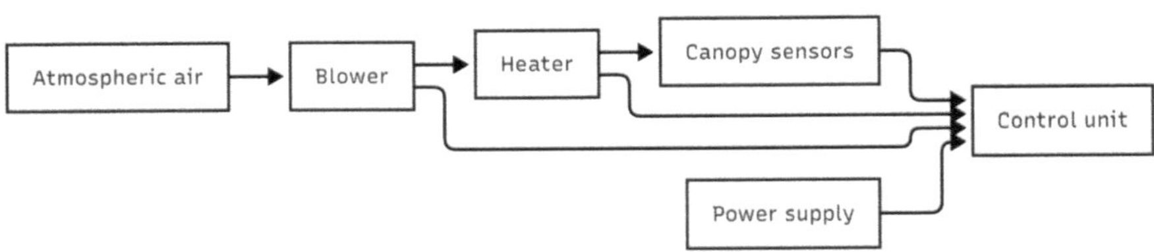


Fig. 2.49 The principle of action of the entire incubator

## Heater

The heater is the most important part of the incubator, so special care must be taken of its design and function (Fig. 2.50).

The radiant warmer is an overhead element placed above the head of the bed. The temperature sensor taped to the baby's skin, and the warmer regulates the heat output to maintain the infant at a constant temperature. The working principle of the radiant warmer can be presented by a block diagram. The power supply and the temperature skin sensor send information to the control unit. After processing the

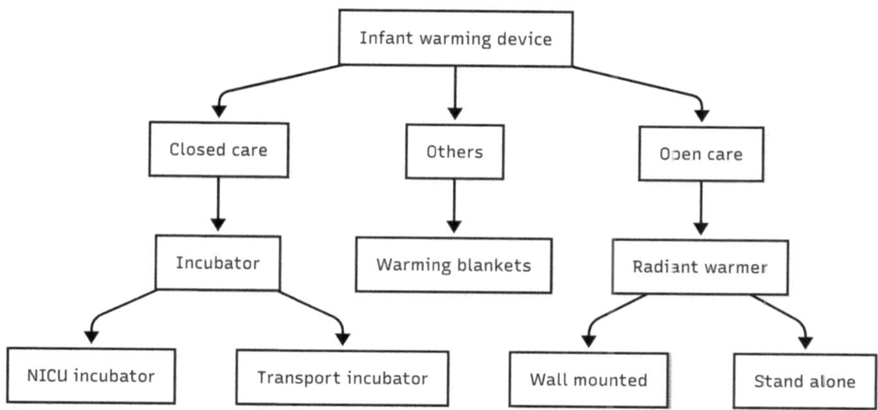


**Fig. 2.50** Classification of infant warming devices

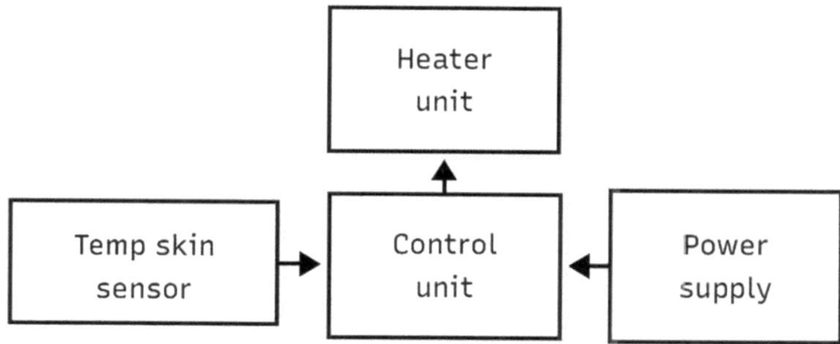


**Fig. 2.51** Radiant warmer work principle

input, the output from the control unit extends to the heater unit, and the temperature is emitted to the baby [144] (Fig. 2.51).

The greatest advantage of the radiant warmer is that, because of its makeup, the infant is easily accessible to doctors and nurses. However, because of that exposure, it is susceptible to a variety of outside influences and eventually bacteria from the neonatal intensive care unit (NICU). In addition, it is very hard to control the temperature in an incubator of this type [331].

### Fan

The fan blows the filtered room air through the heating element and the humidifier. Without the fan, the heat cannot be removed from the heater, and therefore, both the heater and the incubator itself will overheat.

### Temperature Control

Simple incubators are controlled with a thermostat consisting of a sensor and a pressure can. The sensor is a thin capillary tube connected to a pressure can (expansion chamber). The pressure can is equipped with a removable lid or a diaphragm. This closed system has a liquid or gas that expands when heated. Evoked by expansion, the lid moves and activates an electrical switch connected to it. Another type of temperature controller is an electronic controller with a cable sensor instead of the capillary sensor. The sensor's output controls a relay (on-off) or a dimmer (infinitely variable control). The advantage of the electronically controlled type is that an additional temperature sensor can be used. This is the temperature sensor that is used for controlling the amount of heat emitted by the heater unit. The temperature display or a thermometer should be separated from the temperature control unit. Both digital and alcohol glass thermometers can be used. Mercury thermometers are forbidden because of the toxicity of Mercury [332].

### Humidity Control

The container with water is placed just in front of the heating element, and during the transfer of heat from the heating element to the inside of the incubator, the air gets moistened. The container has a deflector plate, and by opening or closing that deflector plate, humidity can be regulated. Water container can be avoided if the incubator is equipped with a wet heater, which creates more humidity due to increased temperature. A hygrometer measures humidity. In order to prevent corrosion of the incubator, only distilled water should be used as the humidifier [332].

### Oxygen Control

Most infant incubators have a hose connection for applying additional oxygen from an external cylinder, oxygen concentrator, or the central gas supply. After being humidified, oxygen supplies the heated air. An alternative to this noninvasive oxygen supply is the invasive oxygen supply via a nasal cannula [333].

### Access Ports

Access ports are the only way to touch the infant inside the incubator. They have a cover that has to be closed every time the procedure is finished so that the infant can be in an environment that is as pure as possible [333].

**Software**

Alarms and Safety Features

To ensure the safety of infants, all electronically controlled incubators are equipped with a monitoring system that tracks the environment's state within the incubator. An alarm is generated if some parameters reach a critical value. There are three main types of alarms for three different failures [334]:

- Overheating
- Fan failure
- Power off

In addition to these alarms, all incubators, even those that are not electronically controlled, are equipped with overheating protection. If the temperature in the cabinet reaches 40 °C, the heater is completely switched off.

### 2.10.3 Types of Devices

Incubators today are much more developed, but the goal and function remain the same. The primary purpose of incubators remains to protect infants during the earliest stages of development. Major distinction is on:

- Intensive Care Incubator (type 100 and type 200)
- Warmer Radiant
- Transport Incubator

Neonatal incubators consist of a rigid box-like structure in which an infant may be kept in a controlled environment for medical care. The device includes an AC-powered heater, a fan to circulate the warmed air, a container for adding water to increase humidity, a control valve for adding oxygen, and access ports for nursing care. It may also contain a servo control to help regulate incubator air temperature.

**Intensive Care Incubators**

The Intensive Care Incubator 100 has been designed to provide the safest and most stable environment for critically ill neonates. The large front opening of the INC 100 provides access for major procedures and easy removal of the baby. The bed may be tilted to 8 degrees at either end [130].

Features of Intensive Care Incubator 200: clear, visibility, double wall canopy to reduce heat loss, unique side doors open from sides, in-built weighing scales temperature, servo humidity and servo oxygen controls, color touch screen, motorized bed tilting and height adjustment from both sides, trend display for temperature and rotatable bed.

Warmer Radiant consists of an open tray (where the baby is kept), and the artificial heating is provided by a heating mechanism mounted overhead. The heating mechanism consists of quartz, which produces the desired heat, and a reflecting mechanism to divert the heat to the baby tray. The skin temperature of the baby can be monitored by a temperature measuring knob that is kept continuously attached to the body. The variation in the skin temperature can be seen on a small LCD panel, which continuously shows the body temperature. Radiant warmers are equipped with alarms to indicate the temperature change and hence attract the attention of medical professionals attending to the baby. Radiant Warmers can be manual or automatic, depending on the temperature control. The heat generated and the skin's temperature can be individually seen, but the fundamental difference between these models will be temperature regulation. The automatic model increases the heat output in small predetermined steps to reach at the desired temperature of the body. The device may seem simple to handle, but it is always recommended to have proper training and read the manufacturer's guidelines for persons handling this equipment. It is necessary to regularly clean and disinfect the instrument [335].

The Transport Incubator provides transport of high-risk, premature, critically ill newborns. It is ménage to control air temperature, oxygen concentrations, and relative humidity. Walls of transport incubators are double protectors that permit complete visibility and provide an effective thermal and sound barrier from the environment. Door panels and arm ports provide front and head access. Transport Incubators are designed to operate from one of three sources. If external AC is not available, it switches to external DC; if it is not available, it switches to its external batteries [335] (Fig. 2.52).

All of these incubators serve the same purpose: providing the best possible conditions for an infant needing a specific type of medical care. It is impossible to say that one type is better than the other; they are designed for specific conditions of the newborn.

Because baby incubators are necessary, there are many different kinds, which differ significantly in their construction and manner of operation. However, they all share one common goal: to help sustain the lives of premature babies. In this part, three different types of baby incubators, together with some of their models, will be presented.

### Closed Incubator

Closed-type incubators have a special function in concentrating fresh air after its filtration. Also, it prevents water loss by radiation and being inside a closed environment; the baby is entirely protected from infection. Two models of closed incubators, which display the properties of this type, are:

1. Fanem 1186 Neonatal Incubator
2. C2000 Isolette Infant Incubator

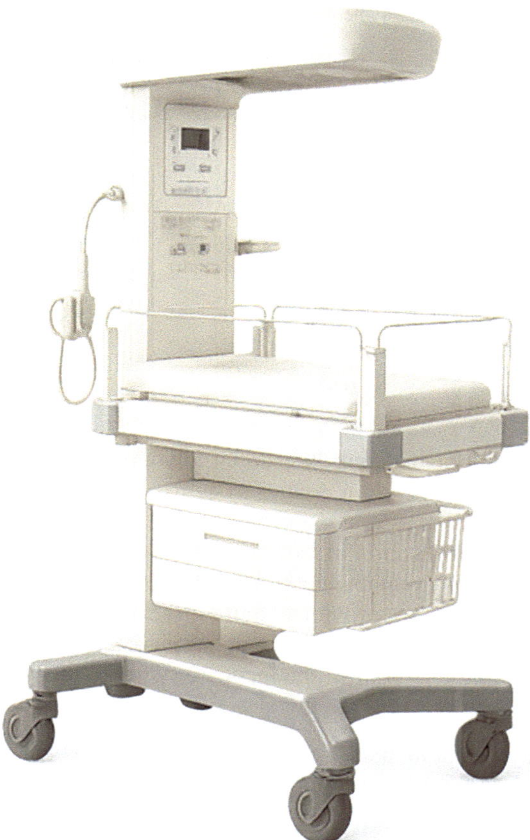

**Fig. 2.52** Radiant warmer

Fanem 1186 Neonatal Incubator

Fanem 1186 Neonatal incubator has been developed to fulfill the most varied requests for models, enabling the assembly from basic equipment to an assortment of optional equipment. This incubator provides easy interaction and lets the user control all operating parameters. There are three kinds of control panels:

(a) Intensive care incubator with the possibility to install all of the available features
(b) Intermediary incubator with an LED display
(c) Basic incubator equipped only with air and skin control and an LED display

The Fanem 1186 Neonatal incubator has the following purposes (Table 2.14):

- Effective insulation of the newborn with respect to the contaminant agents that are transported through the air. This insulation is performed by supplying micro-filtered air to the incubator.

**Table 2.14** Electrical specifications of Fanem 1186 Neonatal Incubator

| | |
|---|---|
| Feeding tension | 127 V ~ or 220 V ~ or 240 V |
| Network frequency | 50/60 Hz |
| Nominal current | 5A-127 V~/3A-220 and 240 V~ |
| Scape current | <100 μA |
| Inlet power | |
| LED panel with no options | 300 W |
| LCD panel with options | 350 W |
| Network outlet power | 150 W (each switch) |
| Motor group power | 50 W |
| Humidifier group power | 120 W |
| Ergometric support power | 180 W |
| Rechargeable battery | 9 V |

- The newborn is warmed using controlled air circulation and uniform distribution of heat. Two possible temperature control systems are internal air temperature monitoring and skin temperature monitoring.
- Enabling ambient humidification in two possible manners: through a humidity passive system or through an integrated micro control active system.
- An integrated pulse oximeter provides continuous, noninvasive monitoring of arterial oxygen saturation and pulse frequency of patients.
- Weight monitoring in the interior of the incubator without the need to move the patient from the incubator or handle it.

The integrated alarming system in the Fanem 1186 is presented by five LEDs whose sounds may be inhibited for 15 min by pressing the "INHIBIT SOUND" key. Five alarms are as follows:

- The Power Failure Alarm is audiovisual. It indicates that the electric power is cut off, the cable is disconnected, or the fuse located on the lateral panel is out.
- The Lack of Ventilation Alarm is audiovisual and indicates that the air flow is interrupted in case of an obstruction in the air ventilation duct. Activation of this alarm triggers the interruption of warming.
- The Sensor Missing Alarm is audiovisual and indicates when the patient sensor plug is disconnected from the lateral panel switch, or in case of sensor failure, when the sensor wire is broken or in a short circuit, the sensor will become detached from the patient's skin.
- The High-Temperature Alarm actuates in three different situations: when the mode selection is at air, when the mode selection is at skin, and when the dome air safety is at high temperature.
- The Low Temperature Alarm is triggered in two different conditions: when the mode selection is in air and when the mode selection is in skin.

**Table 2.15** Electrical specifications of different types of Isolette Infant Incubator

| | |
|---|---|
| Power requirements of an incubator with a fixed height pedestal stand (100 V and 120 V model) | 100 V/120 V ± 10%, 50/60 Hz, 630 W maximum |
| Power requirements of an incubator with a variable height adjustable pedestal stand (100 V and 120 V models) | 100 V/120 V ± 10%, 50/60 Hz, 1900 W maximum |
| Power requirements of an incubator with a fixed height and or a variable height adjustable pedestal stand (220 V and 240 V models) | 220 V or 240 V ± 10%, 50/60 Hz, 500 W maximum |
| Convenience outlets (100 V and 120 V models) | 100 V/120 V ± 10%, 50/60 Hz, 500 W maximum |
| Convenience outlets (220 V and 240 V models) | 220 V or 240 V, 500 W maximum |
| Chassis current leakage (110 V and 120 V models) | 300 μA or less |
| Chassis current leakage (220 V and 240 V models) | 500 μA or less |

### C2000 Isolette Infant Incubator

The Model C2000 Isolette Infant Incubator provides a therapeutic environment for low birth-weight neonates. The Model C2000 Isolette Infant Incubator provides the following features (Table 2.15):

- Data trending—The unit graphically trends critical data, such as air temperature, skin temperature, heater power, oxygen, and humidity, for intervals of 12 to 24 h, and up to 7 days for weight changes.
- Thermal performance—The unit's thermal management capabilities include a patented dual-air curtain that reduces radiant heat loss from the infant by warming the surface of the inner hood.
- Bi-directional airflow minimizes temperature fluctuations within the incubator when the access door is opened.
- Low operating sound levels ensure a developmentally supportive environment for infants.
- Centralized care for multiple births allows the caregiver to track multiple births.
- Integrated X-ray cassette tray is located beneath the mattress.
- The front-side access makes infant access easier, enabling two clinicians to care for the baby while it is still in the incubator.
- Servo-controlled Oxygen simplifies oxygen delivery by selecting and controlling whole-hood oxygen concentrations from 21% to 65%.
- Servo-controlled humidity—The front-loading humidity reservoir requires filling only once every 24 h. The caregiver can set the desired humidity, minimizing the infant's evaporative heat loss.
- The remote monitoring feature enables the user to view all patient parameters on a nearby monitor or a central monitoring system.

- System alarms on the C2000 Isolette Infant Incubator:The power failure alarm is activated to signal the complete failure of the electrical power or inadvertent disconnection from the power source.
- The motor failure alarm is activated when the fan motor's speed falls outside specified tolerances for a period greater than 40 s.
- Various controller failure alarms are triggered when one or more controllers fail in their functions.
- Two types of heater failure alarms are triggered when the heater thermocouple voltage exceeds ±40 mV, and the other is triggered when the heater thermocouple wires are open or shorted.
- Sensor disconnect alarm is activated when the communication with the sensor module fails
- Sensor Out of Position alarm occurs when the sensor module is not in the hood or calibration position.
- The stuck key alarm is activated when a stuck key is detected.
- Skin Mode Disabled alarm occurs when the controller is configured for Air only operation, when the Skin mode is selected.
- The failure of various sensors triggers Various Sensor Module Failure alarms.
- Temperature-specific alarms are triggered by one of the sensors detecting unusual temperature values.
- Humidity Specific Alarm occurs when the humidity has not risen to a predetermined threshold within a designated time. The most likely cause for triggering this alarm is a low water level in the humidifier.
- Oxygen-specific alarms are activated when the displayed oxygen level is either 3% above or 3% below the oxygen set point. Another cause can be a difference in oxygen readings above 3%, which results in interruption of the oxygen flow into the system. Two oxygen-specific alarms are related to the malfunction of the parts providing oxygen to the incubator.
- Special types of alarms are UPS alarms, which are signaled with an audible indication generated by the UPS system. These alarms are related to AC supply failure, low battery, and system fault.

### Open Box Incubator

In open box incubators, the infant is placed on a bed with no particulate special features besides that a radiant warmer can be attached if the child depends on warming. This incubator does not provide a thermoneutral environment if the lids are opened often. Also, it does not filter the air. Its only advantage is that it is easy to handle the baby in this incubator [336]. The model that presents the characteristics of open box incubators is the Ohmeda Giraffe OmniBed.

**Table 2.16** Electrical properties of the Giraffe OmniBed

| | |
|---|---|
| Electrical power | 115 V-50/60 Hz |
| Radiant heater | Approximately 430 W |
| Patient measurement accuracy | ±0.3 °C between 30 °C and 42 °C |
| Air velocity | <10 cm/s |
| Sound level | <50 dBa |
| Humidifier reservoir capacity | 1000 mL |
| Servo Oxygen control display range | Up to 65% |
| Battery | 9 V NiMH |

### Ohmeda Giraffe OmniBed

The Ohmeda Giraffe OmniBed is an incubator and infant radiant warmer in one device. A touch of the switch converts it from an incubator to a radiant warmer.

- Features of the Giraffe OmniBed are (Table 2.16):The rotating mattress allows the clinician to rotate the mattress 360° and enables optimal patient access.
- Centralized display/control unit is accessible from either side of the bed and enables tracking of all equipment and patient parameters.
- Integrated trending for control settings, thermal parameters, and baby weight provides significant data for the physicians.
- The integrated radiant warming system heats the mattress without heating the caregiver. This type of warming enables heating of the baby at all times, even while taking an X-ray.
- Servo-controlled humidifiers provide humidity up to 95%.
- The optional servo oxygen control system maintains a controlled oxygen environment from 21 to 65% and can react quickly during surgical interventions.
- The optional in-bed scale with weight trending enables tracking the baby's weight without removing it from the bed.
- Pressure diffusing mattress promotes improved clinical efficiency.
- Unique Comfort Zone provides a neutral thermal environment by best-practice thermos-regulation.

- Alarm system of the Giraffe OmniBed:High Air Temperature alarm is triggered when the measured temperature exceeds the previously set temperature by more than 1.5 °C.
- The Low Air temperature alarm is triggered when the compartment's temperature falls 3.0 °C below the previously set temperature.
- A fan failure alarm is triggered when the fan is missing or malfunctioning, which leads to the conclusion that there is inadequate airflow.
- A malfunction of the air probe triggers the Air Probe Disconnect or Air Probe failure alarm.
- Check that the Baby alarm is triggered when the radiant heater has been running on 100% for over 12 min.
- Power Failure alarm is triggered when the power to the unit is cut off.

- Service alarms indicate that a repair is required, but the OmniBed can still be used by changing the operating mode. Some service alarms are: Radiant Heater Failure, Heater Doors Not Closed, Canopy Pedal Failure, Bed Up Pedal Failure, Bed Down Pedal Failure, Bed Heater Failure, Motor Drive Failure.
- The option alarms are related to the humidifier and include the Add Water alarm, the Water Reservoir Not Engaged alarm, the Humidity Probe Failure alarm, and the Humidity Failure alarm.

## Transport Incubators

The transport incubator is used for the transport of high-risk, premature, low birth-weight, or critically ill newborns. It is equipped with means to control air, temperature, oxygen concentrations, and relative humidity. Arm ports and door panels allow easy access to the newborn. The model that describes the mechanical properties of this type of incubator is the Isolette TI500.

### Isolette TI500 Incubator

This incubator can be defined as a self-contained, mobile intensive care unit.

- Features of the Isolette TI500 are (Table 2.17):Constant air temperature is maintained through a double wall design, reducing radiant heat loss from the infant during transport.
- Integral humidity pad minimizes the infant's evaporative heat loss by providing 50 to 70% humidity in the hood for up to 12 h.
- The controller is based on a display that is easily read at any distance during transport. All of the essential information about the infant's health status and device status are shown.
- Flexible power sources, including both AC and DC power supplies, make this incubator special. The switchover from DC to AC is based on whether there is an available alternating current source.

**Table 2.17** Technical specifications of Isoltee TI500

| | |
|---|---|
| External power requirements | 110 V/120 V AC, 50/60/400 Hz, 270 W<br>220 V/240 V AC, 50/60/400 Hz, 270 W |
| Internal battery voltage | 12 V DC nominal |
| Operating temperature range | 10 °C to 30 °C |
| Relative humidity range | 0% to 95%, non-condensing |
| Mattress air velocity | 20 cm/s |
| The carbon dioxide level within the hood | <0.5% in normal conditions |
| Oxygen concentration | From 21% to 58% |
| Noise level | <60 dBa |

- Access is made easy through the front access door, head door, or port access doors. An iris port and six tubing ports offer ventilator tubing support and entry possibilities for sensors while keeping the temperature stable.
- Integrated exam light provides equal distribution of light all over the mattress.
- The incubator is designed to fit into small spaces, and the system weight is reduced to enhance mobility and ease access in and out of emergency transport vehicles.

- Alarm system in Isolette TI500:High temperature alarm is signaled when the incubator temperature is equal to or greater than 39 °C ± 0.5 °C.
- High heater temperature indicates that the heater temperature has exceeded 77 °C. When this occurs, the heater and heater indicator turn off.
- Airflow indicator signals an alarm, which means that the fan impeller has stopped rotating or is missing.
- A low DC indicator alarm means that the incubator DC power source has fallen below a predetermined value.
- A power failure alarm means that the AC power is lost, and the device does not have a DC or internal battery.

## 2.10.4 *Clinical Applications*

Premature babies are not fully equipped to deal with life in our world. Their little bodies still have underdeveloped parts that include: lungs, digestive system, immune system, and skin. Most premature babies are born with a weight that is less than normal. They usually find it really hard to adjust to the new environment after being delivered [337]. And that is mainly why they are always at risk of having different infections. Infants who are placed in the incubator are:

- Premature babies who were born underdeveloped and who are not able to endure all the conditions outside the womb. This is why they require extra help and care.
- Infants who suffer from illnesses, ailments, or infections. They require intensive monitoring and care. They are kept in special infant incubators for recovery and safeguarding from other disorders.
- Infants with low birth weight are newborns who are underweight and therefore sensitive to diseases and extremely weak. They are placed into baby incubators in order to monitor their health.

### Care of the Newborn

Methods of feeding depend on the premature newborn's individual needs. We have a division on:

- Intravenous lines: These lines carry nutrition directly into the baby's bloodstream. They are used for premature babies who have immature digestive systems and are unable to suck, swallow and breathe normally. This method is sometimes used when treatment for other health complications is being implemented.
- Umbilical catheter: This painless method involves a tube being surgically placed into a vessel of the umbilical cord. It is normally used only in the most critical cases.
- Oral and nasal feeding: This method utilizes a narrow, flexible tube that is threaded through the nose or mouth. It is a solution for babies who are ready to digest breast milk but are not yet able to suck.
- Central line: This is an intravenous line inserted into a vein, often in the arm, to allow the use of a larger vein.

There are additional ways to provide care for a baby in the intensive care incubator. Both the mother and father are encouraged to interact with their baby. Some of the suggestions are:

1. Touch the baby as much as possible. You can do this by using a gentle touch and stroking motions.
2. Talk to the baby because the baby can recognize parents' voices and be comforted by hearing you.
3. Change diapers.
4. Participate in your baby's first bath.
5. Take your baby's temperature.

**BabyBloom**

Up to now, incubators' design hasn't changed its fundamental function; its appearance, ease, and comfort in use, until the BabyBloom was created. The BabyBloom incubator for babies has been designed using the input of many doctors, nurses, technical staff, and parents of incubator children by the engineer Heleen. Together with her brother-in-law Jeroen van den Hout, she founded BabyBloom. The BabyBloom protects the baby under an innovative integrated shield that reduces noise and light. It also has a very silent working climate system and keeps the environment around the baby quiet. The three side panels and the two smaller observation windows in the hood can be opened or closed independently, allowing a balance between protection and observation of the child's condition.

- BabyBloom offers:The look that is not overwhelming and discomforting to the parents. Its friendly design, colors, and patterns ease parents, thereby indirectly positively affecting their child. The noise and light protective hood is hygienic, can be delivered in different colors and patterns, and can even be designed to fit a specific neonatology ward.

- The possibility to place the incubator over a hospital bed where the mother can be in very close contact with her child.
- The extensive height adjustment; it can be positioned much higher and lower than other incubators. It also offers much legroom underneath. It is the first incubator where any person, regardless of their status, can work sitting or standing in an ideal ergonomic position.
- Advanced accessibility. The patient can be reached from three sides, and the sides can be opened in two parts for regular or extensive access. The complete light and noise protective hood can be removed with a single press of a button.
- An extra-large viewing plane and rubberless doors enable the staff to make clear observation of the child and make eye contact between parents and child.
- A built-in camera to observe the child on a display from a remote location, like the nurses' desk, a computer at home, or even on a mobile phone.
- User-friendly interface that's very intuitive in use. Designed to simplify user interaction, maximize safety, and be self-teaching and easy to remember. Can be adapted to any language.

## Milestones the Newborn Must Pass

While they're in the newborn intensive care unit, premature babies have several milestones to meet before they are allowed to go home with their parents. Before the incubator is discharged, premature babies need to be able to do the following:

1. Breathe Without Oxygen

One of the first milestones that many premature babies meet is being able to keep their oxygen saturation high without needing extra oxygen or other respiratory support. Many preemies need some kind of respiratory support soon after birth. Some babies may need only extra oxygen. Babies who are very small or are born very early are at risk for a chronic condition called bronchopulmonary dysplasia.

2. Take All Feedings by Mouth

Premature babies are not as strong as full-term babies and aren't able to coordinate sucking and swallowing until about 32–34 weeks gestational age. Most premature babies are initially fed with total parenteral nutrition, and they are fed through a feeding tube until they're strong enough to drink from the breast or a bottle. Before babies can be discharged from the incubator, they should eat from a bottle well enough to gain weight and have a feeding schedule. This usually happens around 37 weeks gestational age, although some babies, but those with severe respiratory problems, may take longer.

3. Pass Various Tests

Baby might have to pass a blood test, as well as a hearing test before discharge. Doctors may also want to administer a "car seat test" to check your baby's heart and breathing while the baby sits in a car seat.

4. Maintain a Stable Temperature

Most premature babies must first sleep in an incubator to stay warm. An incubator is an apparatus with an enclosed, clear dome with a heated platform on which babies lie. Premature babies cannot keep themselves warm as well as full-term babies and will get too cold if they are not skin to skin in kangaroo care or kept in an incubator. Staying warm outside an incubator and sleeping in a crib is a significant milestone that preemies must meet before leaving the incubator. It is a milestone based on weight more than gestational age, and most babies can keep themselves warm by the time they weigh about four pounds. While the baby is in the incubator, it must wear a nappy and a hat. Baby needs a hat because they can lose so much body heat through their head.

## Premature Babies at Increased Risk of Depression and Anxiety

Some research has provided evidence that children who are born prematurely are at a higher risk for behavioral problems and even attention-deficit hyperactivity disorder. However, until now, there has been little evidence suggesting that these children are also more vulnerable to mood disorders and mental health problems later in life. According to a new study of Psychology at Melbourne in Australia, children born prematurely and with low birth weights are three and a half times more likely to develop mental health problems such as depression and anxiety. Children born prematurely are already at increased risk for physical health problems, learning disabilities, and other cognitive challenges. In order to examine the relationship between low birth weights and mental health problems, Burnett analyzed previous studies and looked specifically at prematurity, low birth weight, and how it influenced the development of anxiety and depression in adolescence and young adulthood. Burnett discovered that children who were born prematurely and had low birth weights had a significantly higher risk than normal birth weight babies for the development of psychiatric problems later in life. The results of this study have significant clinical implications. Burnett believes that professionals treating the physical and cognitive impairments in low birthweight children should be aware of the negative psychological predisposition that these children possess. Also, coauthor Richard E. Tremblay, a professor of psychology, researches this theme. He stated: "In mammals, separation between mother and child after birth has always been considered a major stressor that can cause behavioral problems well into adulthood". Researchers found that [338]:

- Of the 16.5% of babies placed in incubators, only 5% suffered major depression by age 21.
- Among participants who were not placed in incubators, 9% developed depression, which is the average rate for the general society.
- Correlation between decreased depression and incubator care remained after factoring in participant age, weight at birth, family adversity, or maternal depression.

## 2.10.5 Regulatory Considerations

### FDA

Federal law (Federal Food, Drug, and Cosmetic Act, section 513) defines a classification system of medical devices based on the risk of their usage. There are three regulatory classes in which all of the medical devices are classified in. Class I, Class II, and Class III are medical devices based on the level of control necessary to provide reasonable assurance that they are effective and safe to use. Class I medical devices are subject to the least regulatory control, Class II are subjected to intermediate regulatory control, and Class III devices are subject to the strictest regulatory control. They are briefly defined as:

- Class I (low to moderate risk): general controls
- Class II (moderate to high risk): General Controls and Special Controls
- Class III (high risk): general controls and Premarket Approval (PMA)

Incubators are classified as Class II medical devices, meaning that they are subjected to both General and Special Controls.

General Controls

General controls are regulatory requirements authorized by the FD&C (Federal Drug and Cosmetics) Act, under sections 501, 502, 510, 516, 518, and 520. All devices are subjected to general control unless regulations exempt them. If a particular device is indeed exempted from one of the general controls, that exemption must be stated in the classification regulation for that device. General controls are described in particular sections of the FD&C Act:

501: Adulterated devices
502: Misbranded devices
510: Registration of producers of devices

- Establishment registration and device listing
- Premarket Notification (510k)
- Reprocessed single-use devices

516: Banned devices
518: Notifications and other remedies

- Notification
- Repair
- Replacement
- Refund
- Reimbursement
- Mandatory recall

519: Records and reports on devices

- Adverse event report
- Device tracking
- Unique device identification system
- Reports of removals and corrections

520: General provisions respecting control of devices intended for human use

- Custom device
- Restricted device
- Good manufacturing practice requirements
- Exemptions for devices for investigational use
- Transitional provisions for devices considered as new drugs
- Humanitarian device exemption

#### Special Controls

Special controls are reserved for class II medical devices. The FDA classifies devices as Class II if the general controls alone are insufficient to reasonably ensure the device is effective. They are different from class III devices because exceptional control provides enough assurance that the device is safe and effective. Special controls are specific for each device and include:

- Performance standards
- Postmarket surveillance
- Patient registries
- Special labeling requirements
- Premarket data requirements
- Guidelines

#### Premarket Approval

Premarket approval is reserved only for class III medical devices. Devices not within a type marketed before the Medical Device Amendments of 1976—referred to as pre-amendment devices—are classified into class III automatically under federal law (Medical Device Calibration Program, 2016). Class III medical devices also include the devices constructed to sustain human life, prevent the impairment of human health, or present a potential unreasonable risk of illness or injury. For these devices, it is insufficient to be subjected to general and special control.

## IEC and ISO

IEC (International Electro technical Commission) and ISO (International Organization for Standardization) discuss the following topics in their classification of medical equipment:

- Materials of construction
- Engineering diagrams
- Mode of operations
- Power source
- Heating and cooling mechanism
- Air-controlled versus baby-controlled
- Supplementary gas connectors
- Functionality
- Physical durability and robustness
- Environmental conditions for proper operations
- Performance
- Temperature control
- Accuracy
- Rise Time
- Variability
- Undershoot/Overshoot
- Air Flow
- Velocity
- Flow rates
- Supplementary Gas Control
- Connectors
- Mixing/Concentrations
- Safety features
- Weight capacity
- Electrical
- Restraints
- Alarms
- Fire protection
- Sensors
- Lockout

## Standardization

Standards for incubators that the FDA recognizes:

- IEC 601–2-19 Amendment I Medical Electrical Equipment—Part 2: Particular Requirements for Safety of Baby Incubators
- IEC 601–2-20 Medical Electrical Equipment—Part 2: Particular Requirements for Safety of Transport Incubators

- ISO 10993-1: 1992 Biological Evaluation of Medical Devices—Part 1: Evaluation and Testing

The FDA has not recognized the following draft standards, but they provide helpful guidance for these devices:

- AAMI 1151-D-1994 Transport Infant Incubator (Draft Standard)
- AAMI/CDV-1 II36 1997 Infant Incubator (Draft Standard)

The CDRH (Center for Devices and Radiological Health) does not have to recognize the standards mentioned above.

## Verification and Calibration

Validation and Verification

The process of validation and verification of all medical equipment ought to be made. Validation ensures that there is objective evidence that the device meets the user's needs and intended uses. Tests, inspections, and analysis do validation. The validation target is to ensure that a medical device's user needs are met and that it consistently provides the intended medical benefit in real-time use. Verification is tightly connected to validation, and it ensures that there is objective evidence that the specified requirements are met.
When it comes to verification and validation, specialized human factor testing techniques, such as formative and summative testing, are used. The two standards that provide guidance for the overall usability engineering process, as well as design techniques, are:

- ISO's IEC 62366:2007 "Medical Devices—Application of Usability Engineering to Medical Devices"
- AAMI's ANSI/AAMI HE75: 2009's "Human Factors Engineering—Design of Medical Devices".

Verification and validation cover all phases of product development and many different technologies. For example: electronics, fluids, mechanical/physical, thermal systems, electromechanical product evaluation, biological aspects, instrumentation, etc. The most important stage for considering verification and calibration is the design stage, when the product's requirements and specifications are being developed. For example, adding test points on circuit boards, having accessible connectors, providing data storage/retrieval capabilities, and making products modular can enhance the ability to test a product, which saves time and money.

Incubator Verification

While manufacturing an incubator, the producer must ensure that the device is suitable for use in reference conditions.
Referent conditions are as follows:

- Voltage source: 220–240 V AC, 50 Hz,
- Ambient:
  - Temperature: 20–35 °C,
  - Pressure: 600 hPa—1060 hPa,
  - Relative humidity: 10–95% without condensation.

The incubator sensors have to have the following measurement ranges:

- Air temperature: 13–42 °C
- Skin temperature: 13–43 °C
- Oxygen: 18–99 Vol.%
- Relative humidity 10–99%
- Mass: 0–10 kg.

The metrology requirements include the boundaries of error, which are as follows:

- Air temperature: ± 0.8 °C
- Skin temperature: ± 0.3 °C
- Oxygen: ± 3 Vol.%
- Relative humidity: ± 10%
- Mass:
  - ± 2% for mass from 0 to 2 kg
  - ± 5% for mass from 2 to 10 kg.

If the measurement error in any of the previously mentioned cases is greater than the maximum allowed error, then the incubator must not be used and must be subjected to additional verification. After putting the baby in the incubator, all of the necessary life-sustaining parameters are set up on the device control, and the monitoring values of those parameters are shown on the monitor, which is a basic part of the incubator.

Incubators must be constructed so that, in normal conditions, they guarantee protection against electric shock, overheating, and dust entering the housing of measuring devices. All of the parts of the incubator that are subject to corrosion have to be efficiently protected. That protection must be made of stainless steel.

Incubators must have a tile that displays the following:

- Manufacturer name or label
- Serial number and the year of production
- Label of the measurand type
- Official label of the measurand type

Incubators must pass the validation and verification procedure before first usage. Also, certificates of approval and verification must be obtained before placing the device on the market. Measurand type inspection is performed based on documentation that the manufacturer must supply with approval. Documentation must contain:

1. General, technical, and other documentation related to compatibility with other standards
2. User manual, which includes:
   (a) General information and description of the device with its parts
   (b) Description and function of programmable equipment if the device is equipped with a microprocessor.

The first verification includes a visual inspection of every measurement to ensure compatibility with the approved type. It is performed with the corresponding instruments according to the standard. The maximal error in regular verifications must not be above the maximal allowed error in the first verification. The same inspection resources must be used in both first and regular verifications. The law defines periods of verification.

Besides previously explained verification, the electromagnetic compatibility of the device, harmonized standards IEC 60601-2-19, IEC 60601-2-20, IEC 60601-2-21, and valid law acts have to be taken into account for final approval of the device [48].

Calibration

**Incubator Calibration**

The parameters for the quality of neonatal incubators must comply with the IEC 60601-2-19 "Particular requirements for the safety of neonatal incubators" standard. This standard determines the acceptable range of variations regarding the environment in the neonatal incubator, including temperature, humidity, velocity of air flow, and noise level.

According to this standard, five positions inside the incubator measure temperature and relative humidity. The measurement plane has to be placed 10 cm above the incubator mattress, and a set of five measurement points must exist. The five temperature sensors must be pointed in positions A, B, C, D, and E, while the humidity sensor must be positioned at A, the central point.

According to IEC 60601-2-19, the sensors must be correctly positioned, and six steps must be followed to calibrate the incubator. The steps are:

- The environment temperature must be between 21 °C and 26 °C while testing.
- The incubator temperature control must be set to 11 °C above the environment temperature. The incubator must reach the specified temperature control time with a tolerance of up to 20%. The incubator sensor measures the temperature control.

- The incubator temperature control must be adjusted to two operational points, for example, 32 °C and 36 °C. Stabilization of temperature conditions must be waited for. The measured incubator temperature at point A must not vary more than 1 °C within 1 h.
- The average temperature measured by the sensors at points A, B, C, D, and E in the previous step may not vary by more than 0.8 °C from the average temperature in the incubator within the 1 h. The average temperature cannot differ more than ±1.5 °C from the incubator control temperature. The average temperature of the incubator is obtained by measuring temperatures at regular intervals.
- With the incubator temperature at 32 °C, the temperature control reference in steady state should be set at 26 °C. Verify that the overshoot is below 2 °C and that the setting is reached in <15 min.
- The humidity value shown by the incubator sensor must not differ by more than 13% of the value measured by the sensor at position A during the entire functioning period.

### *2.10.6 Future Perspectives*

Modern days have provided humanity with a variety of innovations that have been shaped to make life better. One of the purposes of medical devices is to provide humans with modern and efficient medical care. Infants are the most sensitive human beings, and caring for them is important. The number of premature deliveries has increased dramatically, and therefore, there is a need for developing a life-sustaining machine for these babies. That machine is an incubator that brings about an "artificial mother's womb", meaning that it mimics the environment of the womb. This is of high importance for babies who do not possess sufficiently developed organs and organ systems to deal with standard environmental conditions. Therefore, these babies are placed in the incubator where the temperature, humidity, pressure, and oxygen levels are set based on their needs.
Incubators have provided mankind with the ability to sustain the life of premature infants and increase the life expectancy of babies who have to undergo various operative procedures in their early days. The incubator acts as an ICU for babies as it is sealed and protects the infant from all of the outer influences. However, the incubator has some risks regarding the mental state of adults placed in the incubator in their childhood. They tend to be more susceptible to depression and anxiety because they were deprived of parental care while being in the incubator. When realizing that risk, obstetricians now tend to provide the baby with as much contact with the family as possible [72].

When considering the engineering aspect of the incubator, it is possible to say that the incubators have evolved significantly. From the first incubator, where a few infants were warmed over a hot-water reservoir attached to an external heating source, to highly sophisticated incubators, where the procedure of controlling the environment is digitized and monitoring the baby's state is possible at all times. The unbreakable bond of engineering and medicine is displayed in the incubator, as in all other medical devices. The obstetricians have defined the need for a container that will be able to sustain the life of infants, and the engineers have developed such a container. The continuous improvements are aimed at developing an incubator that provides the baby with a suitable environment and enables easy handling [266, 339].

Incubators are classified as Class II medical devices, based on the controlling necessity of the device. Incubators are subjected to general and special controlling procedures before being placed on the market. When taking that along with thoroughness and strictness of the medical inspection, it is possible to say that incubators are very delicate, and care must be taken of every part of the controlling mechanism. When comparing three basic types of infant incubators, it is possible to say that every incubator performs its purpose in the best possible way. It is impossible to say that, for example, the open-box type is less efficient than the closed-box type. It is designed to serve a distinct purpose and to help an infant with a specific condition.

## 2.11 Surgical Devices

The last two decades have witnessed surgery revolutionized. Drastic change is not incremental development; it is a real move away from the past. Two are particularly notable. Firstly, there has been significant progress in medical imaging. Secondly, surgical tools have become ever more precise. Together, these two have driven surgery into a new era. This is not an incremental or step-by-step improvement; it is a substantial move in the right direction. The underlying reason for all this progress is self-evident: improved results. That means more accurate procedures, fewer complications, and less invasive techniques.

New imaging methods give surgeons more precise details about the body. They can even specify how tissues are functioning. This enables physicians to plan and conduct surgeries with greater accuracy. At the same time, better equipment enables surgeons to perform delicate procedures with more control. In this, robotics has played a key role in the development of surgery. It provides better control, stability, and accuracy. Robotic systems utilize imaging data from MRI and CT scans to guide tools to the target location. This requires smart software, intuitive interfaces, and accurate sensors to translate what can be seen in the scans into real-time events. Minimally invasive surgery nowadays relies ever more on remotely operated robotic instruments controlled by surgeons. They allow surgeries inside the body using minor cuts. To operate in such confined spaces, the instruments need to be intelligently designed and equipped with sophisticated sensors. Robotic systems are currently applied to a majority of surgical fields. In neurosurgery, they guide instruments for brain biopsies while minimizing harm to adjacent tissues. In orthopedic surgery, robots assist in accurately sculpting the bones during hip replacement operations. Robotics is also on the horizon for heart surgery, eye surgery, and in simulating and training would-be surgeons.

Despite tremendous early success, some challenges persist. Surgeons require time and training to learn new systems. The machinery is expensive. It also requires thorough testing to ensure it is safe and optimal for patients [340].

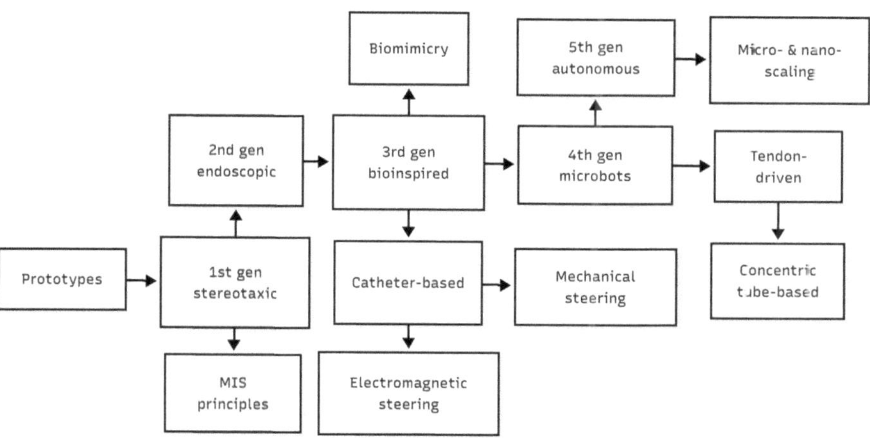


**Fig. 2.53** Five generations of robots

## 2.11.1 *History*

The history of development of medical robots is depicted in Fig. 2.53).

### Historical Trajectory and Foundational Origins

The development of robotics began with mechanical devices designed to handle simple tasks. One of the earliest documented examples is Archytas' steam-powered "Flying Pigeon," created in the fourth century BCE. Another notable invention was Heron of Alexandria's three-wheeled cart, dating back to the first century. The term "robot" did not appear until much later—it was introduced in 1920 by the writer Karel Čapek and is derived from a Slavic word meaning "forced labor." The concept gained broader recognition in the 1940s, mainly due to the writings of Isaac Asimov. By the 1960s, the field of robotics experienced rapid growth, driven in part by the momentum of the Space Race. This period saw robotics branching into medical applications, particularly in procedures that require extreme accuracy, such as brain biopsies. An early step in this direction was the development of an electromagnetic guidance system in 1967. However, it was not until the late 1980s that robotic systems were sufficiently advanced for practical use in surgical settings.

### First Generation

The first robotic system used in surgery was the PUMA 200, introduced in 1985 to assist with needle placement during brain biopsies. Around the same period, surgeons also performed the first laparoscopic cholecystectomy, marking a significant shift toward minimally invasive techniques. Following the PUMA system, more

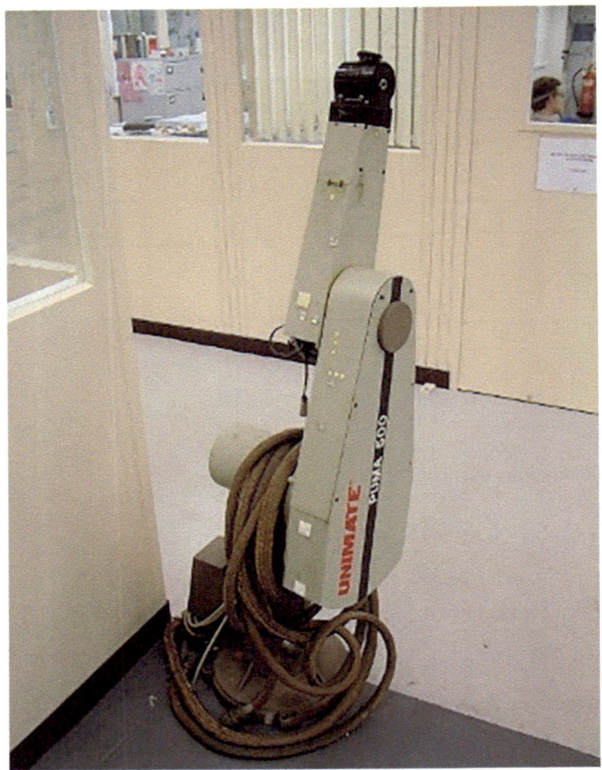


**Fig. 2.54** PUMA 200 (https://commons.wikimedia.org/wiki/File:UNIMATE_PUMA_200_Robot_Arm_(6202074072).jpg)

specialized platforms, such as Neuromate, were developed to support neurosurgical procedures.

In orthopedic surgery, robotic tools such as SCARA, ROBODOC, and AcroBot were designed to assist in joint replacement operations. These systems operated under a master-slave model, where the surgeon remained in complete control and the robot executed specific commands. However, early surgical robots had several constraints: they lacked autonomous capabilities, struggled with manipulating soft tissue, and required constant oversight and input from the surgeon (Figs. 2.54 and 2.55).

## Second Generation

The second generation of surgical robots introduced key advancements, particularly the capability to operate on soft tissues with greater precision. One notable example was PROBOT, developed specifically for prostate procedures. As the preference for minimally invasive techniques grew, new systems emerged to overcome the

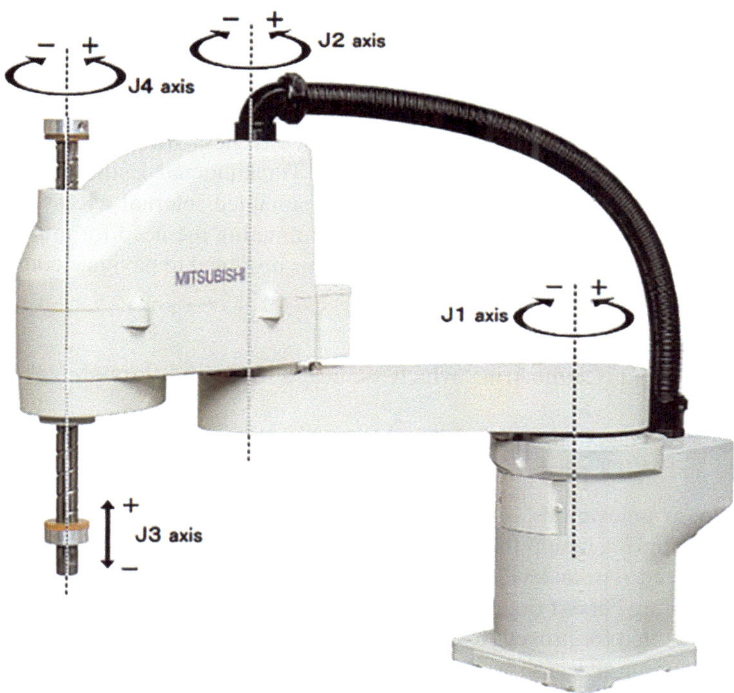


**Fig. 2.55** SCARA robot (https://commons.wikimedia.org/wiki/File:SCARA_robot_2R.png)

limitations of earlier models. Compared to conventional surgical instruments, these robotic platforms provided several advantages:

- Enhanced access to confined anatomical regions such as the pelvic cavity or thoracic space
- Greater precision during intricate tasks like vascular suturing
- Immersive three-dimensional visualization rather than traditional two-dimensional imaging
- Improved instrument dexterity and reduced physical strain on surgeons

Two landmark systems from this period were ZEUS, introduced in 1998, and the da Vinci system, released in 2000. ZEUS played a critical role in pioneering surgeries, including a cardiac procedure in Canada and the first transatlantic remote operation, in which surgeons in New York successfully performed surgery on a patient in France in 2001.

Following a legal conflict, Intuitive Surgical—the developer of the da Vinci system—merged with the company behind ZEUS in 2003. This consolidation solidified da Vinci's position as the dominant robotic surgical system. Other innovative platforms, such as UW Raven and DLR MicroSurge, have contributed additional features, including modular configurations and enhanced haptic feedback, thereby expanding the functional possibilities of robotic-assisted surgery.

## Third Generation

Robotic systems developed during this phase aimed to replicate the natural movements of the human body and introduced more compact, flexible instruments. The primary objective was to further minimize invasiveness in surgical procedures. Emerging techniques such as Natural Orifice Translumenal Endoscopic Surgery (NOTES) and Single Port Laparoscopy (SPL) enabled internal access through a single entry point or natural body openings, eliminating the need for multiple incisions. These advancements relied on robotic arms designed to navigate complex and confined anatomical regions.
Notable systems from this era included:

- i-SNAKE and CardioArm, which achieved mobility through cable-driven mechanisms
- Amigo and Magellan, which utilized steerable catheters for navigation
- Niobe and CGCI, operated using electromagnetic control

Despite these innovations, catheter-based platforms faced challenges in applying precise force during manipulation. To address this limitation, concentric tube robots were introduced. These devices are exceptionally slender and highly flexible, capable of navigating curved trajectories with precision. Their adaptability makes them particularly suited for procedures within narrow passages such as blood vessels and airways. Ongoing research is also evaluating their potential in advanced applications, including fetal diagnostics and imaging.

## Fourth Generation

A breakthrough in the evolution of surgical robotics came with the development of microrobots—miniature machines often just a few millimeters in size. Inspired by concepts once confined to science fiction, such as the 1966 film Fantastic Voyage, these devices have become a reality in modern medicine. One widely used example is the capsule endoscope, like the PillCam (Fig. 2.56), which captures images of the gastrointestinal tract as it naturally travels through the body.

The next generation of microrobots is expected to feature significant advancements, including enhanced mobility, higher-resolution imaging, and magnetic navigation capabilities. Some designs may even mimic the locomotion of small animals,

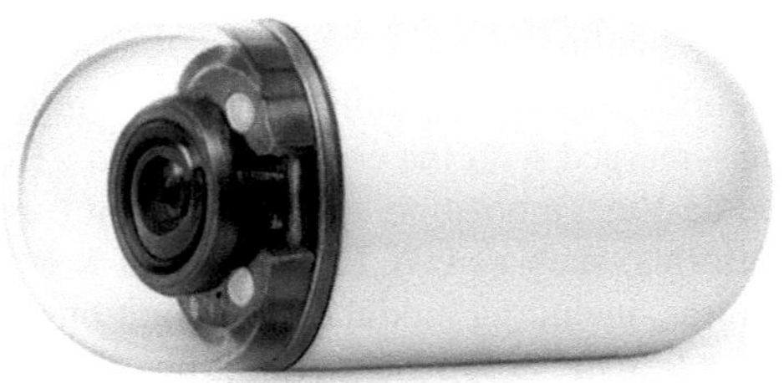

**Fig. 2.56** PillCam capsule

such as fish or insects. In the future, these tiny machines could operate individually or as coordinated swarms, offering highly targeted diagnostics and treatments with extraordinary precision.

#### Fifth Generation

Fifth-generation surgical robots are being designed with the goal of complete autonomy. Unlike previous systems that rely heavily on human input, these advanced platforms are envisioned to operate independently by leveraging artificial intelligence and sophisticated learning algorithms. Their forms may vary widely, from humanoid machines to microscopic swarms capable of navigating the human body. Such robots have the potential to revolutionize both surgical practice and the treatment of complex conditions located deep within the body.

### *2.11.2 Technical Characteristics*

#### Hardware

For research applications, a specialized version of the Da Vinci system, known as the Research Kit, is available. This platform incorporates components from the original Da Vinci model, commonly referred to as the Da Vinci Classic. The kit includes two Master Tool Manipulators (MTMs), two Patient Side Manipulators (PSMs), a high-resolution stereo viewer (HRSV), and a foot pedal interface.

Intuitive Surgical, the company behind the Da Vinci system, has made this kit accessible to various research institutions. However, several components are deliberately excluded. The Research Kit does not come with the proprietary control software or electronics, a decision intended to promote open-source innovation within the research community. As a result, teams develop their own software and control architectures tailored to specific experimental goals. Additionally, the kit lacks other structural and functional elements found in the clinical version of the system, such as the passive setup joints that stabilize the PSMs, the endoscopic camera arm (ECM), the stereo camera, and the external housing and support frame. These omissions allow researchers to focus on software and control development without the constraints of the whole surgical system [341].

#### Software

The Da Vinci Research Kit operates using a centralized computing model, where all core processing tasks are handled on a Linux-based PC. This setup manages data acquisition, servo control loops, and overall robot motion. Hardware communication is established through an IEEE-1394 serial interface, and the system integrates with the Robot Operating System (ROS) for orchestrating various robotic subsystems.

### Low-Level Interface

At the hardware communication level, a C++ library provides direct access to input and output signals via the IEEE 1394 (FireWire) bus, utilizing the Linux library libraw1394. For applications requiring tighter real-time control, an additional driver known as RT Fire can be implemented. Performance tests reveal that the primary source of latency originates from the PC itself, rather than the data link; minor packets experience delays of approximately 30–35 microseconds, while larger packets require slightly more time. Simultaneous transmission and reception can reduce overall delay.
The low-level control is structured around two key classes:

- FireWire port—manages the physical communication port
- AmpIO—handles individual FPGA devices connected to that port

Multiple FPGA boards can share a single FireWire port. During operation, sensor data is read from these boards and stored in memory, while motor commands are transmitted back. Data is stored in numerical formats optimized for FPGA memory constraints.

### Component-Based Control Architecture

The control software is composed of modular components built using the open-source Cisst and SAW libraries. Each module is assigned a specific function, ranging from data I/O and servo control to high-level motion management, and they communicate through well-defined interfaces. Examples include:

- mtsRobotIO1394—interfaces directly with the robot hardware
- Servo modules—issue commands to drive robotic actuators
- Pedal interface—initiates or halts actions based on foot pedal input

All components operate within a single execution thread to maintain precise data synchronization. Two principal modules represent the robotic arms:

- mtsMTM for the Master Tool Manipulator (includes a built-in gripper)
- mtsPSM for the Patient Side Manipulator (supports interchangeable tools like scissors or forceps)

Tools with active end-effectors require dedicated software modules to manage gripping actions.

ROS Interface

ROS is used to facilitate communication between subsystems and across multiple machines when necessary. Although the primary codebase is built on Cisst, a specialized interface allows seamless integration with ROS. This interface publishes robot state information (e.g., joint positions) and subscribes to incoming command messages using ROS-compatible formats. A utility library, sawROS, handles real-time data translation between the two frameworks and operates at a refresh rate of 50 Hz.

Robot models for both MTM and PSM are described using URDF (Unified Robot Description Format), enabling their simulation and visualization within ROS environments. A typical implementation involves using a real MTM and foot pedal to control a simulated PSM in real-time. This flexible framework supports real-time control, simulation, and interoperability across custom and standard robotic tools, making it a robust platform for experimental and developmental research [341].

### 2.11.3 Types of Devices

In conventional surgery, the surgeon is in direct contact with the patient, using handheld tools to manipulate tissues. Sensory feedback in this context is immediate: the surgeon visually inspects the surgical site unaided, physically palpates structures, and receives continuous tactile and force cues through the instruments. Preoperative imaging plays a supporting role, primarily as a mental map that guides intraoperative decisions.

Minimally Invasive Surgery (MIS) redefines this interaction. Rather than working directly on exposed anatomy, the surgeon uses long, slender instruments inserted through small incisions. These tools, often equipped with charge-coupled device (CCD) cameras, transmit images to an external monitor, creating an indirect visual interface. This setup disrupts the surgeon's direct line of sight and significantly reduces haptic feedback, as the instruments increase the physical distance from the target tissues.

Computer-assisted surgical platforms further advance this evolution by embedding intelligence into the surgical process. These systems combine sensor-enabled tools and sophisticated control interfaces that integrate real-time imaging and guidance during surgery. Some provide augmented visualization by superimposing preoperative data on the live operative field, while others dynamically adapt to the surgical environment, adjusting their behavior in response to real-time inputs. Compared to both traditional open surgery and basic minimally invasive surgery (MIS), these technologies introduce more complex interactions between the human and machine, utilizing instrumented tools with built-in sensors and software that align preoperative imaging with intraoperative conditions.

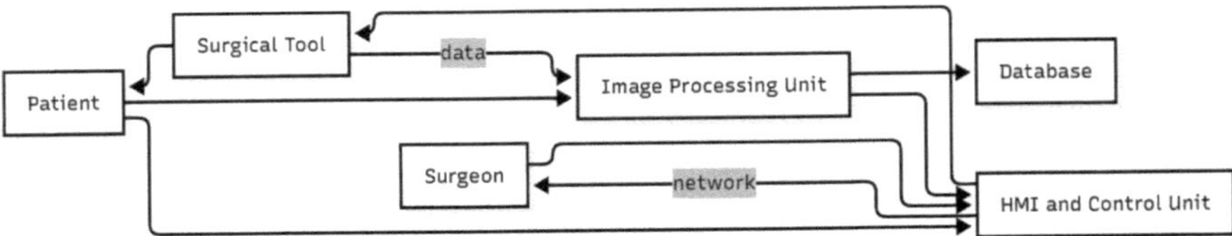


**Fig. 2.57** Block diagram of computer assisted surgery scenario

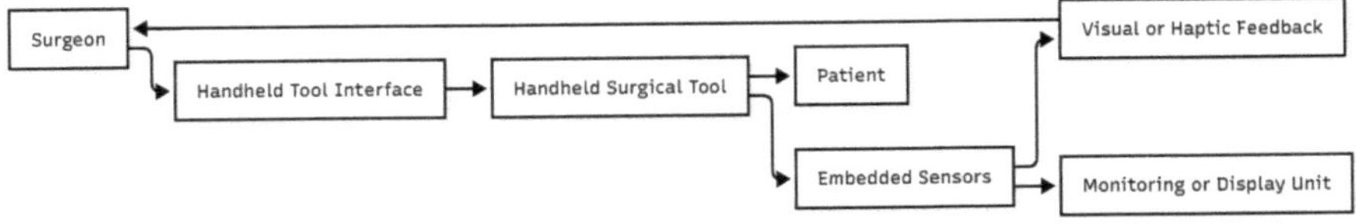


**Fig. 2.58** Block diagram of handheld tools for surgery

This study focuses on robotic surgical systems designed to enhance the accuracy and effectiveness of minimally invasive surgical (MIS) procedures. Three main categories are addressed:

- Handheld robotic instruments that support the surgeon by improving precision, reducing tremor, or enhancing dexterity
- Teleoperated robotic systems, where the surgeon manipulates robotic instruments from a remote console
- Autonomous robotic platforms, capable of executing predefined tasks with varying levels of decision-making ability

These systems are evaluated based on critical features, including their physical dimensions, degrees of freedom (DOF), autonomy level, embedded computational intelligence, and the nature of surgeon-patient interaction. Although CAD/CAM robots are covered in a separate survey within this special issue, the focus here remains on platforms engineered for minimally invasive applications—those designed to make surgical procedures more precise, less traumatic, and better aligned with the complexities of modern operative care [342] (Figs. 2.57 and 2.58).

## Handheld Surgical Tools

Modern handheld robotic tools are increasingly designed with built-in intelligence and autonomous functionalities to assist surgeons during operations. These instruments can correct motion errors, adapt dynamically to the surgical environment, and enhance the precision of manual movements. This category encompasses sensor-equipped catheters, robotic laparoscopic tools, advanced endoscopes, and mechatronic scalpels that offer features like tremor suppression.

### Scientific Instruments: Measurement of Tissue Properties and Surgical Phenomena

A significant subset of handheld robotic devices is dedicated to the intraoperative assessment of tissue properties. Grasping tools integrated with sensors can collect real-time force-deflection data, aiding in tissue modeling and surgical simulation. Instruments such as indentors and tissue stretchers are used to evaluate mechanical properties in situ. Others capture forces and torques at both the tool-tissue and surgeon-tool interfaces, supporting the refinement of robotic systems and contributing to objective assessments of surgical skill.

### Surgical Mechatronics Tools

Although not yet routine in clinical settings, advanced mechatronic tools are being developed to improve tissue interaction. For instance, graspers with sensory feedback can detect pulsations in blood vessels. A force-feedback-enabled grasper designed by Rosen et al. enhances the surgeon's tactile perception. Dario et al. introduced a steerable-tip arthroscopic tool capable of avoiding delicate structures such as cartilage, with contact detection accuracy within 2 mm.

One of the most advanced examples is a tremor-canceling microsurgical instrument developed for ophthalmic surgery. Equipped with six inertial sensors at the distal tip, it detects and suppresses involuntary movements in real time. Evaluations of this device demonstrated a 45% reduction in one-dimensional errors and a 37% improvement in three-dimensional precision.

### Directly Driven Mechanisms

Some robotic systems are designed to modify or constrain the surgeon's hand movements, enhancing control during delicate tasks. The "steady-hand" robot from Johns Hopkins University, for example, stabilizes motion to reduce tremor. Systems may be passive, like those developed by Troccaz, or active, such as Garbini's orthopedic robot, which guides instruments along predefined surgical planes. Salcudean's configuration integrates a force-feedback mechanism and tremor suppression within a tool mounted on a manipulator; however, it does not incorporate motion scaling [342].

## Teleoperated Surgical Tools for Minimal Invasive Surgery

Teleoperation in surgery draws on remote manipulation technologies developed initially in the mid-twentieth century by Goertz for handling hazardous materials. These systems evolved from mechanical linkages to fully electronic platforms, laying the groundwork for surgical telemanipulation. Initially intended for battlefield

use in the 1980s, telesurgical tools were later adapted for civilian minimally invasive procedures.
Telesurgical systems provide enhanced precision in confined anatomical areas and are particularly useful for complex operations such as prostatectomies. They also hold promise for extending expert surgical care to remote or underserved locations. However, challenges remain in ensuring reliable communication networks and emergency responsiveness.

Compared to conventional MIS, teleoperated systems restore critical elements such as fine motor control, depth perception, and ergonomic working conditions. Surgeons control robotic instruments from a console interface, guided by high-resolution, real-time imaging. Early telesurgical robots developed in the 1990s featured dual manipulators with six degrees of freedom and stereoscopic visualization. Today, commercially available systems are utilized in a range of procedures, including cholecystectomies and prostatectomies, with ongoing refinements continually expanding their capabilities [342].

#### Da Vinci System

Developed by Intuitive Surgical, the Da Vinci system is a teleoperated platform designed for minimally invasive surgery (MIS), featuring dual-hand control. Its multi-axis design supports the manipulation of interchangeable instruments, offering three translational degrees of freedom (DOF) and redundant joints that enable optimal tool positioning. The articulated wrist system closely mimics human wrist motion, enabling precise and intuitive instrument movement. A 3D high-definition visualization interface, coupled with motion scaling and tremor reduction features, significantly enhances surgical accuracy and control.

#### Zeus System

The Zeus system, introduced by Computer Motion, is another dual-arm teleoperated robotic platform. It utilizes a compact SCARA-type mechanism to guide surgical tools through three degrees of freedom (DOF) in translation. Although it offers fewer degrees of freedom than Da Vinci, its cable-driven wrist mechanism provides essential yaw movement. Visualization is achieved using a standard endoscope connected to a monitor positioned in front of the surgeon. Despite its simplified architecture, Zeus eliminates the counterintuitive motion seen in conventional MIS setups, preserving fidelity in tool response [342].

#### Autonomous Surgical Robots for Minimal Invasive Surgery

Autonomous surgical robotics emerged with systems like the Unimation Puma 200, which integrated computed tomography (CT) imaging to perform neurosurgical biopsies without the need for stereotactic frames. These systems are tailored for executing predefined, high-precision tasks, particularly within neurosurgery and orthopedic disciplines.

Autonomous platforms leverage preoperative and intraoperative imaging alignment to execute tasks under the surgeon's supervision. While they do not require real-time manual control, they operate under continuous oversight. Advances in medical imaging and processing have enabled patient-specific planning, improving implant fit and procedural accuracy.

A notable example is the Minerva robot, developed at École Polytechnique Fédérale de Lausanne (EPFL) in Switzerland. It performed complex neurosurgical functions—including drilling, incision, and tool exchange—within a CT-guided environment using five motorized DOF. Despite its capabilities, it saw limited clinical adoption due to hesitations around full autonomy in surgery.

In orthopedics, systems such as ROBODOC and CASPAR have been utilized for precise implant alignment based on preoperative imaging. Although they offer measurable gains in accuracy, the clinical advantages of these techniques compared to conventional ones remain a topic of debate.

The CyberKnife system represents a distinct application of autonomous robotics, using a robotic arm to deliver highly targeted stereotactic radiation. It accounts for patient movement in real time and is widely employed for treating tumors located in anatomically complex regions [342].

##### Autonomous Minimally Invasive Robots for Endoscopy

Soft tissue interventions, such as gastrointestinal procedures, present greater challenges due to organ motion and the demand for real-time adaptability. Autonomous systems targeting these areas must continuously adjust to dynamic conditions. Semi-autonomous inchworm-like robots for colonoscopy have been developed to enhance patient comfort and navigation efficiency. Additionally, swallowable capsules such as the M2A provide passive intestinal imaging. More advanced versions, such as NORIKA3, can be guided via electromagnetic fields, but they still lack full autonomy and therapeutic functionality.

Although significant progress has been made—particularly in neurosurgery, orthopedics, and endoscopy—the clinical superiority of fully autonomous systems remains to be investigated. However, rapid innovation in robotics and imaging technologies indicates a promising trajectory for autonomous MIS tools [342].

### 2.11.4 Clinical Application

Surgical devices span a spectrum from basic tools to advanced robotic systems, playing a central role in ensuring precision, efficiency, and safety across various specialties.

#### Orthopedics

In orthopedics, surgical systems assist in diagnosis, preoperative planning, and intraoperative execution. Robotic platforms, such as MAKO, provide exceptional accuracy in implant positioning during joint replacement surgeries, thereby improving outcomes and reducing complications. External fixation systems, such as the Taylor Spatial Frame and Ilizarov apparatus, are widely used for correcting skeletal deformities and managing complex fractures [343].

#### General Surgery

Contemporary general surgery relies heavily on minimally invasive surgery (MIS) tools that enhance precision and reduce trauma. Articulated handheld robotic devices improve maneuverability and ergonomics, reducing surgery time and post-operative complications. Surgical meshes are commonly employed in hernia repairs to reinforce the abdominal wall and prevent recurrence [344].

#### Gynecology

Robotic technologies in gynecology support precise, low-risk procedures, such as hysterectomy and myomectomy, enabling minimally invasive options with faster recovery times. However, specific devices, such as transvaginal meshes for pelvic organ prolapse, have faced scrutiny due to adverse outcomes and increasing regulatory oversight [345].

#### Thoracic Surgery

Thoracic procedures, such as lobectomies, have been revolutionized by techniques like Video-Assisted Thoracoscopic Surgery (VATS), which uses camera systems and specialized instruments to reduce recovery time and postoperative discomfort.

#### Neurosurgery

High-precision microsurgical instruments and neuronavigation tools are essential in neurosurgery. Technologies like stereotactic systems enable the accurate targeting of intracranial structures, minimizing collateral damage and enhancing outcomes in both brain and spinal surgeries.

#### Pediatric Surgery

Devices designed for pediatric surgery are scaled for the anatomical size of infants and children. Miniaturized laparoscopic tools help minimize trauma in the surgical correction of conditions such as esophageal atresia and Hirschsprung's disease, promoting safer procedures and quicker recovery [346].

### *2.11.5 Regulatory Considerations*

Regulation ensures that surgical devices are safe, effective, and compliant with international medical standards. Regulatory bodies, such as the U.S. Food and Drug Administration (FDA) and the European Medicines Agency (EMA), oversee the evaluation, approval, and monitoring of these devices.

#### Classification and Regulatory Pathways

Devices are classified by risk level:

- Class I—low risk
- Class II—moderate risk
- Class III—high risk, requiring stringent clinical trials and detailed documentation

The EU's Medical Device Regulation [224] similarly mandates comprehensive conformity assessments, post-market surveillance, and clinical evaluation for higher-risk categories. Global harmonization efforts, led by the International Medical Device Regulators Forum (IMDRF), aim to standardize regulations and streamline device approvals across markets [347].

#### Quality, Risk Management, and Clinical Evaluation

Manufacturers must implement robust Quality Management Systems (QMS), typically in line with ISO 13485, to ensure consistent product safety and performance. ISO 14971 provides structured risk assessment methods to identify and mitigate device-related hazards, including mechanical failure or software malfunction. For complex devices, especially those involving robotics or AI, thorough clinical evaluations are essential. These studies follow ISO 14155 guidelines, ensuring that they are conducted in an ethical, scientific, and statistically sound manner.

#### Emerging Challenges: 3D Printing, Customization, and Legal Perspectives

The rise of additive manufacturing (3D printing) introduces regulatory complexities, particularly for patient-specific, custom-designed devices. Ensuring material consistency and reproducibility remains a key challenge. Ethical issues, such as data security and informed consent, also become increasingly significant. Legally, robotic systems present new questions around liability, mainly when malfunctions or software errors occur. Legal frameworks are evolving to define accountability and ensure patient protection in the age of intelligent surgical tools [348].

#### Surgical Devices Oversight After Approval

After approval, surgical devices undergo continuous monitoring to ensure long-term safety and performance.

- U.S. Regulations
  The FDA requires manufacturers to report serious adverse events under Medical Device Reporting (MDR) and, in some cases, conduct Post-Approval Studies (PAS). High-risk devices must also be traceable to specific patients via Device Tracking systems.
- EU Regulations
  Under the EU MDR 2017/745, manufacturers are required to implement a Post-Market Surveillance System (PMSS) and generate regular Periodic Safety Update Reports (PSURs). Vigilance systems require immediate reporting of serious incidents or field safety actions.

Healthcare institutions also play a vital role by reporting device issues and participating in follow-up studies. Manufacturers are responsible for updating risk assessments, maintaining technical documentation, and implementing corrective actions when needed. For robotic systems, PMS must address software validation, cybersecurity, and data privacy, particularly when AI or cloud-based components are used.

### *2.11.6 Future Perspectives*

The future of robotic surgery is defined by five interconnected pillars, summarized under the TECAT model:

- Technology: Integration of cutting-edge tools to enhance surgical accuracy and expand clinical scope
- Evidence: Rigorous clinical data supporting safe and effective implementation
- Cost: Economic viability to ensure wide accessibility and system sustainability
- Awareness: Broader public understanding and acceptance of robotic procedures
- Training: Specialized education to equip surgical teams with the skills to operate complex robotic systems

As robotic applications expand across fields such as urology, bariatrics, and plastic surgery, current systems enable surgeons to independently manage multiple robotic arms, effectively replacing the need for a human assistant.

Nonetheless, barriers persist. High upfront costs—such as the Da Vinci system's price tag of nearly $1 million—alongside bulky design and extended setup times, can hinder integration in clinical practice. Additionally, regulatory challenges remain. Agencies like the FDA require extensive validation before approval, and defining risk levels for semi-autonomous and mobile robotic platforms is an ongoing concern. New standards are needed to keep pace with these technological advancements and ensure safe, effective surgical care [349].

## 2.12 Future Trends in Medical Devices

The future of healthcare is intricately tied to the advancements in medical technology, where innovations are enabling transformative shifts in patient care, treatment options, and healthcare delivery systems [350]. Among the most revolutionary developments in the medical field today are miniaturization, wearable technology, and smart devices. These trends are reshaping how healthcare is experienced, making it more personal, accessible, and data-driven [351].

As the demand for healthcare continues to grow globally, integrating these technologies addresses several key challenges, including the increasing burden on healthcare systems, the need for more accurate and efficient diagnostic tools, and the desire for more personalized patient care [352]. These innovations are enhancing medical professionals' capabilities and empowering patients to take more control of their health and wellness in real time [353].

A major catalyst for these changes is miniaturization, which enables the development of compact, portable, and less invasive devices that can monitor, diagnose, and treat a range of conditions. Smaller devices enable clinicians to offer faster, more accurate diagnostics and personalized treatments while simultaneously reducing the need for traditional, more intrusive procedures. Coupled with the growing availability of wearable technologies, these devices pave the way for continuous health monitoring outside clinical settings.

Wearable devices, such as smartwatches, biosensors, and patches, are gaining immense popularity due to their ability to monitor a range of physiological parameters in real-time continuously [354]. These devices offer convenience and facilitate home healthcare, enabling more proactive management of chronic conditions such as diabetes, hypertension, and heart disease [355]. By tracking critical health metrics and providing actionable insights, wearables contribute to early detection, disease prevention, and enhanced patient engagement [356].

In tandem with wearables, the rise of smart devices equipped with artificial intelligence (AI) and the Internet of Medical Things (IoMT) connectivity is unlocking the potential for more intelligent, responsive, and efficient healthcare systems. By integrating IoMT, medical devices can communicate with each other and healthcare providers, creating a seamless flow of information that enhances clinical decision-making, supports remote patient management, and improves overall healthcare outcomes.

This chapter explores these exciting trends, beginning with the pivotal role of wearable technologies in transforming healthcare practices. Following that, we will explore the rise of smart devices and their ability to revolutionize healthcare systems through AI integration and IoMT connectivity. Together, these innovations promise to drive the future of medicine, shifting the focus from reactive to proactive care and ultimately improving the quality and accessibility of healthcare for all.

### 2.12.1 Miniaturization and Wearable Technology

Miniaturization in medical devices has become one of the most transformative trends in modern healthcare, enabling the development of more compact, efficient, and portable tools that deliver high functionality without compromising quality [357]. Over the past few decades, advances in microelectronics, nanotechnology, and biocompatible materials have led to the development of smaller, more precise, and often less invasive devices compared to their predecessors [358]. These innovations have played a crucial role in pushing the boundaries of what is possible in medical diagnostics, treatment, and patient care.

One of medicine's most prominent examples of miniaturization is the implantable pacemaker. Early pacemakers were bulky devices requiring invasive surgical implantation and a considerable recovery period. Today, pacemakers are smaller, lighter, and capable of providing more accurate heart rate regulation. The development of micro-electromechanical systems (MEMS) has also enabled the creation of microsurgical tools that can perform complex surgeries using minimally invasive techniques, thereby drastically reducing patient recovery time and improving outcomes [359]. Similarly, nano-sensors have been developed that can monitor biological processes at a cellular level, providing invaluable data on the body's internal functions in real-time [263, 360].

Miniaturized devices are often employed in point-of-care diagnostics, allowing healthcare providers to conduct tests and perform interventions without relying on large, centralized laboratories. These devices are particularly beneficial for managing chronic conditions such as diabetes, cardiovascular diseases, and respiratory disorders, where continuous monitoring can help in early detection and

**Table 2.18** A variety of wearable devices

| Smartwatches | Fitness trackers | ECG monitors |
|---|---|---|
| 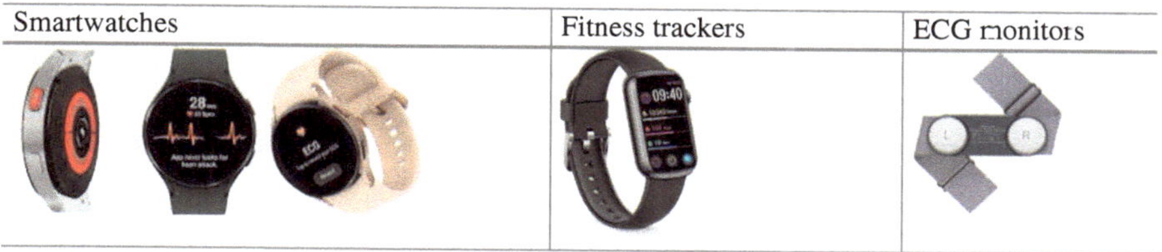 | | |

intervention. The potential for miniaturization extends to areas like personalized medicine, where small-scale technologies can assess genetic, physiological, and environmental factors, tailoring treatments to an individual's unique needs.

The ability to develop and deploy smaller devices that can deliver comprehensive diagnostic and therapeutic capabilities in compact formats is revolutionizing healthcare. As the demand for personalized and precision medicine grows, miniaturization will continue to play a crucial role in delivering more accessible, efficient, and effective medical treatments. Devices integrating advanced diagnostics, therapeutic tools, and monitoring systems will become increasingly ubiquitous, enabling continuous patient monitoring and real-time data collection in outpatient settings [48]. This shift promises not only to enhance the quality of patient care but also to reduce costs and increase overall healthcare accessibility.

Wearable technology has become one of the most significant developments in the healthcare industry. These devices, which can be worn on the body to collect data continuously, are transforming how we approach health monitoring, chronic disease management, and even fitness tracking. Today's wearables are designed for consumers and clinical use, providing healthcare professionals with real-time data on patients' conditions and enabling more proactive care (Table 2.18).

Smartwatches, fitness trackers, biosensors, and bright clothing are wearable technologies that have become increasingly popular in consumer health and clinical settings. These devices have sensors that can track various physiological parameters, including heart rate, blood pressure, activity levels, sleep patterns, and blood glucose levels. Such devices can detect irregularities in a patient's health status, such as abnormal heart rhythms, and send alerts to users or healthcare providers. This capability is particularly valuable in managing chronic conditions where continuous monitoring can significantly improve patient outcomes [48, 117].

For example, continuous glucose monitors (CGMs) have revolutionized diabetes management by enabling patients to monitor their blood glucose levels continuously throughout the day without requiring multiple fingerstick tests. This provides patients with a better understanding of their condition and helps healthcare providers tailor treatment plans in real-time, adjusting medications and lifestyle recommendations based on continuous feedback. Similarly, wearable ECG monitors can detect arrhythmias or other heart-related abnormalities early, enabling timely intervention and reducing the risk of more serious complications.

Wearables are particularly beneficial for patients with chronic conditions, such as hypertension, diabetes, and cardiovascular disease, because they enable ongoing monitoring without requiring frequent hospital visits. By providing patients with real-time feedback on their health status, wearables can help improve adherence to prescribed treatments and lifestyle modifications, ultimately leading to better management of these conditions.

Moreover, wearables have the potential to significantly reduce healthcare costs by minimizing the need for hospital visits and preventing unnecessary hospitalizations. Continuous monitoring through wearables can help detect health issues before they escalate, enabling early interventions that may prevent costly and invasive treatments. This improves patient outcomes and supports healthcare systems by reducing the overall burden on hospitals and emergency care facilities. The future of wearable technology is inspiring, with the integration of artificial intelligence (AI) and machine learning algorithms. These advancements have the potential to unlock even deeper insights from the data collected by wearables, enabling predictive analytics that can identify health risks before they manifest. AI algorithms could analyze patterns in the data, offering early warnings and suggesting interventions that can prevent the onset of severe conditions.

Wearables may evolve into fully integrated health-monitoring platforms, where users can track their health status in real time, receive personalized health recommendations, and even interact with healthcare providers remotely. Such systems could help create a more personalized and patient-centric approach to healthcare, focusing on prevention and early intervention rather than simply treating diseases after they occur. As miniaturized devices and wearables continue to evolve, they have the potential to reshape the healthcare landscape dramatically. The ongoing development of smaller, more efficient, and user-friendly devices will empower patients to take control of their health, reducing the reliance on centralized healthcare facilities and making it easier for individuals to manage their conditions independently.

Integrating AI and machine learning technologies with wearable devices and miniaturized sensors will enable more sophisticated data analysis and real-time decision-making. This could lead to more personalized treatments, faster diagnoses, and improved patient outcomes. Additionally, miniaturized devices have the potential to revolutionize the delivery of healthcare, particularly in remote or underserved areas, by enabling healthcare professionals to provide high-quality care outside traditional clinical settings [48, 222]. The rise of personalized medicine, driven by advancements in miniaturization and wearable technology, will enable treatments to be tailored to each patient's unique genetic, physiological, and environmental characteristics. As these devices improve in accuracy, reliability, and ease of use, they will undoubtedly become indispensable tools in the healthcare toolkit, offering a range of benefits, including increased patient engagement, improved disease management, and reduced healthcare costs.

### 2.12.2 *Smart Devices and Internet of Medical Things*

Smart devices and the Internet of Medical Things (IoMT) have revolutionized the healthcare landscape, offering unprecedented opportunities for real-time monitoring, data sharing, and personalized treatment [361]. IoMT refers to the network of connected medical devices that communicate with each other and centralized healthcare systems via the internet [362]. These smart devices are equipped with sensors, embedded software, and wireless connectivity, enabling them to collect, transmit, and analyze patient data in real-time [363]. This network of interconnected devices holds immense potential to improve patient outcomes, streamline healthcare processes, and reduce costs.

The development of smart devices and IoMT is driven by the growing need for more efficient, accurate, and accessible healthcare solutions. The medical industry is poised to deliver more personalized, data-driven, and proactive care with the rapid advancement of technologies, including artificial intelligence (AI), machine learning (ML), cloud computing, and big data analytics.

By integrating sensors and connectivity into everyday devices, healthcare providers can continuously monitor patients, track their progress, and make timely interventions, thereby preventing complications and improving overall health outcomes (Fig. 2.59).

Smart devices in healthcare refer to a wide range of connected technologies designed to track and monitor a patient's health. These devices include wearables such as fitness trackers, continuous glucose monitors (CGMs), smartwatches, smart implants, and even mobile health applications that integrate with smartphones [350].

The primary function of these devices is to collect real-time health data, such as heart rate, blood glucose levels, oxygen saturation, sleep patterns, and physical activity.

Smart devices can continuously monitor vital signs, which is crucial for patients with chronic conditions like diabetes, hypertension, and cardiovascular diseases.

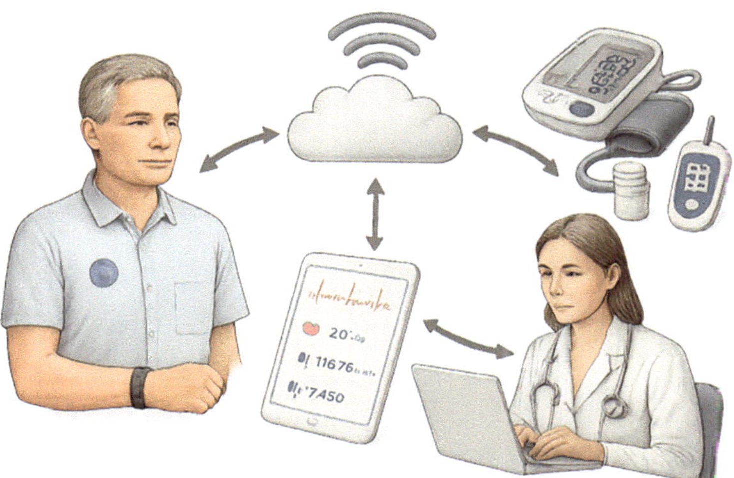

**Fig. 2.59** Diagram showing the IoMT ecosystem

For example, a patient with diabetes can use a continuous glucose monitor (CGM) to track their blood glucose levels in real-time and adjust their insulin doses accordingly. This reduces the need for invasive testing and allows for more precise control over their condition. Similarly, patients with heart disease can wear smart ECG devices to monitor their heart rate and rhythm, alerting them and their doctors to any potential arrhythmias or abnormal patterns.

Integrating AI and machine learning algorithms into smart devices has significantly enhanced their capabilities. These technologies analyze the devices' data to identify patterns, detect anomalies, and make predictions [364]. For example, AI algorithms can detect early signs of an impending heart attack by analyzing ECG data or alerting patients to irregular blood glucose levels before they become dangerous [365]. These predictive capabilities make smart devices invaluable for prevention and early intervention.

Moreover, the ability of smart devices to provide real-time feedback to patients promotes engagement and adherence to treatment plans. For instance, a smart watch that tracks a patient's physical activity and sends notifications to encourage movement can motivate individuals to stay active and manage their weight more effectively. The convenience and accessibility of these devices encourage patients to take a more active role in managing their health, resulting in improved outcomes (Fig. 2.60).

The true potential of smart devices in healthcare is realized when they are connected through the Internet of Medical Things (IoMT). The IoMT ecosystem

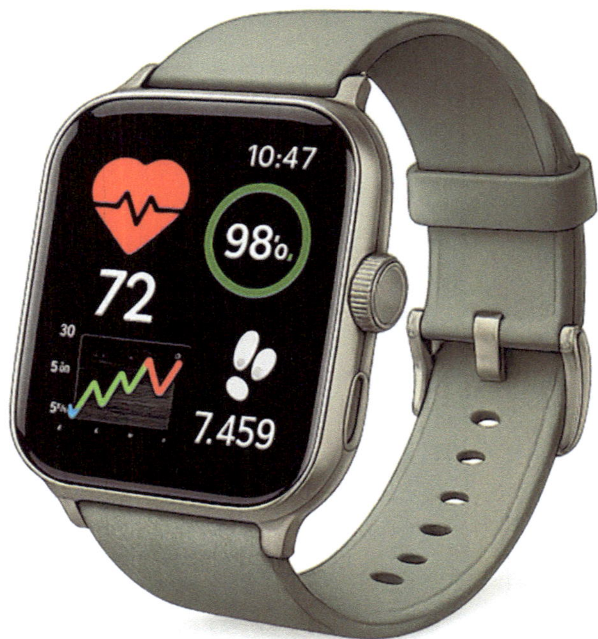


**Fig. 2.60** A smart watch with integrated health tracking features

comprises medical devices, software applications, and healthcare systems, all interconnected by a network that enables seamless communication and data sharing. This connectivity gives healthcare providers a more comprehensive view of a patient's health. It facilitates the tracking of progress, enables real-time intervention, and promotes collaboration across various medical specialties [361].

For example, a hospital might use IoMT to connect patient monitoring equipment, such as heart rate monitors, ECG devices, and oxygen saturation sensors, to a central database where doctors and nurses can access the data remotely. This real-time data sharing allows for faster decision-making, even in critical situations. Additionally, IoMT facilitates remote patient monitoring, which is particularly useful in rural or underserved areas where access to healthcare facilities may be limited (Fig. 2.61).

One of the primary benefits of IoMT is its ability to reduce hospital readmissions and emergency visits. Continuous monitoring of patients in the home setting allows healthcare providers to identify early signs of deterioration, intervene before conditions worsen, and provide patients with timely care without hospital visits [362]. For example, IoMT-connected wearable devices can send real-time data to healthcare providers, alerting them to any significant changes in a patient's condition, such as a sudden drop in blood pressure or an elevated heart rate, which could indicate the need for immediate attention. Additionally, IoMT enables more effective patient management and personalized care. With continuous access to patient data, healthcare providers can adjust treatment plans based on the most current information

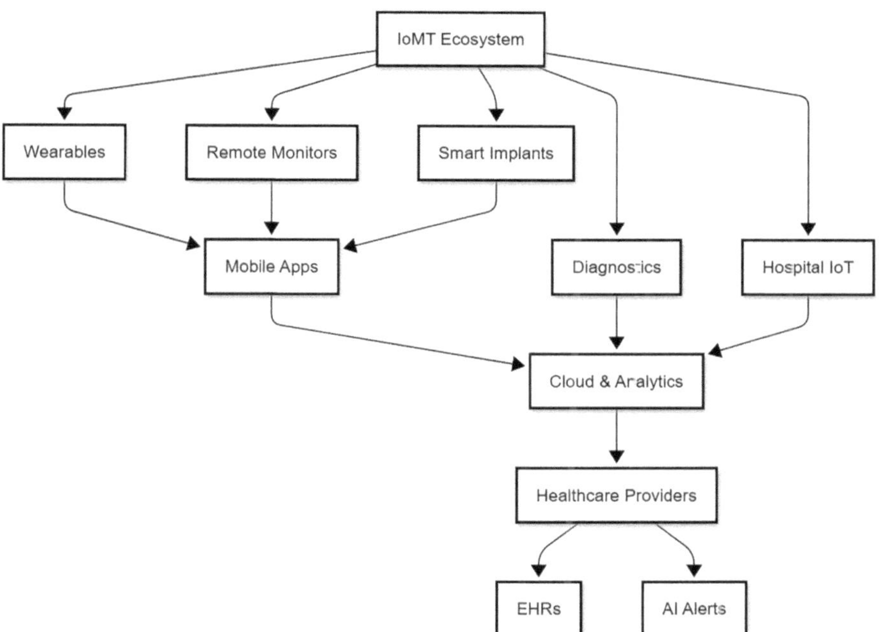


**Fig. 2.61** Diagram of a hospital's IoMT ecosystem with interconnected devices communicating with a central healthcare system

available. For instance, a smart insulin pump can automatically adjust insulin delivery based on a patient's blood glucose levels, and an AI-powered heart monitor can suggest lifestyle modifications based on real-time heart rate variability.

While the potential benefits of IoMT are vast, several challenges must be addressed to realize its potential fully. One of the primary concerns is the security and privacy of patient data. As more devices become connected to the internet, the risk of cyberattacks and data breaches increases. Healthcare organizations must ensure patient data is encrypted, stored securely, and shared only with authorized parties. Implementing robust cybersecurity protocols and adhering to regulations such as the Health Insurance Portability and Accountability Act (HIPAA) is crucial for maintaining patient confidentiality and trust.

Another challenge is the interoperability of IoMT devices. Healthcare organizations use various medical devices from different manufacturers, and ensuring that these devices can communicate with each other and centralized systems is critical for effective patient management. Standardization efforts are underway to create standard protocols and frameworks for IoMT devices, but achieving seamless integration across diverse platforms remains a significant hurdle. The reliability and accuracy of data collected by IoMT devices must be carefully considered. As these devices become more widely used, healthcare providers must ensure that the data they receive is accurate and actionable. Inaccurate or unreliable data could lead to misdiagnosis or unnecessary interventions, potentially harming patients. Rigorous testing, validation, and ongoing monitoring of IoMT devices are necessary to maintain the quality and safety of care.

The future of smart devices and the Internet of Medical Things in healthcare appears bright. The combination of IoMT and AI-powered smart devices will likely lead to a new era of healthcare, where treatments are highly personalized, proactive, and more efficient than ever before. As the technology evolves, we can expect to see even more advanced capabilities in wearable devices, such as non-invasive glucose monitoring, continuous blood pressure tracking, and real-time monitoring of mental health conditions. Integrating IoMT with emerging technologies, such as 5G networks and blockchain, could further enhance the ability to transmit and store data securely and quickly, enabling more reliable remote patient monitoring and faster decision-making. Augmented reality (AR) and virtual reality (VR), in conjunction with IoMT, could enable immersive patient care, allowing doctors to visualize a patient's condition in real-time and provide patients with remote consultations or therapeutic interventions.

## 2.13 Robotic Systems in Medicine

Robotic technologies have become increasingly vital components in modern medicine, particularly in enhancing surgical accuracy, operational workflow, and patient safety. The integration of robotics into minimally invasive procedures began in the early 1980s, initially within neurosurgery, and has since expanded to include specialties like orthopedics and general surgery.

From a hardware standpoint, medical robotic systems typically comprise high-resolution imaging units, articulated robotic arms, and custom-designed instruments for precise surgical manipulation. These robotic arms often offer multiple degrees of freedom, enabling refined, hand-like movements. Surgeons typically control these systems from ergonomically designed consoles, which allow for enhanced maneuverability and comfort throughout procedures. On the software side, advanced computational tools manage real-time visualization, integrate imaging data, and provide dynamic feedback during surgery. These systems often feature intuitive interfaces to support surgeon interaction, training modules for skill development, and regular software updates that ensure optimal functionality and adherence to safety regulations. The synergy between cutting-edge hardware and intelligent software continues to redefine surgical methods and improve outcomes across a wide range of clinical applications.

The progression of surgical robotics has shifted away from the bulky, general-purpose machines once standard in industrial use toward compact, procedure-specific systems tailored for operating room environments. These developments have contributed to greater surgical dexterity, improved ergonomics, and easier access to anatomically challenging regions. Classification of robotic systems in healthcare often centers on their level of autonomy and how they interact with clinicians. Early designs fell into two main categories: fully autonomous systems that carried out specific, pre-programmed tasks with oversight, and semi-active systems that assisted in tool positioning while leaving critical decisions to the surgeon. This collaborative approach—blending human expertise with robotic precision—is particularly beneficial in complex, unpredictable scenarios. More recently, new approaches, such as co-manipulation, where both the robot and the surgeon guide surgical tools in tandem, have emerged to optimize performance. Teleoperated systems, often structured in master-slave configurations, have become the standard for complex tasks that require precise fine motor control and distance.

Innovations such as haptic (force) feedback and image-guided navigation have further enhanced these platforms, allowing for more accurate interventions. Today's systems also focus on specialized, streamlined designs that support specific tasks—such as vascular catheterization or orthopedic implant placement—while minimizing invasiveness and maintaining strict hygiene standards. As the field continues to evolve, robotic surgery is transitioning from a novel technology to a core element of operative care. Future developments are expected to deliver increasingly intelligent, adaptable, and integrated systems that transform surgical capabilities and redefine the boundaries of what is clinically possible.

### *2.13.1 History*

The development of medical robotics has followed a gradual yet impactful trajectory, moving from abstract ideas to transformative technologies that have reshaped surgical practice. The concept of a "robot" first entered the lexicon in the early twentieth century, derived from the Czech word robota, meaning forced labor. This idea gained momentum during the space race, which highlighted the necessity of robotic and telecommunication systems to overcome the physical limitations of human presence in extreme environments [366].

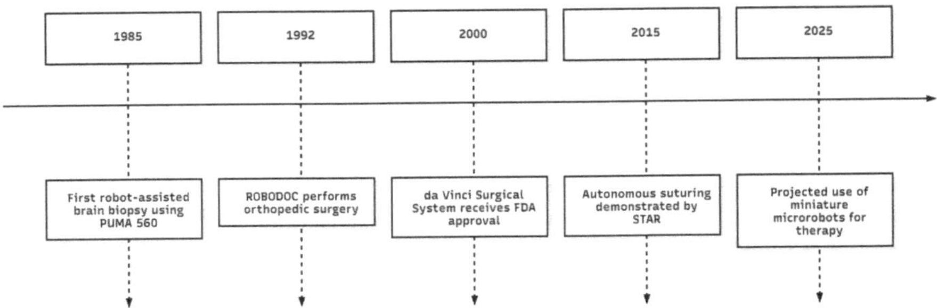


**Fig. 2.62** Medical robots development

Key innovators, such as Phil Green, known for his work on robotic telemanipulation, and Scott Fisher, a pioneer in head-mounted display systems, laid important groundwork. Their contributions played a foundational role in the emergence of telesurgery, where surgeons could operate remotely through robotic interfaces. The first practical application of robotics in medicine took shape in the 1980s. Kwoh and his team used the PUMA 560 robotic arm to assist with neurosurgical biopsies, marking a significant milestone in robotic-assisted surgery. This early use demonstrated the potential of robotic systems to enhance precision in minimally invasive procedures.

Further advancements followed with the creation of the PROBOT®, developed for performing transurethral resections of the prostate. This device expanded the scope of robotic applications and helped establish the feasibility of automated surgical assistance. The field reached a new level of sophistication with the introduction of the Da Vinci Surgical System by Intuitive Surgical (Fig. 2.62). This platform redefined surgical capabilities by offering surgeons refined dexterity, high-definition 3D visualization, and minimally invasive access, setting a new standard in robotic-assisted operations. Over the last 30 years, robotics has evolved from a novel concept to an integral part of surgical practice across numerous medical specialties [367]. The convergence of computer-assisted systems, virtual reality technologies, and automation has significantly enhanced surgical precision, efficiency, and consistency, resulting in improved clinical outcomes. Ongoing advancements continue to reshape the landscape, not only refining established techniques but also opening new frontiers in healthcare. These developments signal a future in which robotic systems are expected to play an increasingly prominent and versatile role in surgical care.

## *2.13.2 Technical Characteristics*

### Hardware

Sensors and Actuators

The foundation of any medical robotic system lies in its hardware—particularly sensors and actuators—which bridge the gap between physical action and computational control. Sensors play a crucial role in monitoring various intraoperative and physiological parameters, including spatial positioning, biomechanical feedback, and biological signals. For example, high-resolution visual systems can assist in surgical navigation by continuously providing spatial orientation data. Optical tracking technologies are frequently used to localize instruments relative to patient anatomy, enabling real-time adaptive responses that enhance both surgical safety and precision [368].

Standard sensor types include accelerometers and gyroscopes for tracking movement and orientation, as well as pressure sensors for measuring applied force, making robotic interactions more intuitive. Actuators, in turn, convert software-driven commands into mechanical motion. Their design is tailored for tasks that range from fine surgical manipulation to broader physical support in rehabilitation settings. The integration of responsive actuators—often built with biomimetic materials—ensures that the robotic output aligns closely with human movement patterns and reaction times, supporting smooth and safe interaction.

The synchronization of sensors and actuators enables robotic systems to operate with high precision, particularly in constrained surgical environments. Innovations in microactuation and adaptive force control have led to the development of compact, agile robots that deliver performance comparable to human dexterity. These systems work in tandem with surgical navigation software to ensure seamless and accurate instrument control. As the field advances, the performance and safety of medical robotic systems will increasingly depend on the continued development of these core hardware components. Multidisciplinary collaboration among clinicians, engineers, and researchers is essential to ensure that these innovations translate into clinically valuable solutions. Long-term studies and comparative analyses with traditional surgical methods will be crucial to validate their effectiveness and safety in real-world settings.

### Robotic Arms

Robotic arms are central to many modern medical robotics platforms, especially in procedures that demand high precision, such as minimally invasive and remote surgeries. These arms are engineered with multiple degrees of freedom (DoF), allowing them to replicate complex movements that mimic those of a human hand. A typical robotic arm system may include four DoF, enabling control over spatial positioning along three axes and rotational movement [369].

Advanced positioning systems, such as those using infrared detection paired with LED arrays and specialized cameras, provide the necessary spatial awareness for accurate arm movement. These systems can achieve high positional accuracy—sub-millimeter resolution in some cases—ensuring that even the smallest motion aligns with surgical intent. Encoder resolutions of approximately 0.4 mm and positional tracking accuracy of less than 0.6 mm per pixel have been reported, providing precise and consistent performance in delicate surgical contexts [370].

The actuation of these arms is commonly achieved through lead screw mechanisms, delivering motion speeds up to 0.28 m/s. Such responsiveness supports the timely execution of complex tasks. Control systems, often based on proportional-integrator (PI) frameworks, provide smooth and stable arm motion. These control architectures yield fast rise times, low steady-state error, and short settling periods, ensuring reliability during critical phases of surgery [371]. Despite challenges like cumulative inertial drift, current designs demonstrate significant potential for expanding the role of robotic arms in both localized and remote surgical applications.

#### End Effectors

End effectors, often referred to as the "hands" of robotic systems, are crucial for executing tasks in medical procedures. They hold and manipulate tools, perform suturing, or interact directly with human tissue. Their design must account for both functionality and safety, particularly when working in sensitive anatomical environments. Teleoperated systems have enabled intuitive control of endoscopes and surgical tools through multi-limbed platforms. For example, some systems use a foot interface to control an endoscope while two hand-controlled instruments perform surgical tasks. With up to 13 degrees of freedom, these platforms enable surgeons to operate with high precision and autonomy, thereby minimizing reliance on human assistants and reducing the risk of miscommunication.

Recent innovations in soft robotics have driven the development of compliant, adaptable end effectors. These devices can conform to the shape and fragility of the object being manipulated without requiring complex control algorithms. Their soft structure minimizes the application of excessive force and protects delicate tissues, making them particularly suitable for medical procedures where the preservation of biological integrity is critical. Additionally, soft grippers reduce cost and energy consumption, contributing to the accessibility and safety of robotic interventions [372].

The evolution of end effectors, from rigid precision grippers to flexible, adaptive systems, reflects the growing need for versatility and safety in surgical robotics. Future development will continue to focus on enhancing the tactile control, sensitivity, and responsiveness of these tools, ensuring their alignment with the complex and variable nature of clinical procedures.

#### Power Supply Systems

A reliable power supply is fundamental to the functionality of robotic systems in medical settings. These systems must maintain consistent performance throughout prolonged procedures, which necessitates a robust, efficient, and often redundant power infrastructure. Power sources may include direct mains connections, advanced battery systems (e.g., lithium-ion batteries), or emerging technologies such as fuel cells.

In surgical environments, power systems must be lightweight yet energy-dense to preserve the mobility and compactness of robotic devices. Lithium-ion batteries are preferred for their balance of capacity and weight, but system design must also account for recharge cycles, heat management, and backup protocols. Redundant power solutions ensure continuity of operation in the event of failure, which is especially critical during complex or time-sensitive procedures. Intelligent power management systems enhance the reliability and efficiency of robotic platforms. These systems regulate energy distribution based on real-time operational demands, prolong battery life, and prevent system overloads. In scenarios with limited access to electricity, such as field hospitals or remote surgical units, energy-efficient designs and emerging technologies like energy harvesting (from motion or body heat) can extend the autonomy of medical robots.

As medical robotics becomes more advanced, the convergence of hardware reliability and smart energy systems will be essential. Software algorithms must actively assess power consumption and predict energy needs to optimize resource allocation. This integration will not only improve safety and performance but also enable more flexible deployment of robotic systems across various clinical settings, from operating rooms to rehabilitation centers.

### Software

Software architecture forms the backbone of medical robotic systems, enabling the seamless coordination between mechanical hardware and computational intelligence. Its primary objective is to enhance system accuracy and reduce the likelihood of procedural errors, critical in the context of clinical environments where precision is non-negotiable. Robotic platforms have already demonstrated superior stability and fine motor control compared to human operators in specific surgical contexts. However, such technical capabilities must be supported by adaptive and intelligent software frameworks that can navigate the dynamic and unpredictable nature of medical procedures [112].

Traditional human-robot interaction models have prioritized user-friendliness but often fall short in process-level control, limiting the ability of robotic systems to manage complex, branching tasks autonomously. A solution to this limitation lies in the adoption of Finite State Machines (FSMs)—architectures designed to model discrete-event systems by clearly defining system states and transitions. By structuring robotic behaviors through finite state machines (FSMs), medical procedures can follow predictable and organized workflows.

Hierarchical Finite State Machines (hFSMs) represent a significant advancement in this area. By allowing the parallel execution of subtasks within a larger procedural context, hFSMs support modular and adaptive task execution, making them particularly suited to the nuanced demands of surgical interventions. The growing interplay between sensing, visualization, and actuation modules further underscores the need to integrate these components within a cohesive software framework [373].

To address the complexity of these interactions, systems such as the Surgical Assistant Workstation (SAW) and the Robot Operating System (ROS) have adopted modular, distributed architectures. These platforms help compartmentalize development efforts and support reliable fault-tolerant behavior by breaking tasks into manageable submodules, especially for perception and actuation tasks. However, for medical robotics to achieve full procedural integration, software architecture must evolve to encompass not only control but comprehensive workflow management. This demands a shift toward reconfigurable, scalable systems that can adapt to various surgical tasks without requiring a complete redevelopment from scratch. As robotic systems become increasingly complex, the underlying software will become increasingly critical in supporting their safe and flexible use in diverse clinical settings.

### Operating Systems for Medical Robotics

Operating systems serve as the operational core of medical robotics, enabling communication between sensors, actuators, and high-level control systems. Platforms like ROS (Robot Operating System) and OROCOS (Open Robot Control Software) have emerged as foundational tools that facilitate the integration of robotic technologies into surgical workflows. These operating environments provide modularity, flexibility, and access to a large ecosystem of pre-built libraries—features that significantly reduce development time and enhance interoperability. ROS, in particular, supports rapid prototyping and deployment by offering a vast collection of software packages that address everyday robotic tasks, from sensor integration to kinematic control. These features enable medical developers to focus on customizing clinical applications without having to reinvent low-level functionalities. Despite these advantages, the widespread adoption of robotic operating systems in clinical practice faces several hurdles. High implementation costs, steep learning curves, and infrastructural limitations—especially in smaller clinics—restrict access to robotic technologies. Transitioning from conventional methods to robotic-assisted techniques also requires specialized training, which is not yet universally available [370, 373].

Nonetheless, advances in collaborative robotics have demonstrated the value of improved operating systems. For example, robots that assist in procedures such as ultrasound-guided needle insertions can operate alongside surgeons, increasing both accuracy and efficiency. Emerging standards, such as Service-Oriented Device Connectivity (SDC), hold promise for making surgical robotics more modular and interoperable, facilitating integration into complex clinical environments and promoting safer, more coordinated care.

### Control Algorithms

Control algorithms are the computational engines that drive the functionality of medical robotic systems. They ensure that the robot responds intelligently to environmental changes, adheres to clinical protocols, and maintains optimal performance across various use cases. By integrating adaptive control strategies, robotic platforms can reduce their reliance on manual input, respond to intraoperative variability, and minimize the risks associated with human error. A prominent strategy in control system design is the use of hFSMs. These allow robots to manage complex procedures by segmenting them into smaller, manageable states, each with defined transition rules. This architecture enables systems to respond in real time to changes in patient condition or surgical context, maintaining procedural flow while allowing for adaptability [112].

Importantly, hFSMs bridge the gap between human expertise and robotic automation. They convert the tacit knowledge of surgeons—such as conditional steps in a procedure—into logical, machine-executable states. This enables robotic platforms to interpret and implement clinical workflows more faithfully and reliably. Moreover, when coupled with a modular design strategy, hFSMs enhance both hardware-software compatibility and development scalability. Developers can isolate and test modules independently, ensuring system robustness and reducing the likelihood of cascading failures [373].

### 2.13.3 Types of Devices

Robotic technologies in healthcare have evolved into a multifaceted domain, addressing a wide range of surgical, diagnostic, and rehabilitative functions. These systems fall into several key categories: telerobotics, surgical robots, rehabilitation robotics, and assistive devices such as prosthetics and telepresence platforms, each tailored to a specific clinical need.

Telerobotic systems have redefined the boundaries of surgical practice by enabling specialists to operate remotely, utilizing high-speed communication networks to transmit video and control signals in real-time. These setups facilitate remote surgeries and consultations, offering access to expert care regardless of geographic location. However, the deployment of telerobotics introduces complex concerns, including cybersecurity for patient data and the ethical responsibilities associated with remote medical interventions [374].

Surgical robotic platforms, such as the da Vinci Surgical System, have become central to many minimally invasive procedures. Through surgeon-controlled articulated instruments, these platforms offer superior precision and dexterity in operations such as prostatectomies and cardiac valve repairs. While they provide remarkable clinical advantages, challenges persist in ensuring robust control mechanisms and system reliability under demanding surgical conditions [375].

Rehabilitation robots support recovery following injury or surgery by guiding patients through repetitive, controlled movements that promote neuromuscular retraining. These systems utilize adaptive algorithms to personalize therapy regimens, thereby enhancing outcomes and improving patient engagement during the recovery process [376].

Looking ahead, the trajectory of medical robotics is expected to include the expanded use of telementoring, enabling real-time remote instruction and surgical support. Ongoing collaboration between academia and industry will likely drive innovations that yield more flexible, AI-integrated platforms capable of adapting to various clinical contexts. However, ethical issues surrounding data privacy, system accountability, and equitable access must remain at the forefront as these technologies become more pervasive.

### Surgical Robots

The advent of surgical robots has fundamentally reshaped operative care, steering the field toward less invasive, more precise techniques. Since the first robotic-assisted neurosurgery in 1985 and the pioneering laparoscopic cholecystectomy in 1987, robotic systems have steadily advanced in capability and adoption. Contemporary platforms commonly utilize master-slave configurations, where the surgeon operates from a console while robotic arms execute finely controlled maneuvers within the surgical site. Early systems, such as PROBOT®, revealed the potential of robotic precision but were limited in scope, lacking functionalities like coagulation. Innovations such as ROBODOC®, the first FDA-approved orthopedic robot, and the da Vinci system marked turning points by introducing advanced imaging, haptic feedback, and multi-DoF articulation.

Today's surgical robots can replicate intricate manual gestures while offering enhanced stability and visualization, effectively extending a surgeon's capability beyond human physical limits. The integration of machine learning, real-time analytics, and virtual reality environments is expected to revolutionize operative care further, providing decision support, predictive modeling, and augmented surgical navigation. These developments are moving robotic systems from mere assistive tools toward collaborative, semi-autonomous platforms capable of redefining surgical protocols across disciplines (Fig. 2.63).

### Rehabilitation Robots

Rehabilitation robotics has emerged as a transformative approach to therapy, particularly in the recovery of motor function following injuries, surgeries, or neurological disorders. These systems guide patients through controlled, repeatable exercises designed to strengthen muscles, improve coordination, and retrain neural pathways. Rehabilitation platforms include wearable exoskeletons, robotic limbs, and robot-assisted treadmills. Exoskeletons support individuals with spinal cord injuries or post-stroke conditions, enabling upright movement and locomotor training. Robotic arms aid in upper limb therapy by offering adjustable resistance and real-time feedback, while treadmill systems provide gait training that simulates natural walking, accelerating ambulation recovery [377, 378] (Fig. 2.64).

These technologies often incorporate sensors and adaptive algorithms that monitor performance and adjust assistance levels dynamically, preventing overexertion and tailoring the therapy to each patient's progress. Research continues to explore

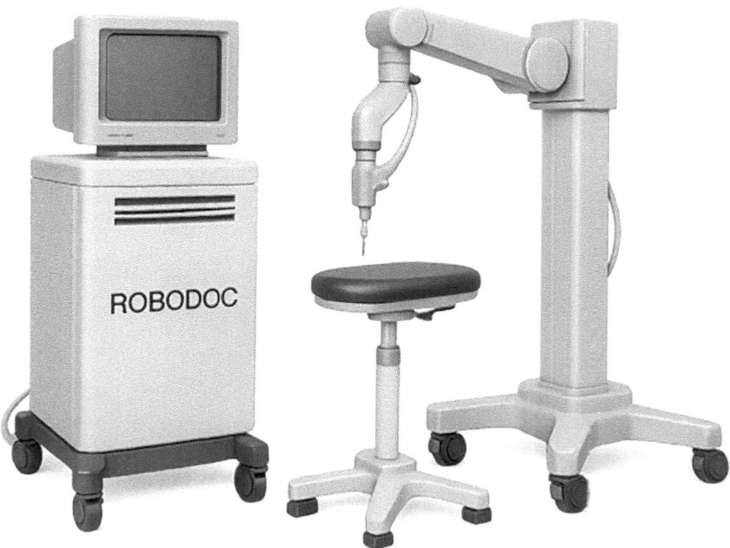


**Fig. 2.63** The ROBODOC surgical system

the use of robotics for cognitive rehabilitation, suggesting broader applications in neurorehabilitation and integrative care. As these systems mature, they promise to enhance therapeutic outcomes, reduce the burden on therapists, and promote more personalized, patient-centered recovery.

## Telepresence Robots

Telepresence robots have become a vital component of remote healthcare delivery, facilitating virtual face-to-face interactions between clinicians and patients. Typically mounted on mobile platforms, these systems include high-definition video conferencing tools, microphones, and sensors, enabling physicians to communicate, observe, and even examine patients remotely [379].

These robots can navigate autonomously or be remotely steered through hospital corridors or home environments, offering flexibility in care delivery. Their functionality can be enhanced with diagnostic attachments, such as digital stethoscopes or otoscopes, allowing for more comprehensive assessments. Telepresence robots are especially valuable in rural or underserved regions, where access to specialized care may be limited (Fig. 2.65).

The global push for telehealth, accelerated by recent pandemics, has highlighted the importance of such technologies. In addition to improving access, they also reduce hospital traffic and the risk of infections. As AI and machine learning are integrated into telepresence platforms, future models may offer intelligent triage, automated reporting, and tailored patient communication. These innovations will

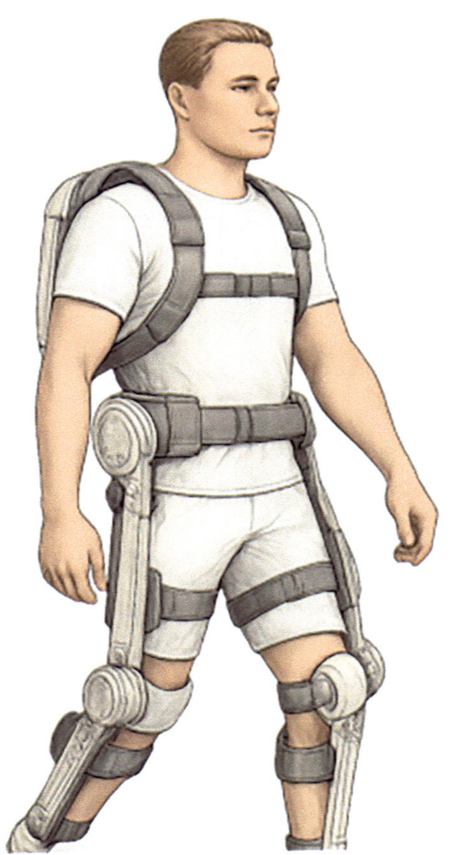

**Fig. 2.64** Exoskeleton

likely extend their utility into elder care, mental health, and post-operative monitoring, redefining what constitutes accessible and responsive medical care.

## Robotic Prosthetics

Robotic prosthetics represent one of the most significant intersections of human-centered design and robotics, aiming to restore function and autonomy to individuals who have lost a limb. These advanced devices simulate the natural biomechanics of limbs by integrating sensors, actuators, and intelligent control systems, providing users with greater freedom in their daily lives.

Modern prosthetics can perform complex, multi-joint motions with high precision. Powered prosthetic arms, for instance, enable fine motor tasks such as grasping fragile objects or manipulating tools, thereby vastly expanding functional independence. Sensor arrays within the prosthetic detect myoelectric signals—muscle activity from the residual limb—which are translated into real-time control

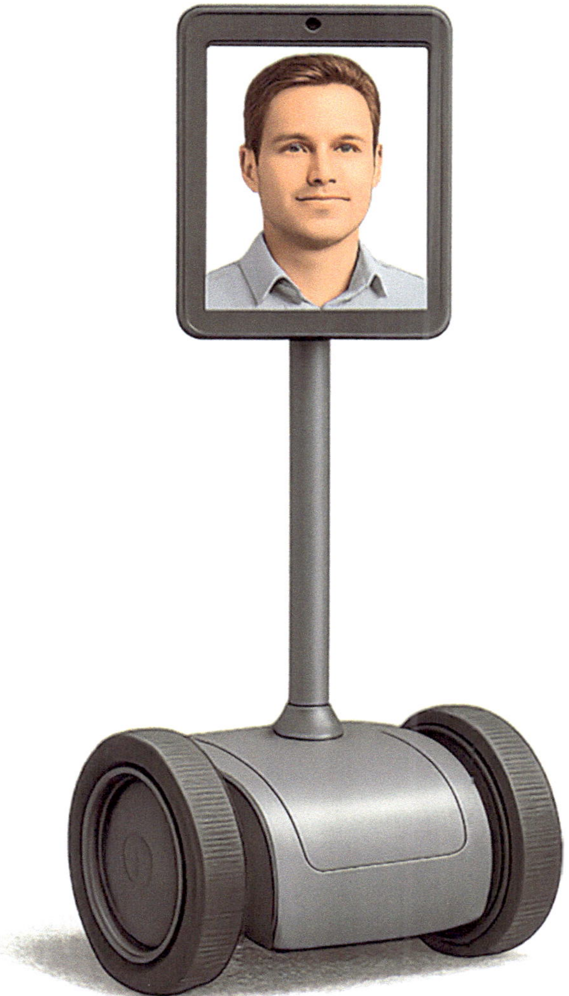

**Fig. 2.65** Telepresence robot

commands. This biofeedback loop enables intuitive interaction, aligning prosthetic movement with the user's intent. Material innovations have led to lighter, more durable designs, minimizing fatigue while enhancing comfort. In parallel, AI-based systems are being introduced to learn user preferences and adapt in real time, creating a more personalized experience. Robotic prosthetics are also contributing to the emerging field of neuroprosthetics, where direct neural interfaces may 1 day allow for seamless control of artificial limbs via brain signals (Fig. 2.66).

As these technologies continue to advance, robotic prosthetics are expected to go beyond functional replacement, offering enhanced abilities, improved aesthetics,

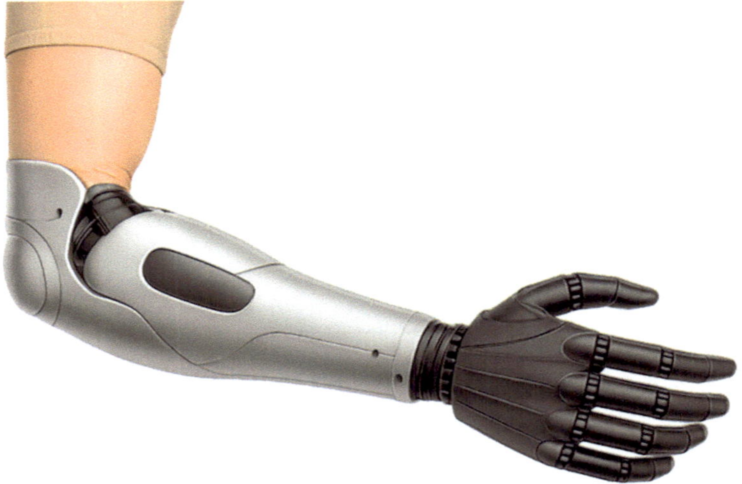

**Fig. 2.66** Powered prosthetic arm

and deeper integration with biological systems. The shift toward customized, data-driven prosthetic solutions reflects a broader trend in medicine toward individualized care, underscoring the importance of combining technological innovation with human-centered design.

## *2.13.4 Clinical Applications*

Robotic technology has become a transformative force in modern surgical medicine, reshaping how procedures are performed and significantly enhancing clinical outcomes. Among its most impactful applications is minimally invasive surgery (MIS), where robotic platforms enable surgeons to perform complex operations through small incisions. This approach reduces trauma, shortens recovery times, and lowers the risk of infection and postoperative scarring. A leading example, the da Vinci Surgical System, has become a mainstay across numerous surgical specialties, offering unparalleled instrument control and 3D visualization that allow for refined, high-precision techniques in operations ranging from prostate removal to heart valve repair [380].

Beyond MIS, robotic systems have demonstrated significant value in orthopedic surgery, particularly in joint replacement procedures. Tools such as the MAKO system enhance both preoperative planning and intraoperative precision by using 3D imaging and robotic guidance to ensure exact bone resection and implant positioning. This level of accuracy contributes to better functional outcomes and extends the lifespan of prosthetic implants, while also minimizing complications. Robotic technology is also advancing the field of neurosurgery, where exactitude is critical. Robotic-assisted systems for stereotactic procedures enable targeted interventions within the brain, minimizing disruption to surrounding tissue. Such precision is essential in applications like tumor removal or deep brain stimulation, where even slight deviations can have profound clinical implications. As robotic innovations continue to progress, their role in surgical practice is expected to grow substantially, ushering in a new era of enhanced safety, reduced invasiveness, and expanded procedural possibilities.

### Minimally Invasive Surgery (MIS)

Minimally invasive surgery has revolutionized operative care by achieving therapeutic goals while minimizing trauma to the patient. Unlike traditional open procedures that require large incisions and extensive recovery, MIS utilizes minor access points—typically just a few millimeters wide—through which cameras and instruments are inserted. The precision offered by robotic-assisted minimally invasive surgery enables surgeons to perform intricate operations with greater control, visibility, and safety. Modern robotic systems designed for MIS are equipped with articulated instruments that mimic wrist-like movements, providing enhanced dexterity within confined anatomical regions [375]. Surgeons operate these tools from a remote console, gaining access to a high-definition, three-dimensional view of the surgical field. This not only improves depth perception but also supports more accurate dissection and suturing in procedures such as prostatectomies, hysterectomies, and minimally invasive cardiac surgeries.

Additional capabilities, such as haptic feedback—which conveys tactile sensations like tissue resistance—further refine the surgeon's control. By integrating these features, robotic MIS platforms enhance both technical performance and patient outcomes, resulting in reduced pain, shorter hospital stays, and faster recovery to normal activities.

### Robotic-Assisted Surgery

Robotic-assisted surgery represents a convergence of human expertise and robotic precision, empowering surgeons to perform complex procedures with improved accuracy and reduced physical strain. These systems typically consist of a surgeon-controlled console, robotic arms equipped with precision instruments, and a high-resolution camera system. The robotic arms mirror the surgeon's movements, translating them into refined, stable motions that are often superior to what can be achieved by hand alone. This approach has shown substantial benefits across multiple specialties. For instance, in urological, gynecological, cardiovascular, and gastrointestinal surgeries, robotic assistance improves operative control in delicate anatomical areas. Enhanced visualization, maneuverability, and reduced invasiveness translate into fewer complications, lower blood loss, and faster recovery times.

From the patient's perspective, robotic-assisted surgery often results in less postoperative discomfort, minimal scarring, and shorter hospital stays. However, several barriers still limit widespread adoption. These include the high capital and maintenance costs of robotic systems, as well as the need for extensive training to operate them effectively. Moreover, while short-term outcomes are promising, long-term data comparing robotic and traditional techniques are still under active investigation. Ongoing research is crucial for validating the benefits and optimizing the implementation of robotic systems in various clinical contexts.

## Training and Simulation

As robotic surgery becomes increasingly sophisticated, practical training and simulation programs are critical to preparing clinicians for the demands of robotic-assisted procedures. High-fidelity simulators now replicate complex surgical environments with remarkable realism, enabling trainees to develop technical proficiency without risking patient safety.

These platforms often incorporate tactile (haptic) feedback, visual cues, and performance tracking, allowing users to practice nuanced skills such as tissue manipulation, suturing, and navigation within confined anatomical spaces. In addition to technical skills, simulation supports decision-making under pressure, helping surgeons gain confidence in managing unexpected challenges. The integration of virtual reality (VR) and augmented reality (AR) has further advanced medical training. These technologies offer immersive, interactive environments that allow trainees to explore three-dimensional anatomy, interact with virtual instruments, and engage in scenario-based simulations. Performance metrics and analytics enable instructors to assess progress, deliver targeted feedback, and tailor instruction to meet the individual needs of students.

Simulation-based education promotes a culture of continuous improvement, accelerating skill acquisition and ensuring that surgical teams are proficient and adaptable. As robotic systems evolve, training methodologies will also need to keep pace, ensuring that practitioners are well-equipped to harness the full potential of robotic technology in clinical practice.

## Robotics in Rehabilitation

This section provides a comprehensive overview of the integration of robotics in various aspects of healthcare, with a focus on rehabilitation, telemedicine, surgical support, diagnostics, and biopsy procedures. It highlights the profound impact of robotic technologies in enhancing precision, efficiency, and accessibility across the medical field.

#### Physical Rehabilitation

Robotic systems, particularly exoskeletons, have revolutionized physical rehabilitation by facilitating high-intensity, task-oriented training. These systems are particularly beneficial for patients recovering from strokes and injuries, as they provide personalized therapy that promotes neuroplasticity. Notable devices, such as MIT-MANUS and ARMin III, offer upper-limb rehabilitation, integrating haptic feedback and adjustable difficulty levels to maintain patient motivation. The importance of ergonomic design in exoskeletons ensures comfort during therapy, thereby enhancing patient adherence and facilitating more effective rehabilitation [378].

#### Cognitive Rehabilitation

Robots in cognitive rehabilitation provide consistent, repetitive task-based training that helps restore cognitive functions in individuals with neurological impairments. Devices for upper-limb rehabilitation guide patients through movements that help prevent muscle atrophy, while collaborative robots assist therapists in providing structured support. Remote rehabilitation systems, such as those enabling upper-limb exercises at home, have made therapy more accessible and flexible, addressing the growing demand for care, particularly among the aging population [377].

### Telemedicine and Robotic Systems

Telemedicine has been significantly enhanced by robotic systems, enabling remote surgeries and consultations. Telesurgery improves surgical precision by eliminating human tremors and fatigue. The use of telerobotics, such as the da Vinci system, has already transformed surgical practices by enabling complex procedures to be conducted remotely; however, challenges, including cybersecurity, regulatory issues, and communication stability, still need to be addressed.

#### Remote Consultations

Teleoperated robotic systems, such as the one developed by Boschetti et al., have made remote surgeries more feasible by integrating haptic feedback and real-time interaction, enabling surgeons to operate from distant locations. Systems such as MELODY, which integrates robotic ultrasonography, enhance the accessibility and quality of remote consultations, supporting healthcare professionals in maintaining optimal care standards [374].

Surgical Support

Robotic-assisted surgery has advanced significantly with the introduction of systems like the da Vinci Surgical System, which enables minimally invasive surgeries and provides greater precision. However, challenges remain, including high operational complexity and the need for seamless integration into existing clinical workflows. Future advancements aim to enhance automation in robotic-assisted surgery, thereby reducing the cognitive load on surgeons and improving surgical outcomes [379].

### Robotic Systems for Diagnostics

Robotic systems in diagnostics have played a pivotal role in enhancing the accuracy and accessibility of imaging technologies. Robotic ultrasound systems are enabling remote diagnostics, particularly during the COVID-19 pandemic, reducing exposure risks while maintaining imaging quality [148]. The integration of robotic arms in sonography also enhances diagnostic precision, which is particularly valuable in prenatal care.

Imaging Systems

Robotic systems integrated with imaging modalities, such as MRI and ultrasound, provide real-time imaging, which is crucial for precision in surgeries and diagnostics. The da Vinci system, for example, supports minimally invasive procedures, while the development of autonomous scanning systems in techniques like confocal laser endomicroscopy shows promise for further improving diagnostic accuracy [381].

Biopsy Robots

Biopsy robots, particularly for lung and breast biopsies, are enhancing the precision of needle placement during image-guided procedures. Robotic systems are addressing challenges such as limited reach in lung biopsies and tissue deformation in breast biopsies, providing enhanced accuracy and safety. The integration of optical tracking capabilities and motorized steering in breast biopsy procedures exemplifies the potential of robotic systems in improving diagnostic workflows. These advancements underscore the transformative role of robotic systems in modern medicine, improving both the technical and patient experience aspects of healthcare. As research and innovation continue, these technologies are expected to further refine the quality of care, increase efficiency, and expand access to critical medical services [370].

## 2.13.5 Regulatory Considerations

Implementing robotic systems in medicine—particularly in surgical applications—presents a range of challenges, both technological and organizational. One of the primary obstacles is the disruptive nature of robotic-assisted surgery (RAS). While RAS offers clear benefits such as enhanced precision, superior ergonomics, and improved intraoperative visualization, its integration demands considerable shifts in medical practice and training paradigms. This transformation can provoke resistance among healthcare professionals accustomed to conventional surgical methods [380].

To ensure successful adoption, healthcare institutions must prioritize comprehensive training programs and restructure clinical pathways to equip surgeons and staff with the competencies required to work effectively with robotic platforms. Additionally, the regulatory landscape poses significant hurdles. Demonstrating the clinical utility of robotic systems requires robust comparative evidence, typically in the form of long-term, controlled studies that compare them against existing surgical standards [382]. These requirements, coupled with the substantial cost and time investments needed for validation, can discourage healthcare providers from adopting robotic solutions.

Another concern lies in public perception and the risk of "early adoption bias," where enthusiasm may outpace evidence-based understanding of a system's capabilities and limitations. As such, a balanced and informed approach—one that critically evaluates both benefits and risks—is crucial for sustainable integration.

### Technical Considerations

Robotic systems in medicine must meet stringent safety, reliability, and compatibility criteria to function effectively in clinical environments. One major challenge involves developing MRI-compatible robotic platforms. These systems must operate within strong magnetic fields and high-frequency radio environments, rendering traditional electric motors and ferromagnetic materials unsuitable. Designing miniaturized and non-magnetic robotic mechanisms thus becomes essential for integration with MRI-based procedures. Another challenge is ensuring that medical robots can deliver reliable performance in confined surgical environments while maintaining ease of use and clinical value. More miniature and more task-specific robots offer the potential to improve workflow efficiency; however, they must compete with established surgical navigation systems, which often come at lower costs and have proven utility [369, 371].

To justify their adoption, robotic systems must demonstrate quantifiable improvements in surgical outcomes, such as fewer complications, shorter recovery times, or enhanced surgical precision. This evidence must be generated through multidisciplinary collaboration between clinicians, engineers, and industry developers. Additionally, blending traditional instruments with robotic enhancements, such as actuators and sensors, may bridge the gap between legacy systems and next-generation robotic tools, thereby fostering broader clinical acceptance.

#### Ethical Considerations

The introduction of robotic systems into clinical practice raises profound ethical considerations that extend well beyond functionality. One of the most pressing concerns is the potential erosion of human interaction in patient care. While robotic precision offers numerous benefits, it also introduces the risk of dehumanizing healthcare encounters, particularly in areas such as rehabilitation and elder care [376].

The ethical deployment of robotics requires safeguarding patient autonomy, ensuring informed consent, and preserving the human dimension in medical interactions. Moreover, the development of robotic systems—especially those incorporating artificial intelligence—raises questions about the transparency and accountability of decision-making. It is essential to establish clear protocols defining who is responsible when robotic systems make errors or produce unintended outcomes.

Cybersecurity and data privacy also form critical areas of concern, particularly as robotic systems increasingly integrate with AI-driven health information systems. These platforms must be designed to prevent data breaches and algorithmic bias, ensuring equitable treatment across diverse patient populations. A proactive, ethical framework, grounded in patient-centered values and developed collaboratively across disciplines, is key to ensuring that robotic systems enhance, rather than undermine, the quality and integrity of healthcare delivery.

### 2.13.6 Future Perspectives

The field of medical robotics is poised for unprecedented growth, driven by innovations that aim to enhance surgical precision, improve rehabilitation outcomes, and enhance patient engagement. Among the most notable trends is the miniaturization of surgical robots, which are tailored for specific clinical applications. These smaller, more specialized platforms are designed for seamless integration into existing surgical workflows, offering enhanced safety profiles.

Telerobotics continues to gain traction, enabling highly accurate and less invasive interventions across vast distances. These systems not only improve access to specialized care but also minimize surgical trauma, contributing to faster recovery and better overall outcomes. Robotic solutions in rehabilitation are also expanding, facilitating both physical and cognitive therapy while empowering patients with real-time feedback and adaptive training environments.

Socially assistive robots represent another exciting avenue. These platforms, designed to support cognitive and emotional health, have shown promise in promoting adherence to therapeutic regimens and improving overall patient well-being. As technology continues to converge with healthcare needs, the integration of artificial intelligence, robotics, and personalized medicine is expected to redefine the therapeutic landscape.

#### Artificial Intelligence Integration

The integration of artificial intelligence into robotic systems is redefining healthcare operations, particularly through enhanced automation, decision support, and predictive analytics. AI-enabled robots can assist with clinical decision-making, reduce human error in medication administration, and optimize hospital logistics by predicting patient needs and allocating resources effectively.

Natural Language Processing (NLP) tools embedded within robotic systems facilitate clinical documentation, transcribing voice notes, and streamlining record-keeping tasks. AI also enables robotic systems to retrieve and analyze patient data, helping clinicians make more informed and timely decisions. Applications of AI-integrated robotics are increasingly diverse. Internally, microrobots perform delicate interventions within blood vessels or the gastrointestinal tract. Externally, robots assist with infection control by minimizing direct human contact [376]. On-body systems, including exoskeletons and prosthetics, provide enhanced mobility and improved quality of life. Collectively, these technologies demonstrate the enormous potential of AI-enhanced robotics in transforming patient care across a spectrum of clinical scenarios.

#### Wearable Robotics

Wearable robotics—including exoskeletons, smart orthotics, and robotic prostheses—represents a transformative shift in assistive and rehabilitative care. These systems aim to restore lost motor functions, enhance mobility, and improve the quality of life for individuals with disabilities or age-related impairments.

Key design priorities include comfort, reliability, and unobtrusiveness. Recent innovations have explored hybrid systems that blend augmented reality with physical actuation to reduce physical bulk and enhance user interaction. This could redefine user experience and increase daily adoption of wearable robots [372]. Technological advancements in soft robotics, intelligent control systems, and adaptive materials have enabled devices that respond in real time to users' needs. Multimodal sensors allow these systems to monitor user intent and environmental conditions, offering dynamic and personalized support. Looking ahead, wearable robotics has the potential to become a scalable solution for an aging population, offering not only mobility support but also integrated health monitoring and preventive care functions.

## 2.14 Implantable Drug Pumps and Insulin Pumps

Implantable drug-delivery systems are being designed to provide continuous drug release into the bloodstream, offering an alternative to hospitalization for intravenous infusions or frequent injections. One common approach involves implanting a drug-containing pellet in subcutaneous tissue, where it gradually releases the drug through surface erosion. Another strategy utilizes silicone rubber capsules for diffusion-based delivery; however, only select materials, such as polyacrylamide, are capable of releasing larger molecular compounds.

Implantable pump systems present several significant advantages. They bypass the gastrointestinal tract, offer greater convenience compared to repeated needle-based injections, and ensure patient compliance. Unlike diffusion-limited devices, pump systems can achieve higher release rates. For targeted therapy, these systems may be implanted directly at the therapeutic site or connected via a catheter, while the pump itself remains accessible subcutaneously. These systems can be broadly categorized into two types: degradable and non-degradable. Both categories typically rely on polymer-based components, which not only serve as delivery vehicles but also contribute structural support, biocompatibility, and stability. Insertable drug systems are especially valuable for their ability to be placed in specific anatomical locations and removed once depleted, allowing for both localized and systemic treatment depending on the site of insertion [383].

Drug delivery implants have been successfully positioned in diverse body regions, including ocular, vaginal, transurethral, and intrauterine locations. Ocular inserts, for example, facilitate local drug delivery to the eye, while other implants enable systemic absorption through permeable biological surfaces. Some devices are engineered to function continuously for up to 5 years, requiring minimal maintenance. Additional benefits include the protection of drugs from premature metabolic degradation and the ability to terminate therapy promptly in the event of adverse reactions or toxicity. Implantable drug-delivery systems are generally classified into two principal types: drug implants and pump-based implants. The first category, drug implants, utilizes polymer matrices or membranes to regulate the kinetics of drug release. These systems are further divided into biodegradable and non-biodegradable variants. The second category encompasses mechanical pump implants, which control drug release using infusion-based mechanisms. A third, emerging category includes atypical delivery systems such as sustained-release intraocular devices for glaucoma, hydroxyapatite cement for local antibiotic delivery in osteomyelitis, and transurethral injection systems for treating erectile dysfunction.

A notable application of implantable technology is the insulin pump—a compact, battery-powered, programmable device that administers rapid-acting insulin in minute doses into the subcutaneous tissue. This mode of delivery mimics the physiological insulin secretion of pancreatic beta cells, often resulting in better glycemic control, increased lifestyle flexibility, and enhanced quality of life. Insulin pump therapy, also known as Continuous Subcutaneous Insulin Infusion (CSII), is a dynamic and increasingly prevalent method of insulin administration. It provides a steady basal infusion of rapid-acting insulin with the option for patient-controlled boluses for meals or glucose correction. CSII is approved for individuals with type 1 diabetes and select patients with type 2 diabetes. However, careful patient selection remains essential for optimal outcomes. As pump technology evolves, integrated systems combining insulin delivery with Continuous Glucose Monitoring (CGM) are becoming standard, offering more precise glucose management and real-time therapeutic adjustments.

### 2.14.1 History

The foundational research on implantable drug delivery systems dates back to 1938, when Deansby and Parkes demonstrated the effects of subcutaneous implantation of compressed crystalline estrone pellets in castrated male chickens. This early investigation laid the groundwork for controlled-release drug formulations. In the 1960s, Folkman and Long pioneered a new era of implantable delivery by introducing polymer-based control mechanisms, specifically using silicone rubber (Silastic®), to achieve sustained systemic drug administration.

Parallel to the advancements in implantable systems, the field of diabetes technology has experienced significant evolution. What began with simple insulin syringes has expanded into a range of sophisticated tools, including insulin pens, external pumps, sensor-augmented pumps, and, more recently, hybrid closed-loop systems. These innovations have been further empowered by integration with consumer electronics and cloud-based data platforms, enabling personalized and precise glucose management.

The first portable insulin pump was developed in 1963 by Dr. Arnold Kadish. Although groundbreaking, the initial model faced limitations due to its size and operational complexity. This was followed in 1974 by the "Biostator," a closed-loop system developed by Dr. Ernst Friedrich Pfeiffer at Miles Laboratory in the United States. The Biostator integrated continuous intravenous insulin infusion with real-time glucose monitoring, providing early proof of concept for automated glucose regulation despite its bulky form factor.

In 1978, Dean Kamen introduced the first wearable insulin pump, initially dubbed the "blue brick" and later marketed as the "AutoSyringe." Due to its complexity and size, early adoption was limited to patients awaiting pancreatic transplantation. In 1979, Seoul National University Hospital conducted clinical testing of the SOOIL insulin pump, and the first commercial insulin pump became available in the United States the same year. MiniMed Technologies, initially established as Pacesetter Systems in 1980, launched its first model, the MiniMed 502, in 1983. By 1986, MiniMed introduced an implantable insulin pump designed for intraperitoneal insulin delivery. The 1990s ushered in the next generation of insulin pumps, featuring more compact and user-friendly designs. These models incorporated bolus calculators, portable diabetic management tools, and visual/audio alerts. In 1992,

MiniMed released the MiniMed 506, which included bolus memory, followed by programmable basal-rate enhancements in models 507, 507C, and 508 [384].

Advancements continued into the 2000s, particularly in battery life, device memory, and algorithmic control. Following its acquisition of MiniMed in 2001, Medtronic introduced the MiniMed Paradigm series, with iterative improvements in the 511, 512, and 515 models, including integration with wired continuous glucose monitoring systems. In 2002, Smiths Medical launched the Deltec Cozmo pump, which was discontinued in 2009 due to financial challenges. In 2003, Medtronic advanced insulin pump design by pairing the Paradigm 512 with the Paradigm Link glucose monitor, enabling wireless data transmission between the glucometer and pump. Roche Diabetes Care entered the market in 2006 with the Accu-Chek Spirit, while Medtronic announced the discontinuation of its implantable insulin pumps in 2007. By 2012, Tandem Diabetes Care had released the t:slim insulin delivery system, and Roche introduced the Accu-Chek Combo. A significant shift came in 2015 with the launch of the Omnipod, a tubeless insulin pump, followed by the Omnipod DASH in 2019 [385].

Today, several insulin pump platforms have achieved international approval, including Medtronic MiniMed, Omnipod, Tandem, DANA R, Cellnovo, Roche's Accu-Chek Solo Micropump, and Ypsomed. These systems continue to evolve, offering users increasingly sophisticated options for maintaining glycemic control, often in conjunction with real-time glucose monitoring and cloud-connected data systems (Fig. 2.67).

## 2.14.2 *Technical Characteristics*

Selecting an insulin pump involves evaluating both user-specific needs and the technical features of available devices. Patient characteristics such as low vision, arthritis, neuropathy, or age extremes (e.g., pediatric or geriatric users) must be carefully considered to ensure usability and safety. Key features influencing pump selection include the availability of advanced functionalities, watertight design, compactness, user interface clarity, backlit screens with strong contrast, intuitive iconography and terminology, and ease of infusion site management.

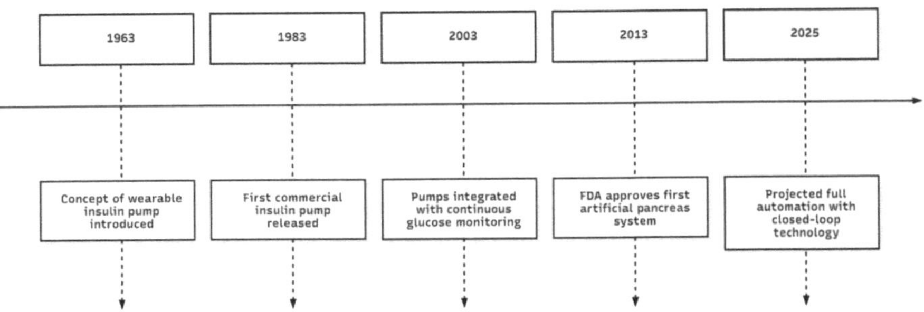


**Fig. 2.67** Evolution of insulin pumps

Effective insulin pump use requires robust troubleshooting skills to prevent potentially serious complications. Users and their support systems must be adequately trained and prepared to handle unexpected operational issues. Troubleshooting competence is essential for ensuring both patient safety and optimal therapeutic outcomes. Modern insulin pumps are designed to be compact, lightweight, and wearable, providing support for mobility and user comfort. These design goals necessitate the use of miniaturized, energy-efficient components, such as ultra-chip-scale packaging (UCSP) and wafer-level packaging (WLP). Advances in materials science and component integration have further contributed to reducing pump size and weight, enhancing daily usability [386].

One of the most impactful innovations for type 1 diabetes management has been the integration of continuous glucose monitoring (CGM), which provides real-time data on glucose trends and trajectories. CGM systems have demonstrated clinical effectiveness in improving glycemic control and have shown psychosocial benefits, such as increased confidence in self-management. However, the extent of benefit varies across individuals and is often linked to the frequency and consistency of use. Limitations of current CGM technology include sensor reliability issues, alarm fatigue, frequent sensor replacements (every 6–7 days), and the visibility of disease management devices, which may increase psychological burden. Recent developments, such as long-term implantable sensors with lifespans of three to 6 months and smartphone integration, aim to address some of these concerns by improving wearability, longevity, and discretion [387] (Fig. 2.68).

From a design perspective, there is growing emphasis on customizable user interfaces that allow individuals to tailor alarms, visual displays, and interface complexity to their personal needs. Future systems should support variable alarm tones and volumes, intuitive menu structures, and automatic synchronization with continuous glucose monitors (CGMs) and glucometers. Resolving time discrepancies across devices, as done in smartphones, would enhance reliability. Additionally, incorporating dietary and activity data entry features, alongside visual bolus counters, would support more informed decision-making and improve insulin dosing accuracy.

- *Implantable Insulin Delivery and Artificial Beta-Cell Systems*
  The intraperitoneal (IP) route of insulin administration in implantable systems offers distinct advantages over subcutaneous (SC) delivery. IP delivery provides faster pharmacokinetics, reduced variability, and improved glycemic control,

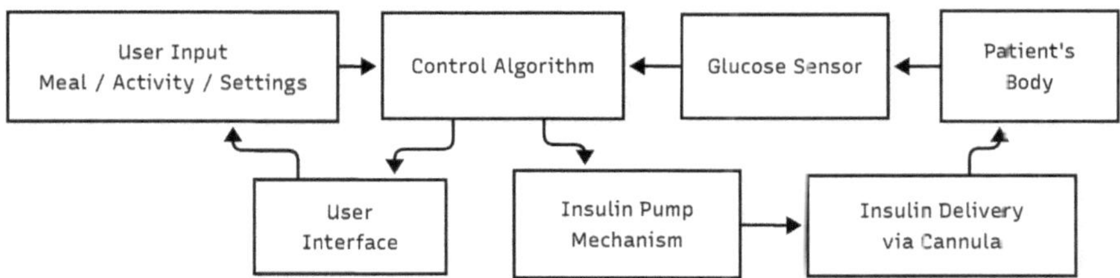


**Fig. 2.68** A block diagram for insulin pumps

while also eliminating the discomfort and visibility associated with SC catheters. Patients often report greater satisfaction and improved quality of life with implantable systems [385].

Although intravenous (IV) sensing initially raised concerns, long-term trials have revealed minimal complications. However, IV sensors often lose structural integrity within 12 months, necessitating regular replacement. This limits their practicality for continuous monitoring. Additionally, delays in glucose sensing with IV sensors can impair the timely delivery of insulin during meals, thereby diminishing the efficacy of closed-loop systems. Comparative studies have shown that systems using IP insulin delivery and IV glucose sensing achieve similar outcomes to those employing SC-SC combinations [388].

- *Technical Requirements and Design Principles for Implantable Pumps*

  Implantable infusion systems can be categorized by their actuation mechanisms into passive (e.g., osmotic or propellant-driven) and active (e.g., battery-powered) systems. Regardless of the mechanism, an ideal implantable drug delivery pump must consistently deliver medication across a range of programmed rates, accommodate both basal and bolus delivery, and allow for adaptability throughout therapy. Pumps must also withstand variable backpressure, enabling drug delivery into solid tissue or high-pressure environments, such as arteries, while maintaining sufficiently low flow rates to avoid hydraulic injury or tissue edema [389].

  Monitoring features are critical and should include real-time feedback on delivery rate, cumulative volume delivered, and remaining drug reservoir. Safeguards must be in place to prevent dose dumping and other forms of inaccurate dosing. The internal and external components of the pump must be sterilizable and biocompatible—non-inflammatory, non-immunogenic, non-thrombogenic, non-carcinogenic—and compatible with a wide range of pharmaceutical compounds [390]. Durability and ease of maintenance are also essential. Pumps should offer long reservoir lifespans, allow for simple refilling procedures, and be designed for both clinical reliability and patient convenience. Together, these features ensure that implantable insulin delivery systems can provide safe, effective, and user-friendly solutions for long-term diabetes management.

## Hardware

The fundamental hardware architecture of insulin pumps has mainly remained consistent since their introduction. These devices are typically composed of three core elements: a motor to actuate insulin delivery, a battery to provide power, and a control interface managed by a microcontroller. Insulin pumps are marketed as integrated systems that include both hardware and proprietary software.

Traditionally, a stepper motor drives a plunger mechanism to subcutaneously dispense insulin. Control is facilitated via a printed circuit board (PCB) and a minimal user interface comprising physical buttons for command input [391]. These components are housed in a compact unit designed for continuous wear. Emerging trends aim to decouple computational functionality from the pump itself, shifting processing tasks to commonly carried smart devices such as smartphones, tablets, or laptops. Offloading computation in this way could streamline pump hardware design and significantly reduce manufacturing costs. Despite the existence of open-source insulin pump projects, none currently offer the same level of portability, robustness, or clinical functionality as commercial devices [384].

Prototyping efforts have also explored the use of mechanical insulin pumps with off-the-shelf components. One such prototype utilized a custom-machined aluminum housing, demonstrating the feasibility of a simplified drive mechanism. Future versions are expected to incorporate Bluetooth connectivity, enabling remote control and monitoring via mobile devices.

#### Software

Modern closed-loop insulin delivery systems comprise three interconnected components: a subcutaneous glucose sensor, a control algorithm, and an intraperitoneal insulin infusion pump. In this configuration, the glucose sensor transmits data to a control system—typically a laptop—using radiofrequency communication. The control system processes the data using a mathematical model based on the biphasic insulin response of pancreatic β-cells, including feedback inhibition mechanisms. The resultant dosing commands are relayed to the pump via Bluetooth. Despite advancements in hardware, software update mechanisms for insulin pumps have not kept pace with the evolution of consumer technology. Software embedded in commercial pumps often remains static throughout the device's warranty period (typically 4 years), limiting the opportunity to implement feature updates or user-requested improvements [391, 392].

Human factors research has revealed that users desire a software update experience comparable to smartphones—intuitive, regular, and optional. Understanding the contextual use of insulin pumps and the environment in which users are likely to use them (i.e., at home vs. in a clinic) is crucial for designing user-friendly software interfaces. This underscores the importance of incorporating user expectations, needs, and limitations into early design iterations, ensuring that software updates enhance usability without compromising safety in a regulated healthcare environment (Fig. 2.69).

### *2.14.3 Types of Devices*

Implantable insulin pumps deliver insulin directly into the peritoneal cavity, a highly vascularized space that facilitates rapid and efficient absorption. The first use of implantable pumps for type 1 diabetes began in 1989, primarily in France, with programmable systems delivering insulin through intraperitoneal (IP) catheters.

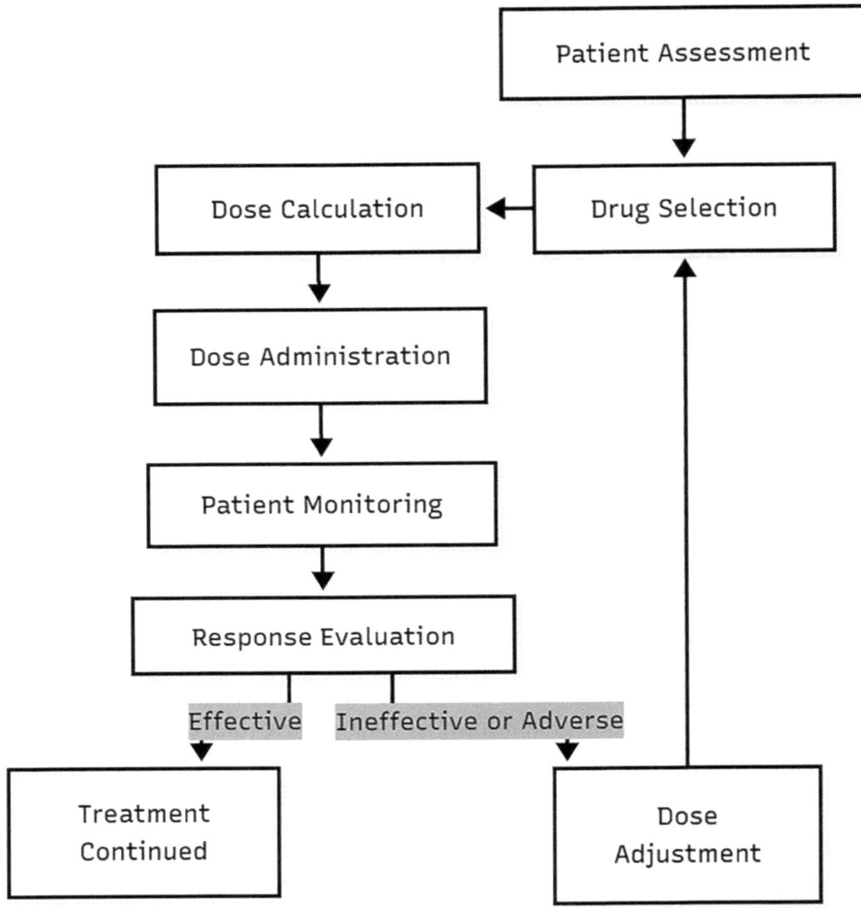


**Fig. 2.69** Decision-making process of drug dosing

The current-generation MIP 2007 model by Medtronic MiniMed integrates improved electronics and offers extended battery life (7–10 years). Insulin delivery mimics that of external pumps and is managed through a Personal Pump Communicator (PPC). The pump is implanted subcutaneously in the abdominal wall, while the catheter enters the peritoneal space. Initially, semi-synthetic insulin formulations, such as Insuplant 400 IU/mL, were used; however, these have since been replaced with stabilized recombinant formulations, like Insuman Implantable 400 IU/mL, to prevent degradation within the pump [385].

One common issue in insulin pump use is back pressure, often caused by occlusions in the infusion set. These may result from fibrillation, cannula kinks, inflammation, or mechanical displacement. Air bubbles in the infusion system may also contribute to delivery inconsistencies. Devices like the Medtronic 670G dynamically adjust insulin delivery in response to glucose levels, but this functionality may exacerbate back pressure. Adjustments in device settings and regular monitoring are essential to mitigate these risks. Notably, manufacturers seldom define back pressure as a critical performance parameter due to its variability among users and conditions. Implantable pumps typically employ one of two mechanisms: fluorocarbon-based vapor pressure systems, which deliver insulin at a fixed rate, and peristaltic motor-driven systems, which are programmable and offer variable dosing. Examples include models from Medtronic and Codman & Shurtleff. The motorized systems provide enhanced flexibility and are powered by long-lasting batteries (4–7 years). Both types are refillable through percutaneous injections [384].

While these systems occupy approximately 200 cm$^3$, only a quarter of that volume is allocated to the drug reservoir. Next-generation miniaturized pumps aim to increase the drug-to-device volume ratio while improving flow rate accuracy, power efficiency, and flexibility in dosing regimens. Some systems now incorporate wireless power transfer and communications, further extending the operational lifespan and clinical functionality of the pump.

### SynchroMed™ III Drug Infusion System

The SynchroMed™ III is an implantable infusion system designed for targeted drug delivery to manage chronic pain, cancer-related pain, and severe spasticity. Unlike oral or systemic treatments that must traverse the blood-brain barrier, this system delivers medication directly into the intrathecal space, enabling effective relief at significantly lower doses and with reduced side effects. The SynchroMed™ III is an advancement over its predecessor, incorporating improved pump electronics, firmware-upgradable implants, and enhanced cybersecurity features. The updated "refill-only" workflow streamlines programming and minimizes clinical intervention time. This next-generation system offers wireless firmware updates, robust patient data protection, and higher reliability. It maintains the durable design enhancements from SynchroMed™ II, achieving a 99% pump survival rate, thus offering long-term performance confidence for clinicians and patients alike.

### Codman Implantable Drug Delivery Device

The CODMAN 3000 Series Constant Flow Implantable Pump features a titanium and silicone rubber body, along with a bolus safety valve, for long-term, ambulatory medication delivery. It includes an integrated silicone rubber catheter and delivers drugs at a constant preset rate. Refills and bolus injections are performed percutaneously with specialized needles, and a built-in safety mechanism ensures secure administration during bolus dosing [393]. The pump's dual-chamber architecture includes an inner drug chamber and an outer chamber containing a thermally activated propellant. Body heat causes the propellant to apply consistent pressure on the bellows, driving drug flow through a filter and flow restrictor into the catheter. Each refill resets the infusion cycle, maintaining continuous drug delivery.

**Osmotic and Intravesical Drug Delivery Systems**

The Medici Drug Delivery System, utilized in ITCA 650, enables long-term exenatide release for the management of type 2 diabetes. Designed for 6- to 12-month dosing, this formulation utilizes a supersaturated osmolyte to maintain a stable release rate. To enhance delivery efficiency, new designs incorporate osmotic flow from urine rather than interstitial fluid, as exemplified by the TARIS System used in GemRIS and lidocaine-releasing implants. These dual-lumen implants offer sustained local drug release without moving parts, thereby improving patient comfort and reducing the treatment burden [394]. However, risks such as device rupture or difficulty in removal underscore the need for cautious deployment.

### *2.14.4 Clinical Applications*

Insulin pumps, also known as continuous subcutaneous insulin infusion (CSII) systems, marked a transformative step in diabetes management by improving glycemic control beyond what was achievable with multiple daily injections (MDI). These devices, initially paired with capillary glucose self-monitoring, have undergone substantial evolution over the past four decades and are now a standard component of advanced diabetes therapy.

Modern insulin pumps are compact, programmable systems that continuously deliver rapid-acting insulin over 24 h, closely mimicking physiological insulin release compared to traditional methods. Each system consists of a disposable insulin reservoir and an infusion set comprising tubing and a subcutaneous cannula. Pumps offer precise basal insulin infusion, which can be adjusted in hourly increments but typically shows optimal performance in 3–4 h blocks, aligning with the pharmacokinetics of rapid-acting analogs. They also support user-defined bolus dosing, both for meals based on carbohydrate content and for correcting hyperglycemia. Integrated bolus calculators help determine optimal doses by taking into account insulin on board and individual insulin action durations. Once insulin enters the bloodstream, it distributes rapidly, with circulation occurring in about 1 min [395]. Drug distribution depends on the compound's chemical properties. Water-soluble agents, like atenolol, remain primarily in plasma and interstitial fluid, while fat-soluble agents, such as clorazepate, preferentially accumulate in adipose tissue. Some drugs localize to specific tissues due to selective affinity. Binding to plasma proteins further influences distribution; bound drug is pharmacologically inactive but can serve as a reservoir, releasing active drug as plasma levels decline.

Therapeutic drug monitoring (TDM), traditionally performed at fixed intervals, plays a central role in maintaining drug concentrations within a defined therapeutic range. While historically used for small molecules, recent applications have extended to monoclonal antibodies. However, conventional TDM methods, including high-performance liquid chromatography-tandem mass spectrometry (HPLC-MS) and enzyme-linked immunosorbent assays (ELISA), are time-consuming, labor-intensive, and reliant on centralized laboratory infrastructure [387]. These constraints hinder real-time decision-making in acute care settings, yielding sparse data points for pharmacokinetic/pharmacodynamic (PK/PD) modeling.

In contrast, implantable insulin delivery systems and drug pumps offer sustained, programmable, and precisely controlled drug administration. This improves treatment stability, reduces dosing errors, and enhances adherence—particularly in the management of chronic diseases—by minimizing the burden of frequent injections. These systems deliver therapeutic agents via pressure differentials, rather than relying on passive diffusion or erosion, which allows for broader and deeper tissue perfusion and more consistent plasma concentrations. Insulin pumps typically use rapid-acting insulin analogues, such as lispro, aspart, and Glulisine. Regular insulin, now seldom used in pumps, has a slower onset (~30 min) compared to analogues (5–15 min), which can delay postprandial control if the bolus is not timed correctly.

Recent innovations include smart insulin pens, simplified patch pumps, advanced pen needle designs, and integrated continuous glucose monitoring (CGM) systems. These technologies, combined with machine learning algorithms and real-time analytics, contribute to more effective and personalized care for individuals with diabetes. The concept of a fully automated artificial pancreas—an autonomous closed-loop system—is nearing clinical reality. Early generations of sensor-augmented pumps provided hypoglycemia shutoff features. Current hybrid closed-loop systems autonomously adjust basal insulin but require manual boluses. The anticipated third generation integrates multihormonal feedback loops for fully automated glucose regulation. Despite these advances, insulin pumps still require user engagement and decision-making. Success with CSII depends on the patient's technical aptitude, self-management skills, and willingness to engage in device training. Not all patients are ideal candidates; individuals with cognitive limitations or resistance to self-directed care may benefit more from a multidisciplinary approach. Eligibility assessments should be conducted by healthcare professionals, taking into account both psychosocial and physiological factors. Insulin pump therapy is typically considered for individuals aged 10 and older.

Implantable pumps capable of variable-rate delivery—without repeated surgical intervention—offer unique advantages in specialized applications. These devices are handy when localized drug perfusion is necessary or when conventional implantable systems are too large or insufficiently responsive. Advances in microfluidics and nanotechnology have led to the development of smaller, more efficient pumps that offer enhanced precision and scalability. These systems support preclinical research and emerging therapeutic paradigms, enabling drug developers to fine-tune delivery kinetics and explore new administration routes. Ultimately, the integration of implantable systems with real-time drug monitoring and smart analytics presents a transformative opportunity in personalized medicine, offering clinicians continuous feedback and patients safer, more adaptive treatment options.

### *2.14.5 Regulatory Considerations*

In the European Union, insulin pumps are classified as Class IIb devices, requiring CE certification via Notified Bodies. These bodies assess technical documentation by MDR Annexes II and III. For combination products, the EMA evaluates the medicinal component while Notified Bodies assess the device aspects. Devices must meet MDR 2017/745 standards, including requirements on biocompatibility, electrical safety, and long-term mechanical reliability. Annex I specifies materials selection, compatibility with biological tissues, and integration with other implant components. Devices that administer medication must demonstrate compatibility with the intended drug and sustain performance across their intended use duration. Compliance with general safety and performance requirements, supported by MDCG guidance and harmonized standards, is mandatory for market access.

### *2.14.6 Future Perspectives*

Despite significant progress, key challenges remain in drug delivery, particularly regarding patient compliance and achieving consistent therapeutic levels. Ideal future systems aim for zero-order release kinetics, extended in vivo performance, and use of advanced biodegradable and biocompatible materials [384].

Next-generation insulin pumps may utilize MR elastomer-based actuators, machine learning algorithms, and integrated smart sensors to enable real-time, adaptive insulin dosing. Advances in micropump design and materials science will enhance reliability, biocompatibility, and patient safety. Intraperitoneal insulin delivery remains an area of interest due to its physiological advantages and improved pharmacokinetics. However, clinical adoption is limited by outdated evidence, lack of fast-acting analogues for IP use, and commercial disinterest. An open-source approach to pump development could accelerate innovation by enabling community-driven enhancements to both hardware and software [390, 391]. Establishing a national registry for insulin pump use and adverse events would provide a clearer understanding of clinical outcomes and support evidence-based improvements in therapy.

## 2.15 Smart Pills

With the accelerating convergence of medicine and digital innovation, the advent of "smart pills" marks a pivotal advancement in precision healthcare and real-time physiological monitoring. Also referred to as ingestible sensors or digital pills, these formulations integrate miniature electronic components capable of transmitting

data from within the gastrointestinal tract to external receivers. Positioned at the intersection of conventional drug delivery systems and emerging diagnostic technologies, smart pills offer a minimally invasive solution for monitoring patient adherence, gastrointestinal parameters, and disease progression.
The impetus behind innovative pill development stems from the urgent need to improve therapeutic adherence, enhance diagnostic accuracy, and mitigate the economic burden of ineffective treatments. Nonadherence remains a persistent challenge in managing chronic conditions such as hypertension, diabetes, and psychiatric disorders. Integrating sensors into oral medications introduces an objective mechanism for tracking ingestion events and providing actionable insights to healthcare providers and caregivers. A notable example is Abilify MyCite®, an FDA-approved digital version of aripiprazole designed to monitor medication intake in patients with schizophrenia and bipolar disorder [396]. Technologically, smart pills comprise components such as micro-scale sensors, chips, power sources, and wireless transmitters, all encapsulated in a biocompatible shell that can withstand gastric conditions. Some devices extend beyond monitoring, incorporating imaging systems, temperature or pH sensors, and controlled drug release mechanisms, enabling dual diagnostic and therapeutic functionalities.

In the realm of biomedical instrumentation, smart pills exemplify ongoing trends toward device miniaturization and instantaneous data analytics. These devices transmit data to smartphones or cloud platforms, enabling continuous remote patient monitoring and facilitating rapid clinical responses. As integral elements of the broader Internet of Medical Things (IoMT) ecosystem, smart pills are poised to significantly influence the future architecture of healthcare delivery [397]. Despite their promise, the adoption of smart pills is accompanied by several challenges. Ethical issues surrounding data privacy, informed consent, and potential misuse must be rigorously addressed. Additionally, questions related to regulatory pathways, insurance reimbursement models, and the long-term safety of ingestible electronics remain critical to their broader implementation.

### *2.15.1 History*

The emergence of smart pills is the product of a dynamic convergence among biomedical engineering, pharmacology, and information technology. The conceptual foundation of ingestible electronics can be traced back to the 1970s, when initial efforts focused on developing capsules capable of recording basic physiological parameters, most notably, core body temperature. These early devices were rudimentary in design and function, primarily serving research applications in gastroenterology [398]. Progress in miniaturization and sensor technology during the 1980s and 1990s paved the way for more advanced ingestible capsules. These iterations could monitor additional physiological variables such as pH, intraluminal pressure, and intestinal motility. Despite offering improved diagnostic capabilities, these capsules lacked real-time wireless communication and integration with external data platforms, which limited their utility to passive data collection rather than interactive or therapeutic use.

A transformative milestone occurred in the early 2000s with the advent of capsule endoscopy, pioneered by Given Imaging. Their PillCam® system integrated a miniature camera within a swallowable capsule, enabling high-resolution imaging of the gastrointestinal tract. This innovation provided a non-invasive, patient-friendly alternative to traditional endoscopic procedures and became widely utilized in the diagnosis of conditions such as Crohn's disease and obscure gastrointestinal bleeding. The 2010s marked a turning point in smart pill development, driven by rapid advancements in wireless communication, low-power microelectronics, and mobile health infrastructure. A notable breakthrough was the 2017 FDA approval of Abilify MyCite®, the first digital medication that combined the antipsychotic agent aripiprazole with an ingestible sensor. This system enabled the tracking of medication ingestion events and wirelessly transmitted the data to a mobile application, significantly enhancing adherence monitoring in patients with schizophrenia and bipolar disorder [399]. This approval represented a paradigm shift, legitimizing digital pills as a component of mainstream clinical care.

Since that time, the scope and capabilities of smart pills have expanded considerably. Contemporary prototypes are being developed with multifunctional platforms that incorporate imaging, biosensing, controlled drug release, and autonomous locomotion via magnetic or motorized propulsion. Ongoing research is also exploring the use of biodegradable electronics, advanced biocompatible materials, and secure wireless protocols to address concerns related to safety, functionality, and data privacy. The evolution of smart pills exemplifies a remarkable trajectory of interdisciplinary innovation, progressing from simple diagnostic tools to fully integrated digital health systems. As these technologies mature, smart pills are expected to play a crucial role in personalized medicine, telehealth delivery, and remote physiological monitoring, ultimately redefining how healthcare is accessed and delivered across various clinical settings (Fig. 2.70).

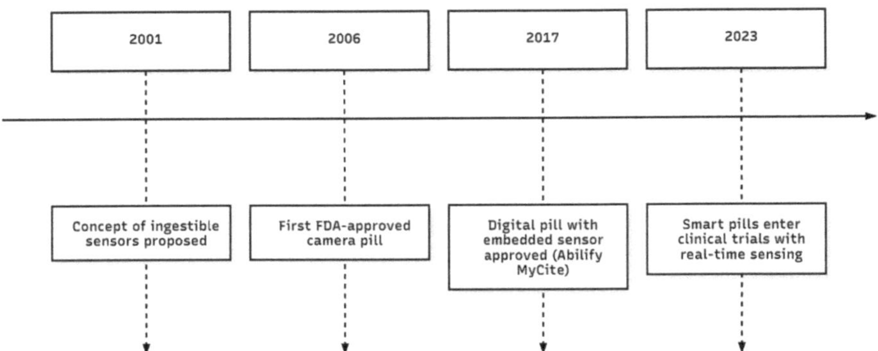


**Fig. 2.70** Timeline of smart pill development

## 2.15.2 Technical Characteristics

### Hardware

Smart pills, also referred to as ingestible sensors or digital pills, represent an emerging class of biomedical devices engineered to function within the human gastrointestinal tract. These devices integrate miniaturized electronics with biocompatible materials to perform a spectrum of tasks, including physiological monitoring, diagnostic imaging, and localized drug delivery [400]. Their hardware design is critical to their effectiveness, demanding compact form factors, energy efficiency, and structural integrity to withstand the chemically aggressive environment of the GI tract.

#### Processing Unit and Sensors

At the core of each smart pill is a microcontroller or embedded processor that orchestrates the device's operations. These processors manage data acquisition from onboard sensors, sequence operational tasks, perform basic data processing, and facilitate wireless data transmission. Due to strict power and size limitations, these computational units are typically ultra-low-power system-on-chip (SoC) designs tailored for biomedical applications. Integrated sensor arrays allow for comprehensive physiological assessment. pH sensors provide positional data by detecting pH transitions between the gastric and intestinal regions. Temperature sensors may help detect pathological conditions, such as inflammation, while pressure sensors assist in assessing gut motility. Imaging capsules, such as capsule endoscopes, contain complementary metal-oxide-semiconductor (CMOS) image sensors and LED arrays for capturing internal mucosal visuals [40, 130, 401] (Fig. 2.71).

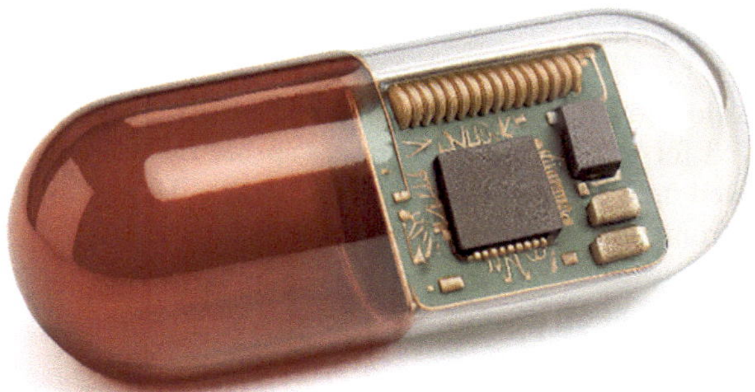

**Fig. 2.71** Internal structure of a smart pill

Power Supply

Powering smart pills is a fundamental engineering constraint. Most devices are equipped with biocompatible coin-cell batteries—typically lithium or silver oxide variants—capable of sustaining device functionality for 8–48 h. Research into bioenergy harvesting, such as generating electricity from gastric fluids, and wireless power transfer methods is also underway, offering potential for extended operational lifespans.

Wireless Communication

Smart pills transmit collected data via embedded wireless modules. Standard communication protocols include radio frequency (RF), Bluetooth Low Energy (BLE), and near-field communication (NFC). Wearable or external receivers receive these signals for further analysis or cloud upload. A miniaturized antenna, optimized for the high-dielectric, lossy medium of the human body, is crucial for successful data transmission.

Housing and Data Storage

Internal components are encapsulated in biocompatible casings made from materials like polycarbonate or polyethylene glycol. Enteric coatings are often applied to control the site of capsule activation or disintegration. This casing not only shields sensitive electronics from harsh digestive fluids but also ensures patient safety [402]. In instances where real-time transmission is compromised, onboard memory such as flash storage or EEPROM is used to store data, which can later be extracted, ensuring continuity in data collection.

Advanced Functionalities

Beyond diagnostics, advanced smart pills include therapeutic capabilities. Actuators can be employed for localized drug release, capsule retention in specific GI segments, or targeted delivery using microneedle arrays. These developments transition smart pills from passive monitors to multifunctional treatment platforms [403].

### Software

A sophisticated integration of embedded software, control logic, and data processing algorithms enables smart pills. These systems facilitate adherence tracking, monitoring of physiological parameters, and seamless communication with healthcare providers [323].

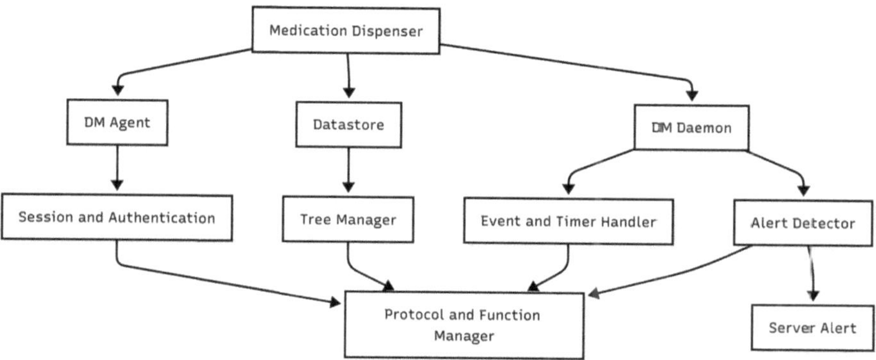


**Fig. 2.72** Software architecture of the smart medication dispenser

## Core Software Design

The software architectures of smart pills employ a modular approach to support scalability and flexibility. For example, there is a layered design composed of a Device Management (DM) Agent, Function Manager, and Daemon. These components coordinate tasks such as session handling, medication status reporting, update management, and error logging (Fig. 2.72).

## IoT and AI Integration

The integration of Internet of Things (IoT) and Artificial Intelligence (AI) technologies has enhanced the functionality of smart pills. SPEC 2.0 comprises a smart dispenser, a sensing-enabled cup, and an Android application—all connected via Bluetooth Low Energy (BLE). The system enforces fail-safe logic, such as verifying the presence of a smart cup before releasing medication, to prevent operational errors [69].

## Context-Aware Reminders

To improve user adherence, context-aware systems utilize AI-driven modules to deliver medication reminders based on behavioral and environmental inputs. It uses a framework that includes an activity recognition engine, a reminder scheduler, and a compliance tracking module. This system customizes alerts based on user habits, thereby enhancing engagement and reducing the likelihood of missed doses (Fig. 2.73).

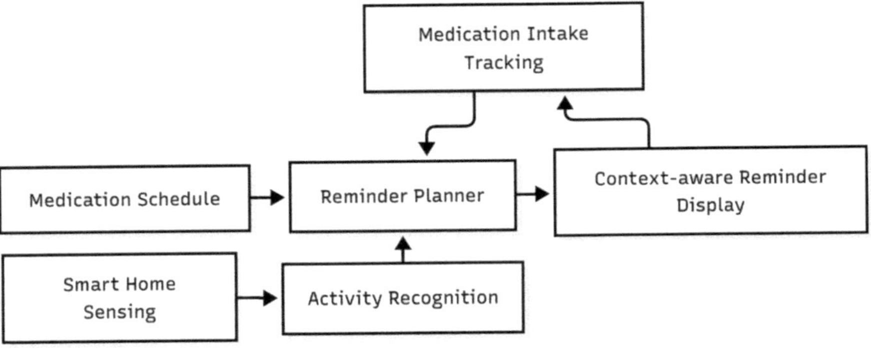


**Fig. 2.73** Conceptual framework of the smart pillbox system

Ingestible Sensor Software

Ingestible sensors embedded in smart pills measure internal parameters, such as pH, temperature, and pressure. For instance, Proteus Digital Health's IEM system emits signals when exposed to gastric fluid, confirming medication ingestion. Software must ensure efficient power use and accurate, lossless data transmission under challenging conditions.

Security and Privacy Protocols

Smart pill systems handle sensitive health data, necessitating stringent cybersecurity measures. These include end-to-end encryption, device and user authentication, and compliance with healthcare privacy regulations like HIPAA. The CAMMS model exemplifies how context-aware monitoring and secure feedback loops can simultaneously ensure system responsiveness and safeguard patient confidentiality.

### 2.15.3 *Types of Devices*

Smart pills—pioneering tools in the realm of ingestible electronics and digital therapeutics—are revolutionizing the practice of medicine by enabling non-invasive diagnostics, continuous physiological monitoring, precision-targeted drug delivery, and real-time medication adherence tracking. These capsule-based devices bring capabilities that were once confined to clinical settings into the hands (and stomachs) of patients, supporting decentralized, personalized healthcare [100].

Smart pills are generally classified by their primary function, which includes imaging, physiological sensing, controlled drug release, adherence monitoring, and integrated (hybrid) operations.

### Imaging Capsules

Imaging capsules represent one of the earliest and most mature applications of smart pill technology. These devices integrate compact optical systems—typically CMOS cameras—alongside LED lighting, batteries, and wireless transmitters. Upon ingestion, they traverse the gastrointestinal (GI) tract while capturing thousands of high-resolution images.

The PillCam™ SB 3, developed by Medtronic, is a leading product in this category. It has been widely adopted for the non-invasive diagnosis of small bowel disorders, particularly in cases of obscure GI bleeding, Crohn's disease, and iron-deficiency anemia. Its ability to replace conventional endoscopy with a swallowable, disposable capsule marks a significant leap in patient comfort and diagnostic reach.

### Physiological Monitoring Capsules

Sensing capsules focus on acquiring in vivo data on physiological parameters, including pH, pressure, temperature, and motility patterns. These metrics are essential for diagnosing disorders related to GI function and motility. The SmartPill™, also by Medtronic, is a prominent example. It evaluates gastric emptying and whole-gut transit times, providing a minimally invasive diagnostic option for patients with suspected gastroparesis or chronic constipation. The sensor suite allows for detailed analysis of digestive tract dynamics without the need for catheters or imaging-based studies [404].

### Drug Delivery Capsules

Smart pills designed for drug delivery enable precise, programmable release of therapeutic agents at specific sites within the GI tract. These capsules typically contain embedded microcontrollers, sensors, and release mechanisms that activate in response to specific locations or times.

IntelliCap®, developed by Philips, exemplifies this innovation. The device integrates environmental sensing, real-time control, and programmable release profiles, making it ideal for targeted delivery of medications where local drug concentration is crucial, such as in inflammatory bowel disease or localized infections. This precision reduces systemic exposure and enhances therapeutic outcomes [402].

### Adherence Monitoring Capsules

Poor medication adherence is a pervasive challenge in managing chronic illnesses such as schizophrenia, hypertension, and diabetes. Adherence monitoring pills incorporate tiny ingestible sensors that activate upon reaching the stomach and transmit confirmation of ingestion. Abilify MyCite, developed by Otsuka Pharmaceutical, is the first FDA-approved digital medicine system that combines the antipsychotic aripiprazole with a sensor. Once ingested, the sensor communicates with a wearable patch, which then relays ingestion data to a mobile application. This ecosystem enables clinicians to remotely track and support patient adherence, particularly beneficial in behavioral health, where nonadherence is common.

#### Hybrid Capsules

Hybrid smart pills combine two or more functionalities—such as sensing, imaging, and drug delivery—within a single device. These platforms represent a step toward autonomous, closed-loop therapeutic systems capable of diagnosing, reporting, and initiating localized treatment without external intervention. While still largely experimental, hybrid capsules exemplify the next wave in ingestible medicine. Challenges such as miniaturization, power consumption, multi-modal integration, and regulatory hurdles remain significant. Nonetheless, such multifunctional systems are poised to revolutionize the detection and treatment of diseases within the body.

### *2.15.4 Clinical Applications*

Smart pills, a subset of ingestible electronic systems, are reshaping the landscape of modern medicine. Their use spans a wide range of clinical applications—from diagnostics and physiological monitoring to precision drug delivery and real-time adherence tracking—addressing persistent gaps in patient care through minimally invasive, data-driven solutions.

#### Diagnostics and Disease Detection

One of the most impactful applications of smart pills lies in diagnostic imaging, particularly within gastroenterology. Capsule endoscopy devices such as the PillCam™ enable high-resolution, non-invasive visualization of the gastrointestinal (GI) tract, facilitating the early detection of obscure GI bleeding, Crohn's disease, and small bowel neoplasms. These capsules house miniature optical sensors and transmitters that wirelessly relay thousands of images as they transit through the digestive tract, replacing the need for invasive endoscopic procedures and significantly improving patient comfort and compliance. In parallel, advanced diagnostic smart pills are being developed with biosensor arrays capable of detecting specific biomarkers [119, 404]. These biosensors monitor local pH, temperature, and pressure conditions, offering real-time physiological insights that aid in the early

detection of colorectal cancer, inflammatory bowel disease, and other gastrointestinal disorders.

### Physiological Monitoring

Continuous, internal monitoring of physiological parameters is crucial for managing chronic and functional disorders. Ingestible sensors embedded within smart pills track variables such as intraluminal pH, pressure, and temperature, providing clinicians with detailed data throughout the entire GI tract. The SmartPill™ by Medtronic is one such device, offering quantifiable metrics on gastric emptying and colonic transit times, key indicators in diagnosing motility disorders. Recent innovations have expanded physiological monitoring capabilities beyond the GI system. Celero Systems, for example, has developed an ingestible capsule that monitors core body temperature, heart rate, and respiratory rate directly from within the stomach. These data have shown high accuracy when compared to standard hospital-based monitors, supporting remote diagnostics in conditions such as sleep apnea or opioid-induced respiratory depression [401].

### Targeted Drug Delivery

Smart pills are also advancing oral drug delivery by enabling site-specific release of therapeutics within the gastrointestinal tract. The IntelliCap® system, for instance, integrates environmental sensing and programmable release mechanisms, enabling the delivery of pharmaceuticals at precise time points or pH-defined locations. This is particularly beneficial for localized diseases such as ulcerative colitis or Crohn's disease, where systemic drug exposure is less effective or poorly tolerated [405]. Emerging research into stimulus-responsive systems—such as those triggered by temperature shifts, enzymatic activity, or magnetic fields—further enhances the potential for smart pills to support personalized and dynamic therapy regimens.

### Medication Adherence Monitoring

Nonadherence to medication regimens remains a significant obstacle in effective disease management. Smart pills provide a novel solution by incorporating ingestible sensors that activate upon reaching gastric fluids, transmitting a signal to external receivers. Abilify MyCite® combines the antipsychotic agent aripiprazole with a sensor-based ingestion tracking system. Once activated, the signal is captured by a wearable patch and logged in a companion mobile application, allowing healthcare professionals to verify whether medication has been taken and intervene when adherence lapses are detected. This approach is particularly valuable in the management of psychiatric disorders, where adherence is often inconsistent yet critical to treatment efficacy [406, 407].

**Remote Monitoring and Chronic Disease Management**

The integration of smart pills into remote patient monitoring platforms enables more proactive and continuous care for individuals with chronic diseases. These ingestible devices transmit real-time physiological data to healthcare systems, thereby reducing the need for in-person visits and enabling timely adjustments to treatment. In conditions such as hypertension, diabetes, and cardiovascular disease, the ability to continuously assess patient status supports earlier intervention and better disease control. Additionally, when combined with artificial intelligence, smart pill data streams can be analyzed to uncover behavioral patterns, predict clinical deterioration, and tailor therapies to individual needs [408]. This enhances both clinical outcomes and healthcare system efficiency by reducing hospitalizations and optimizing resource utilization [409, 410].

## *2.15.5 Regulatory Considerations*

The convergence of pharmaceuticals, electronics, and software in smart pills has created a unique regulatory and ethical environment. These devices blur the traditional boundaries between medicinal products and medical devices, raising complex questions related to safety, data security, classification, and patient autonomy. Regulatory authorities such as the U.S. Food and Drug Administration (FDA) and the European Medicines Agency (EMA) are increasingly tasked with overseeing not only clinical efficacy but also cybersecurity, software integrity, and ethical compliance [396].

**Regulatory Classification and Pathways**

Smart pills are typically regulated as combination products due to their hybrid nature, incorporating drug substances, ingestible electronics, and digital components. Regulatory classification depends on their primary intended function, such as diagnosis, therapy, or monitoring [79].

U.S. FDA Regulatory Framework

In the United States, diagnostic smart pills—such as capsule endoscopy and GI motility monitors—are generally regulated as Class II or Class III medical devices, depending on their level of invasiveness and associated risk (FDA n.d.). Therapeutic smart pills that combine active pharmaceutical ingredients with embedded sensors, such as Abilify MyCite, fall under the category of combination products. These require coordinated oversight from multiple FDA centers, including the Center for Drug Evaluation and Research (CDER) and the Center for Devices and Radiological Health (CDRH).

Smart pills follow one of several FDA regulatory pathways:

- Premarket Approval (PMA): Required for high-risk, novel devices, necessitating comprehensive clinical trials.
- 510(k) Clearance: Suitable for devices that demonstrate substantial equivalence to already-approved products.
- De Novo Classification: For low-to-moderate risk devices with no existing predicate; used to establish new regulatory categories.
- New Drug Application (NDA): Required when pharmacologically active substances are involved, alongside evaluations of sensor technology, wireless communication, and associated software.

The FDA's approval of Abilify MyCite® in 2017 was a landmark case, as it necessitated the simultaneous review of a drug, an ingestible sensor, a wearable patch, and a smartphone application.

### European Union Regulatory Framework

In the European Union, smart pills are governed by the Medical Device Regulation [224] and, when applicable, Directive 2001/83/EC on medicinal products. Combination smart pills that contain both drug and device components must obtain a CE mark, indicating conformity with EU safety, performance, and quality standards (EMA n.d.). Manufacturers must conduct:

- Clinical evaluations and biocompatibility testing,
- Software verification and validation,
- Cybersecurity risk assessments, and
- Ongoing post-market surveillance and adverse event reporting.

As many smart pills incorporate artificial intelligence (AI) for real-time decision-making, EU regulators increasingly emphasize algorithm transparency, validation using real-world evidence, and compliance with AI-specific ethical guidelines.

### Cybersecurity and Data Protection

Smart pills collect, store, and transmit sensitive health information, making data security and privacy fundamental regulatory concerns. In the U.S., developers must adhere to the Health Insurance Portability and Accountability Act (HIPAA), which mandates technical and administrative safeguards for electronic protected health information (ePHI).

In the EU, smart pill systems fall under the General Data Protection Regulation (GDPR). Requirements include:

- Data minimization and encryption,
- Access controls and audit logging,
- Transparent user consent, and
- Accountability for third-party data sharing.

Devices must demonstrate secure wireless protocols, encrypted data storage and transmission, and the ability to track access. Regulatory authorization may be denied or revoked if these requirements are unmet.

### Ethical and Legal Dimensions

The introduction of ingestible digital systems into healthcare raises profound ethical questions. While the potential benefits of smart pills are considerable, issues of autonomy, consent, coercion, and surveillance must be addressed to ensure ethically sound implementation [411].

#### Autonomy and Informed Consent

Smart pills, especially those monitoring medication adherence, can blur the line between support and surveillance. For instance, in psychiatric treatment, digital tracking tools like Abilify MyCite® may undermine a patient's sense of control, particularly when data are shared with third parties such as family members or caregivers. Informed consent must go beyond clinical explanations to include:

- Technical understanding of how data is captured and transmitted,
- Awareness of potential data recipients,
- Understanding of risks associated with data misuse or misinterpretation.

Legalistic user agreements filled with dense terminology further compromise the concept of meaningful consent.

#### Privacy and Data Ownership

The granular data collected by smart pills—covering everything from ingestion events to physiological states—raises significant concerns about privacy and data ownership. Patients often remain unaware of how their data is stored, who has access to it, and how it may be used for purposes beyond clinical care. Clear governance structures, patient-centric data policies, and transparency in data usage are necessary to preserve trust in digital health interventions.

Coercion and Power Dynamics

Smart pills may be used coercively, particularly among vulnerable groups. Patients with mental illness or those under institutional care may feel compelled to use these devices as a condition for treatment, release, or social benefits. This shifts the therapeutic relationship from one of collaboration to control. It is crucial that the introduction of smart pills never supersede voluntary participation or become a substitute for patient engagement and trust-building in care plans.

Ethical Oversight and Policy Development

The ethical landscape surrounding smart pills remains underdeveloped. As these technologies evolve, so too must the regulatory and ethical frameworks guiding their deployment. Robust, interdisciplinary collaboration among engineers, clinicians, ethicists, legal scholars, and policymakers is necessary to develop responsive guidelines that strike a balance between innovation and the protection of human rights.

### *2.15.6 Future Perspectives*

The intersection of biomedical engineering, nanotechnology, and artificial intelligence is redefining the capabilities of smart pills, shifting their role from passive diagnostic tools to dynamic agents of precision medicine. Innovations in device architecture, bioresponsive systems, and data-driven intelligence are laying the groundwork for smart pills capable of real-time diagnostics, adaptive therapy, and autonomous clinical support, reshaping the future of personalized healthcare.

#### **Miniaturization and Biodegradable Electronics**

Continued advancements in micro- and nanofabrication are enabling the development of ultra-compact, energy-efficient smart pills. A key research focus is the integration of biodegradable electronic components that can safely disintegrate after completing their function, minimizing the need for retrieval and reducing both patient burden and environmental waste. These bioresorbable platforms are particularly suited for vulnerable populations, such as pediatric and geriatric patients, as well as for transient applications like short-term disease monitoring or post-operative assessment [400].

### Active Locomotion and Guided Navigation

Most current ingestible devices rely on natural peristaltic movement to navigate the gastrointestinal tract, which limits precision in spatial targeting. Emerging designs incorporate magnetic actuation and micro-robotic propulsion systems to enable controlled navigation. These actively mobile capsules can pause at specific sites for detailed imaging or localized drug delivery and can potentially perform in situ tasks such as mucosal biopsies or targeted ablation [130]. Enhanced navigation dramatically increases diagnostic accuracy and ensures precise therapeutic deployment in pathologies with focal involvement.

### On-Demand Drug Synthesis and Adaptive Delivery

Smart pills of the future may incorporate onboard microreactors or biosynthetic modules that allow for real-time synthesis or titration of drugs based on sensed physiological conditions. This would enable context-sensitive interventions—such as localized release of anti-inflammatories in response to detected biomarkers—creating a closed-loop system of diagnosis and therapy. Such systems can dynamically adjust treatment regimens, optimizing therapeutic outcomes while minimizing side effects and systemic exposure [402].

### Artificial Intelligence and Predictive Analytics

Integrating artificial intelligence (AI) and machine learning (ML) into smart pill systems will significantly elevate their analytical capabilities. AI-driven models can identify complex physiological patterns and detect subtle deviations suggestive of disease onset, often beyond the discernment of human interpretation. Predictive algorithms may enable early warnings for flare-ups in chronic inflammatory diseases, gastrointestinal dysmotility, or even detect signs of malignancy [39, 406]. These capabilities promise to shift healthcare from a reactive to a proactive management approach.

### Integration with Digital Health Ecosystems

Smart pills are expected to become integral components of broader digital health ecosystems, functioning alongside wearable devices, implantables, and remote monitoring platforms within the Internet of Medical Things (IoMT). Seamless interoperability between these systems enables continuous, multimodal monitoring of patient health, providing clinicians with a holistic and longitudinal view [397, 412]. Cloud-based analytics platforms can synthesize these data streams to support real-time clinical decision-making, population health management, and personalized treatment strategies.

### Remaining Challenges and Considerations

Despite their promise, several critical challenges must be addressed to realize the full potential of smart pill technologies:

- Cost and accessibility: High development and production costs currently limit the widespread deployment of this technology [413].
- Ethical implications: Issues surrounding surveillance, autonomy, and informed consent remain unresolved, especially in psychiatric and geriatric care.
- Regulatory evolution: Regulatory frameworks must adapt to encompass emerging hybrid technologies without compromising safety or slowing innovation.
- Cybersecurity risks: The transmission and storage of sensitive patient data must be protected through robust encryption, secure protocols, and strict data governance practices.

Addressing these issues will require a multidisciplinary approach, involving collaboration between engineers, clinicians, ethicists, regulatory bodies, and patients. Only through this coordinated effort can smart pills transition from experimental tools to trusted instruments of mainstream medicine.

## References


1. Pandian MSA, Rashika M, Mohammed SS, Sudherson M. Innovations in biomedical engineering: advancing healthcare devices on recent technology. i-manager's J Embed Syst. 2024.
2. Akkaoui A, Zahidi Y, El Moufid M, Dachry W, Gziri H, Medromi H. Developing medical devices with emerging technologies: trends, challenges, and future directions. F1000Res. 2024;13:1007.
3. Shobeiri S. The innovation of medical devices. In: The innovation and evolution of medical devices. Springer; 2018.
4. Fischer GA, Wells S, Rebuffoni JF, Peterson B, Lebien T. A model for overcoming challenges in academic pediatric medical device innovation. J Clin Transl Sci. 2019;3:5–11.
5. Arney D. Medical device interoperability with provable safety properties. PhD thesis, University of Pennsylvania; 2019.
6. Pathak N, Misra S, Mukherjee A, Kumar N. HeDI: healthcare device interoperability for IoT-based e-health platforms. IEEE Internet Things J. 2021;8:16845–52.
7. Kasparick M, Köny M, Andersen B, Riech K, Keller A, Kämmer S, Guth A, Mündermann L, Stickel A, Klöckner S, Golatowski F, Timmermann D. Service-oriented medical device connectivity: particular interoperability standards for high-frequency surgical equipment and external control devices. Curr Dir Biomed Eng. 2021;7:523–6.
8. Sastri VR. Materials used in medical devices. In: Plastics in medical devices. 3rd ed. Elsevier; 2022.
9. Valente V. Evolution of biotelemetry in medical devices: from radio pills to mm-scale implants. IEEE Trans Biomed Circuits Syst. 2022;16(3):580–99.
10. Nichyi S, Nichyi B. The history of the use of wireless devices in medicine. Curr Issues Soc Sci Hist Med. 2020;2(26):102–6.
11. Filippi L. COVID-19 lessons learned: medical devices at the core of global healthcare. Expert Rev Med Devices. 2023;20(1):1–3.

12. Lübbeke A, Smith J, Prieto-Alhambra D, Carr A. The case for an academic discipline of medical device science. EFORT Open Rev. 2021;6(3):160–3.
13. Nagornov NN, Lyakhov PA, Bergerman MV, Kalita D. Modern trends in improving the technical characteristics of devices and systems for digital image processing. IEEE Access. 2024;12:44659–81.
14. Anselmo C, Attili M, Horton R, Kappe B, Schulman J, Baird P. Hey you, get on the cloud: safe and compliant use of cloud computing with medical devices. Biomed Instrum Technol. 2021;55(1):1–15.
15. Bolkhovskaya O, Elokhin A, Kokarev AO, Sergeev VS, Sorokin I, Spirin A, Maltsev A. Software-hardware complex for design, full-scale and model testing the broadband systems in radio communications, radars and navigation of high-speed objects. Instrum Exp Tech. 2021;64(3):363–9.
16. Spahić L, Kurta E, Ćordić S, Bećirović M, Gurbeta L, Kovačević Ž. Machine learning techniques for performance prediction of medical devices: infant incubators. In: CMBEBIH 2019. Springer; 2020. p. 356–60.
17. Choi H. Investing in hardware vs. software of digital systems for innovation outcomes: a contingency view. Technol Forecast Soc Change. 2024;202.
18. Giordano N, Rosati S, Balestra G. Medical device software: from requirements to certification. Stud Health Technol Inform. 2023;309:139–40.
19. Ravizza A, Sternini F, Giannini A, Molinari F. Methods for preclinical validation of software as a medical device. In: Proceedings of the 13th international joint conference on biomedical engineering systems and technologies (BIOSTEC 2020). Science and Technology Publications; 2022. p. 648–55.
20. Papademetris X, Quraishi AN, Licholai G. Introduction to medical software. Cambridge Univ Press; 2022.
21. Zapata KAC, Patil R, Ward TE, Loughran R, McCaffery F. Analysis of the classification of medical device software in the AI Act proposal. Eur Med Device Regul J. 2023.
22. Eldin WS, Kaboudan A. AI-driven medical imaging platform: advancements in image analysis and healthcare diagnosis. ACS Adv Comput Sci. 2023;14(1).
23. Hampiholi N. Medical imaging enhancement with AI models for automatic disease detection and classification based on medical images. Int J Eng Appl Sci Technol. 2023.
24. Cavanagh P. Advances in imaging. In: The changing role of the hospital in European health systems. Cambridge University Press; 2020.
25. Agostini A, Borgheresi A, Granata V, Bruno F, Palumbo P, De Muzio F, Giovagnoni A. Technological advances in body CT: a primer for beginners. Eur Rev Med Pharmacol Sci. 2022;26(21):7918–37.
26. Kamel RJ, Naeem SA, Musa MM, Karim SN. Advancements in medical imaging technologies: ultrasound, X-ray, and MRI. Eur J Theor Appl Sci. 2024;2(5):149–56.
27. Nayak G, Bolla V, Balivada S, Prabhudev P. Technological evolution of ultrasound devices: a review. Int J Health Technol Innov. 2022;1(03):24–32.
28. Balter M, Leipheimer J, Chen A, Shrirao A, Maguire T, Yarmush M. Automated end-to-end blood testing at the point-of-care: integration of robotic phlebotomy with downstream sample processing. Technology. 2018;6(2):59–66.
29. Alp A. Recent advances in molecular point-of-care tests. Mikrobiyol Bul. 2022;56(3):580–91.
30. Liu D, Wang Y, Li X, Li M, Wu Q, Song Y, Zhu Z, Yang C. Integrated microfluidic devices for in vitro diagnostics at point of care. Aggregate. 2022;3.
31. Mosoyan M, Fedorov D. Modern robotics in medicine. Transl Med. 2020;7(5):91–108.
32. Kenanoglu CU, Le Mesle V, Luarasi G, Sadeghian H, Haddadin S. Design and evaluation of a surgical tool drive unit for sustainable training in robot-assisted minimally invasive surgery. In: 10th IEEE RAS/EMBS int conf biomed robot biomechatron (BioRob). IEEE; 2024. p. 1555–60.
33. Seah TET, Do TN, Takeshita N, Ho K, Phee S. Future of flexible robotic endoscopy systems. arXiv:1703.05569. 2017.

34. Mittelstein D, Deng J, Kohan RM, Sadeghi M, Maarek J, Zada G. Novel technique of a multifunctional electrosurgical system for minimally invasive surgery. J Neurosurg. 2017;126(3):997–1002.
35. Hamilton A. The future of artificial intelligence in surgery. Cureus. 2024;16(7):e63699.
36. Pandey A. Advances in 3D printing of orthopedic implants: a paradigm shift in personalized medicine. J Orthop. 2024.
37. Kulkarni VS, et al. Advancements in otology: hearing restoration and cochlear implant innovations. Int J Recent Innov Trends Comput Commun. 2023.
38. Shekar K, Brodie D, Barrett N. Appraising extracorporeal life support: current and future perspectives. Crit Care Med. 2017;45(9):1470–80.
39. Badnjevic A, Pokvić LG, Hasičić M, Bandić L, Mašetić Z, Kovačević Ž. Evidence-based clinical engineering: machine learning algorithms for prediction of defibrillator performance. Biomed Signal Process Control. 2019;54:101629.
40. Hrvat F, Spahić L, Pokvić LG, Badnjević A. Artificial neural networks for prediction of medical device performance based on conformity assessment data: infusion and perfusor pumps case study. In: 9th Mediterranean conf embedded comput (MECO). IEEE; 2020. p. 1–4.
41. Pandey SK, Mishra P. Quality of life during one-year follow-up after intensive care unit discharge: a study from a tertiary care hospital. Indian J Crit Care Med. 2020;24(6):456–62.
42. Sari D, Ekinci D. Barriers to end-of-life decisions and care objectives in intensive care units: a systematic review. Palliat Support Care. 2023;21(3):390–8.
43. Rackley C. Monitoring during mechanical ventilation. Respir Care. 2020;65:832–46.
44. Deumić S, Crnčević N, Zolota I. Respiratory system dynamical mechanical properties: modeling in time and frequency domain. In: Int Conf Med Biol Eng; 2021. p. 47–57.
45. Vennela M, Kumar VK. Design tracking system for at-home medical equipment during natural disasters. Int J Res. 2017;4:1042–5.
46. Vegas A. Mechanical support, heart transplant. Kardiol Pol. 2018.
47. Chishti A, Walker IA. Patient monitoring techniques. Surgery (Oxford). 2019;37:450–9.
48. Badnjević A, Gurbeta L, Deumić A. A novel method for conformity assessment testing of infant incubators for post-market surveillance purposes. Technol Health Care. 2023;31(1):389–99.
49. Crisafulli J. Patient monitoring replacement forecast. J Clin Eng. 2022;47(1):39–43.
50. Leahy RA, Davenport E. Home monitoring for cardiovascular implantable electronic devices: benefits to patients and to their follow-up clinic. AACN Adv Crit Care. 2015;26:343–55.
51. Kupsad BV. IoT-based remote patient monitoring system. Int J Sci Res Eng Manag. 2024;08:1–11.
52. Ip JE. Wearable devices for cardiac rhythm diagnosis and management. JAMA. 2019;321(4):337–8.
53. Silverio AA, Suarez C, Silvério L, Dino JY, Duran JB, Catambing GEG. An unobtrusive, wireless and wearable single-site blood pressure monitor based on an armband using electrocardiography (ECG) and reflectance photoplethysmography (PPG) signal processing. Electronics. 2023;12(7):1538.
54. Suryawanshi AS. Pulse oximeter: as a tool against COVID-19. J Emerg Technol Innov Res. 2020;7:2120–33.
55. Golpaygani AT, Mehdizadeh A. Future of wearable health devices: smartwatches vs smart headphones. J Biomed Phys Eng. 2021;11:561–2.
56. Aggogeri F. Special collection on advances in rehabilitation engineering with robotics and mechatronic devices. Adv Mech Eng. 2020;12.
57. Granulo E, Becar L, Gurbeta L, Badnjevic A. Telemetry system for diagnosis of asthma and chronic obstructive pulmonary disease (COPD). In: Ahmed MU, Begum S, Raad W, editors. Internet of things technologies for HealthCare. Springer; 2016. p. 113–8.
58. Keerthana R, Jochan MC, SuryaDharshini M, SunilKumar S, Kalidindi S, Vidhya S. A review on prosthetics and orthotics for amputees and disabled. J Biomed Res. 2020.

59. Makwanda AB, Ikhile AO. Advancements of upper limb prostheses can improve patient quality of life: a technology review. URNCST J. 2023.
60. Choo YJ, Chang M. Use of machine learning in the field of prosthetics and orthotics: a systematic narrative review. Prosthet Orthot Int. 2023.
61. Nayak S, Das R. Application of artificial intelligence (AI) in prosthetic and orthotic rehabilitation. In: Serv Robot; 2020.
62. Mombaur K. Optimal prostheses, orthoses and exoskeletons for physical activity. In: 33rd International conference on biomechanics in sports, International Society of Biomechanics in Sports, Jun 2015, Poitiers, France. ISBS; 2016. p. 33.
63. Bednarska V, Czyz H, Jasinski T. Advances in hearing prosthetics. Phys Econ. 2018;1:5–20.
64. Jimbu D, Cristea A, Iliescu D, Oprea D, Iliescu M, Caraban B, Bordei P. The importance of advanced technologies in functional rehabilitation of the hand. Balneo PRM Res J. 2024;15:664.
65. Febriani RA. Utilization of artificial intelligence in image-based medical diagnosis. Jurnal Komputer Indonesia. 2023;2:41–6.
66. Welch HMKF. Artificial intelligence-powered diagnostic tools, networked medical devices, and cyber-physical healthcare systems in assessing and treating patients with COVID-19 symptoms. Am J Med Res. 2021.
67. Kovacevic Z, Gurbeta Pokvic L, Spahic L, Badnjevic A. Prediction of medical device performance using machine learning techniques: infant incubator case study. Health Technol. 2020;10(1):151–5.
68. Holmes J, Sacchi L, Bellazzi R, Peek N. Artificial intelligence in medicine AIME 2015. Artif Intell Med. 2017;81:1–2.
69. Badnjevic A, Avdihodzic H, Gurbeta Pokvic L. Artificial intelligence in medical devices: past, present and future. Psychiatr Danub. 2021;33(Suppl 3):101–6.
70. Wang ML, Yeon P, Chamberlayne CF, Mofidfar M, Xu H, Annes J, Zare R, Arbabian A. A wireless implantable potentiostat for programmable electrochemical drug delivery. In: IEEE Biomed Circuits Syst Conf (BioCAS). IEEE; 2021. p. 1–4.
71. Talmale R, Sonwane S. Biomedical devices: development & performance in healthcare system. In: 2024 2nd DMIHER Int Conf Artif Intell Healthc Educ Ind (IDICAIEI). IEEE; 2024. p. 1–4.
72. Spahic L, Sredovic U, Kurpejovic Z, Mrdanovic E, Pokvic G, Badnjevic A. Machine learning for improved medical device management: a focus on infant incubators. Technol Health Care. 2025;33(4):2034–40.
73. Dong Y, Siu C. Analysis of biomedical applications in embedded systems devices. J Biomed Sustain Healthc Appl. 2021.
74. Yuvaraj R, Giri S, Gupta S. IoT-based applications in healthcare devices. IJCRT. 2023;11(6):e435.
75. Hocaoglu A, Topuz F, Ozkan G, Suna B. The processes in medical device clinical investigations. Eurasian J Health Technol Assess. 2022.
76. Manita D, Vikram A, Rana A, Yadav M, Marwaha R. Regulation of medical devices and their clinical trials studies in the USA: An update. Rice. 2020;13:94–109.
77. Mishra S. FDA, CE mark or something else?—thinking fast and slow. Indian Heart J. 2016;69(1):1–5.
78. Badnjevic A, Pokvic LG, Spahic L. Clinical engineering. In: Iadanza E, editor. Clinical engineering handbook. Academic Press; 2020. p. 491–7.
79. Badnjevic A, Pokvic LG, Deumic A, Becirovic LS. Post-market surveillance of medical devices: a review. Technol Health Care. 2022;30(6):1315–29.
80. Zettler PJ, Lietzan E. Regulating medical devices in the United States. In: Oxford handbook of comparative health law. Oxford University Press; 2020.
81. Mooghali M, Rathi V, Kadakia K, Ross JS, Dhruva S. Medical device risk (re)classification: lessons from the FDA's 515 program initiative. BMJ Surg Interv Health Technol. 2023;5.

82. FDA. Procedures for Class II Device Exemptions from Premarket Notification (Guidance for Industry and CDRH Staff). 2018.
83. Page R. The US Food and Drug Administration premarket approval process and the 515 program initiative: view from a panel chair. JAMA Cardiol. 2016;1(2):119–20.
84. Geller J. FDA approves devices, publishes guidance, issues classifications. J Clin Eng. 2018;43:3–6.
85. McDermott O, Kearney B. A review of the literature on the new European medical device regulations requirements for increased clinical evaluation. Int J Pharm Healthc Mark. 2024.
86. Machal M. Impact of Class I software as medical devices (SaMDs) on public health. Stud Health Technol Inform. 2022;295:33–6.
87. Melvin T. The European medical device regulation – what biomedical engineers need to know. IEEE J Transl Eng Health Med. 2022;10:1–5.
88. Carl A-K, Hochmann D. Impact of the new European medical device regulation: a two-year comparison. Biomed Eng Biomed Tech. 2023;69:317–26.
89. Malvehy J, Ginsberg R, Sampietro-Colom L, Ficapal J, Combalia M, Svedenhag P. New regulation of medical devices in the EU: impact in dermatology. J Eur Acad Dermatol Venereol. 2021;36:360–4.
90. Sandhya M, Madhumitha R, Sankar S. Analysis of threats in interoperability of medical devices. World Acad Sci Eng Technol Int J Med Health Biomed Bioeng Pharm Eng. 2017;11:282–5.
91. Singh J. Challenges with medical devices connected to hospital network. Int J Res Appl Sci Eng Technol. 2024;12:735–49.
92. Oliveira MB, Li F, Choi J, Mano J. Nanomaterials for biomedical applications. Biotechnol J. 2020;15.
93. Alzoubi L, Aljabali A, Tambuwala M. Empowering precision medicine: the impact of 3D printing on personalized therapeutic. AAPS PharmSciTech. 2023;24:228.
94. Chen S, Li R, Li X, Xie J. Electrospinning: An enabling nanotechnology platform for drug delivery and regenerative medicine. Adv Drug Deliv Rev. 2018;132:188–213.
95. Odaibo SG. Risk management of AI/ML software as a medical device (SaMD): on ISO 14971 and related standards and guidances. ArXiv. 2021.
96. Chothani F, Movaliya V, Vaghela K, Zaveri M, Deshpande S, Kanki N. Regulatory prospective on software as a medical device. Int J Drug Regul Aff. 2022.
97. Mahler M, Auza C, Albesa R, Melus C, Wu JA. Regulatory aspects of artificial intelligence and machine learning-enabled software as medical devices (SaMD). In: Precision medicine and artificial intelligence. 2021. pp. 237–65.
98. Youssef A, Fronk BD, Grimes JN, Cheuy L, Larson DB. Beyond the black box: avenues to transparency in regulating radiological AI/ML-enabled SaMD via the FDA 510(k) pathway. 2024. https://doi.org/10.1101/2024.07.12.24309602.
99. Wagner R. AI, EHR, SaMD and hospitals — US, German and Australian regulation make AI immediately available with non-SaMD pathway for hospitals and doctors. 2024.
100. Spahić L, Hundur M, Bećirović F, Gurbeta Pokvić L, Badnjević A. Advancement of post-market surveillance of medical devices leveraging artificial intelligence: ECG devices case study. Technol Health Care. 2023.
101. Qamar SUR, Spahić L, Benolić L, Živanović M, Filipović N. Treatment of peripheral artery disease using injectable biomaterials and drug-coated balloons: safety and efficacy perspective. Pharmaceutics. 2023;15(7):1813.
102. Badnjević A, Zebić EZ. Bosnia and Herzegovina's e-identity initiative: a technological leap in digital solutions and governance. Technol Health Care. 2024;32(5):2853–8.
103. Choi J, Kim S, Lee H, Park K. Analog-to-digital conversion challenges in biomedical signal processing. J Med Electron. 2016;15(2):125–36.
104. Rudra P. Developing electronic devices for clinical applications: challenges and future directions. Biomed Instrum Technol. 2020;28(3):205–19.

105. Ejiyi C, Ahmed R, Patil D. Certification standards and restrictions of wireless electronic devices in clinical environments. Int J Med Electron. 2023;32(4):567–82.
106. Garcia J, Brown S, Patel R. Adaptive filtering techniques for mitigating movement artifacts in biomedical signal processing. IEEE Trans Med Electron. 2021;59(2):345–60.
107. Zhu E. Optimization of low power consumption in wearable health monitoring devices and algorithm design. Applied and Computational Engineering. 2024;41(1):269–74.
108. Jones B, Martin L, Robinson P. Positive pressure ventilation and its effects on lung function. Intensive Care Med. 2022;35(4):155–68.
109. Yu J, Li F, Chan A. Translational biosignal processing: bridging physiological signals and electronic health monitoring. J Biomed Syst. 2019;33(5):452–67.
110. Peruničić Ž, Lalatović I, Spahić L, Ašić A, Pokvić LG, Badnjević A. Enhancing mechanical ventilator reliability through machine learning based predictive maintenance. Technol Health Care. 2025;33(3):1288–97.
111. Singh R, Ahmed P. Battery life and power management strategies for wireless health monitoring systems. IEEE Trans Biomed Eng. 2021;69(5):349–66.
112. Liu M, Patel S, Kim H. Power efficiency in wireless medical monitoring: performance assessment of different communication protocols. IEEE Trans Biomed Circuits. 2023;72(3):178–93.
113. Zhou J, Wang K, Xu T. Design considerations for battery-powered wireless medical systems: a review of challenges and solutions. J Health Technol. 2020;38(1):102–19.
114. Kim S, Wang Y, Chen P. Artifact reduction techniques in biosignal monitoring: advances and future trends. Med Signal Process J. 2021;52(4):213–29.
115. Huang L, Zhou H, Lin W. Wearable biosensors and signal processing: a review of challenges and solutions. IEEE Trans Biomed Eng. 2021;68(6):1442–55.
116. Wu L, Zhang X. Analog filtering and interference suppression in biosignal monitoring. IEEE Trans Biomed Circuits Syst. 2019;45(4):201–16.
117. Hafizović L, Čaušević A, Deumić S, Bećirović LS, Pokvić LG, Badnjević A. The use of artificial intelligence in diagnostic medical imaging: systematic literature review. In: 2021 IEEE 21st Int Conf Bioinf Bioeng. IEEE; 2021. p. 1–7.
118. Mahmood AI, Gharghan SK, Eldosoky MA, Soliman AM. Energy harvesting–based biomedical applications: a review. AIP Conf Proc. 2023.
119. Badnjević A, Gurbeta L, Omanović-Mikličanin E, Sejdić E. A telehealth system for automated diagnosis of asthma and chronic obstructive pulmonary disease. J Am Med Inform Assoc. 2018;25(9):1213–7.
120. Wu L, Zhao X. Privacy and security concerns in wireless health monitoring systems. IEEE Trans Inf Secur Healthc. 2022;44(2):201–16.
121. Liu R, Patel S. Advances in noninvasive medical imaging technologies: a review of current innovations. IEEE Trans Biomed Imaging. 2020;39(2):112–30.
122. Hiware MS, Jirvankar PS. Wearable technology and its effect on the provision of healthcare. In: 2024 2nd DMIHER Int Conf Artif Intell Healthc Educ Ind (IDICAIEI). IEEE; 2024. p. 1–6.
123. Krey M, Schlatter U, Mahadevan D, Derungs K, Oehler J. Wearable technology in healthcare. J Adv Inf Technol. 2020;11(3):172–80.
124. Charan G, Khurana MS, Kalia R. Wearable technology: how healthcare is changing forever. J Chitwan Med Coll. 2023.
125. Rukundo I. The impact of wearable technology on health monitoring and preventive care. In: 2024 2nd DMIHER Int Conf Artif Intell Healthc Educ Ind (IDICAIEI). IEEE; 2024. p. 1–6.
126. Obianyo I, Ezeamii E, Chukwu N. The future of wearable health technology: from monitoring to management. HealthTech Innov J. 2024;14(1):23–35.
127. Arnold T. The role of wearable health technology in monitoring and bridging gaps in global healthcare. Int J Telemed Appl. 2025.
128. Chen Y, Lou H. Application of cloud-driven intelligent medical imaging for early disease detection. Healthc Inform J. 2024;18(1):45–63.

129. Al Khateeb H, Saleh M. Electrical safety standards in neonatal incubators. Med Saf J. 2020;14(2):145–52.
130. Zhang D, Zhu D, Zhao T. Big data monitoring of sports health based on microcomputer processing and BP neural network. Microprocess Microsyst. 2021;82:103939.
131. Nurmaini S, Partan RU, Caesarendra W, Dewi T, Rahmatullah MN, Darmawahyuni A, Bhayyu V, Firdaus F. An automated ECG beat classification system using deep neural networks with an unsupervised feature extraction technique. Appl Sci. 2019;9(14):2921.
132. Thangaraju SK, Munisamy KM. III lead ECG pulse measurement sensor. IOP Conf Ser Mater Sci Eng. 2015;88:012047.
133. Francis J. ECG monitoring leads and special leads. Indian Pacing Electrophysiol J. 2016;16(2):92–5.
134. Kumar P, Ramasamy M, Kallur KR, Rai P, Varadan V. Personalized LSTM models for ECG lead transformations led to fewer diagnostic errors than generalized models: deriving 12-lead ECG from lead II, V2, and V6. Sensors (Basel). 2023;23.
135. Bodini M, Rivolta M, Sassi R. Classification of ECG signals with different lead systems using AutoML. Comput Cardiol Conf. 2021.
136. Takeshita T, Yoshida M, Ouchi A, Hinoki A, Uchida H, Kobayashi T. Development of multi-lead ECG measurement wear using electrostatic flocking technology. In: 2018 Int Conf Electron Packag iMAPS All Asia Conf (ICEP-IAAC). IEEE; 2018. p. 145–6.
137. Namdar M, Chmelevsky M, Hachulla A, Shah D. Precise noninvasive ECG mapping derived localization of the origin of an epicardial ventricular tachycardia. Circ Arrhythm Electrophysiol. 2016;9:e003949.
138. Pepe M, Napoli G, Brindicci G, Carulli E, Nestola PL, Santoro C, Biondi-Zoccai G, Giordano A, D'Ascenzo F, Cirillo P, Saracino A, Favale S. Prognostic value of 12-leads admission electrocardiogram in low-risk patients hospitalized for COVID-19. Minerva Med. 2021.
139. Nguyên UC, Cluitmans M, Strik M, Luermans J, Gommers S, Wildberger J, Bekkers S, Volders P, Mihl C, Prinzen F, Vernooy K. Integration of cardiac magnetic resonance imaging, electrocardiographic imaging, and coronary venous computed tomography angiography for guidance of left ventricular lead positioning. Europace. 2019;21(4):626–35.
140. Saif A, Khan R, Malik F. Portable ECG technologies: a review of mobile healthcare innovations. Digit Health Telemed J. 2022;14(2):66–78.
141. Kashou AH, Palanisamy T, Ramaswamy H. Evaluation of PC-based electrocardiograph systems in remote cardiac care. J Cardiac Technol. 2022;58(3):198–205.
142. Reichlin T, Abächerli R, Twerenbold R, Kühne M, Schaer B, Müller C, Sticherling C, Osswald S. Advanced ECG in 2016: is there more than just a tracing? Swiss Med Wkly. 2016;146:w14303.
143. Chang A, Cadaret L, Liu K. Machine learning in electrocardiography and echocardiography: technological advances in clinical cardiology. Curr Cardiol Rep. 2020;22(3).
144. Xu HR, An B, He X. Filter design for ECG signal processing. Int J Front Eng Technol. 2022;10(4):67–80.
145. Bui N, Phan DT, Nguyen TP, Hoang G, Choi J, Bui QC, Oh JM. Real-time filtering and ECG signal processing based on dual-core digital signal controller system. IEEE Sens J. 2020;20(8):6492–503.
146. Hadjiantoni A, Oak K, Mengi S, Konya J, Ungvári T. Is the correct anatomical placement of the electrocardiogram (ECG) electrodes essential to diagnosis in the clinical setting? A systematic review. Cardiol Cardiovasc Med. 2020.
147. Yang J, Zhang K, Yu J, Zhang S, He L, Wu S, Liu C, Deng Y. Facile fabrication of robust and reusable PDMS supported graphene dry electrodes for wearable electrocardiogram monitoring. Adv Mater Technol. 2021;6.
148. Zhang X, Zhang Z, Li Y, Liu C, Guo YX, Lian Y. A 2.89 μW dry-electrode enabled clockless wireless ECG SoC for wearable applications. IEEE J Solid-State Circuits. 2016;51:2287–98.
149. Magjarevic R, Badnjević A. Inspection and testing of electrocardiographs (ECG) devices. In: Springer biomedical engineering handbook. Springer; 2018. p. 59–79.

150. Hammer A, Scherpf M, Ernst H, Weiß J, Schwensow D, Schmidt M. Automatic classification of 12-, 6-, 4-, 3-, and 2-lead electrocardiograms using morphological feature extraction. Comput Cardiol Conf. 2021.
151. Bulkova V. Long-term ECG monitoring. Vnitr Lek. 2021;67(1):16–21.
152. Nikolsky A, Levanov V, Drozdov D, Kozlov AA. Patients' self-operated telemedical solutions for ECG screening. Medical alphabet. 2019;2:25–8.
153. Rajanna S, Patel H, Prakash R. A review of electrode placement standardization in long-term ECG recording. Biomed Eng Adv. 2021;3:27–38.
154. Landman G, Sarkar S. Optimizing electrode placement for long-term ECG monitoring: a review. Eur Heart J Digit Health. 2019;20(3):123–35.
155. Mellado CM, Rodríguez LF, González E. Frequency-domain analysis in Holter ECG: a novel approach for artifact reduction. Comput Cardiol. 2021;48:112–20.
156. Gersak B, Podlogar V, Kalinšek TP, Jan M. Long-term outcome after convergent procedure for atrial fibrillation. J Clin Med. 2023;13.
157. Silajdžić A, Trkulja A, Muharemović A, Gurbeta-Pokvić L, Begić E, Badnjević A. A brief review on wearable ECG devices and processing techniques for fall risk assessment. In: 2022 11th Mediterranean conference on embedded computing (MECO). IEEE; 2022. p. 1–4.
158. Milstein N, Verma R, D'Souza R. Holter monitoring in high-risk cardiac patients: real-time applications and future perspectives. Int J Cardiol. 2019;275:85–92.
159. Eggett CJ. Advances in event recorders and their clinical applications. J Cardiovasc Electrophysiol. 2015;26(4):387–95.
160. Hughes M, Denison T, Hill R. Advances in subcutaneous implantable loop recorders for cardiac arrhythmia detection. Heart Rhythm. 2015;12(5):845–52.
161. Ali A, Nadeem M, Chaudhry MA. Advancements in implantable cardiac monitoring devices: A review of next-generation ECG technologies. J Cardiovasc Innov. 2022;12(1):33–41.
162. Lynn B, et al. ECG analysis in long-term monitoring: challenges and developments. J Cardiol Res. 2015;48(2):55–68.
163. Nowotny F, Dürst U, Wyss C. Exercise training in contemporary cardiovascular diagnostics. Praxis (Bern 1994). 2020;109(15):1189–93.
164. Marzoog B, Abdullaev M, Suvorov A, Chomakhidze P, Gognieva D, Gagarina N, Mozzhukhina N, Kostin SV, Bestavashvili AA, Fominykha E, Kopylov P, Abdullah B, Marzoog M. Single channel electrocardiography optimizes the diagnostic accuracy of bicycle ergometry. medRxiv. 2024. https://doi.org/10.1101/2024.04.20.24306122.
165. Poderys J, Bikulčienė L, Trinkūnas E, Poderiene K, Buliuolis A, Vainoras A. Matrix analysis of ECG parameters may be a way to improve quality of functional state monitoring during exercising. Balt J Sport Health Sci. 2015;4:39–45.
166. Urban M, Klum M, Pielmus AG, Liebrenz F, Mann S, Tigges T, Orglmeister R. GRU neural network improved bioimpedance-based stroke volume estimation during ergometry stress test. Sensors (Basel). 2022;22.
167. Chaudhari H, Patil N, Sinha V. Online suppression of motion artifacts during treadmill ECG. 2018.
168. Sheleg DO, Bogachev R, Mikhailova L. Induction of cardiac arrhythmias during bicycle ergometry in the diagnosis of coronary heart disease. Complex Issues Cardiovasc Dis. 2023.
169. Siraiy B, Trobec R, Ilic V. Quality of one-channel telemetric ECG sensor signal in maximum exercise stress tests. Meas Sci Rev. 2019;19:79–85.
170. Kenn C, May A. Ergometry - step by step. Dtsch Med Wochenschr. 2018;143(17):1252–7.
171. Vanhees L. The prognostic strength of gas analysis measurement during maximal exercise testing. Eur J Prev Cardiol. 2018;25:770–1.
172. Kang JS, Wen H. A study on several critical problems on arrhythmia detection using varying-dimensional electrocardiography. Physiol Meas. 2022;43:064007.
173. Smulyan H. The computerized ECG: friend and foe. Am J Med. 2019;132(2):153–60.
174. Gitsioudis G, Marwan M, Schneider S, Schmermund A, Korosoglou G, Hausleiter J, Schroeder S, Rixe J, Leber A, Bruder O, Katus H, Senges J, Achenbach S. A systematic

report on non-coronary cardiac CTA in 1097 patients from the German cardiac CT registry. Eur J Radiol. 2020;130:109136.
175. Hundur M, Spahić L, Bećirović F, Gurbeta-Pokvić L, Badnjević A. Advancement of post-market surveillance of medical devices leveraging artificial intelligence: ECG devices case study. Technol Health Care. 2025.
176. Leontsinis I, Kasiakogias A, Mantzouranis M, Fragoulis F, Andrikou I, Tzcrovili E, Tsioufis C. Exercise duration as a predictor of cardiovascular disease in arterial hypertension: data from a 6-year follow-up study. Eur Heart J. 2020;41.
177. Desai N, Sanjay HS, Sinha A, Vishnu Prasad R, Kunnikkullayya K. Automated assessment of the electrocardiogram-aided pulse transit time in healthy individuals - a pilot study. In: IEEE Int Conf Electron Comput Commun Technol (CONECCT). IEEE; 2021.
178. Ermolaev N, Willixhofer R, Kronberger C, Rettl R, Binder C, Duca F, Badr-Eslam R. Cardiopulmonary exercise testing in correlation with magnetic resonance imaging in patients with cardiac amyloidosis. Eur J Prev Cardiol. 2024.
179. Young B. New standards for ECG equipment. J Electrocardiol. 2019;57:S1–4.
180. Mahabadi A, Lehmann N, Kälsch H, Pundt N, Dykun I, Moebus S, Möhlenkamp S. Parameters of exercise stress testing are associated with incident major cardiovascular events independent of risk factors and coronary artery calcification - The Heinz Nixdorf Recall Study. Circulation. 2015.
181. Bisaccia G, Swoboda P, Bucciarelli-Ducci C, Plein S, Greenwood J. Comparative and incremental diagnostic and prognostic yield of exercise ECG, CMR and SPECT in patients with suspected ischaemic heart disease: a CE-MARC sub-study. Circulation. 2023.
182. Ibrahim N, Ann CW, Sari S. Analysis on MET value due to the relation between echocardiogram (ECG) signal and human physical activities. In: 6th International conference on the development of biomedical engineering in Vietnam (BME6). BME 2017. IFMBE Proceedings. Springer; 2018.
183. Fallon N. The challenge of measuring blood pressure accurately. Br J Card Nurs. 2015;10(3):132–9.
184. Rao V. Blood pressure measurement in clinical practice methods and emerging options. Hypertens J. 2019;5:92–8.
185. Goodman C, Kitchen G. Measuring arterial blood pressure. Anaesth Intensive Care Med. 2020.
186. Pielmus AG, Mühlstef J, Bresch E, Glos M, Jungen C, Mieke S, Orglmeister R, Schulze A, Stender B, Voigt V, Zaunseder S. Surrogate-based continuous noninvasive blood pressure measurement. Biomed Tech (Berl). 2021;66:231–45.
187. Hosanee M, Chan G, Welykholowa K, Cooper R, Kyriacou P, Zheng D, et al. Cuffless single-site photoplethysmography for blood pressure monitoring. J Clin Med. 2020;9.
188. Vakulenko D, Zaspa H, Lupenko S. New application of blood pressure monitor with software environment Oranta-AO based on arterial oscillography methods. In: IDDM-2021: 4th International conference on informatics & data-driven medicine, November 19–21, 2021 Valencia, Spain. CEUR-WS; 2021. p. 161–71.
189. Kapoor M, Holman B, Cohen C. Contactless and calibration-free blood pressure and pulse rate monitor for screening and monitoring of hypertension: cross-sectional validation study. JMIR Cardio. 2024;8.
190. Shihab KM, Perdana D, Sussi S. Design and implementation of IoT based blood pressure monitoring tools. Int J Simul Syst Sci Technol. 2020.
191. Vischer A, Burkard T. Principles of blood pressure measurement - current techniques, office vs ambulatory blood pressure measurement. In: Adv Exp Med Biol, vol. 956; 2016. p. 85–96.
192. Babadağ K, Zaybak A. Comparing intra-arterial, auscultatory, and oscillometric measurement methods for arterial blood pressure. Florence Nightingale J Nurs. 2021;29:194–202.
193. Moreno IG. Validation of blood pressure measurement by the complex for daily monitoring of ECG and blood pressure "Medicom-Combi" by oscillometric and auscultatory methods in pediatric population. Med Alphabet. 2021.

194. Fedulaev VA, Kharitonov NG, Sitdikov RA. Influence of vascular tone on blood pressure variability. Biomed Eng. 2020;54(6):367–73.
195. Hanover J. Assessing the strengths and limitations of non-invasive blood pressure measurement. J Clin Hypertens. 2023;25:965–6.
196. Vigato ES, Lamas JLT. Blood pressure measurement by oscillometric and auscultatory methods in normotensive pregnant women. Rev Bras Enferm. 2019;72(suppl 3):162–9.
197. Picone D. Accurate measurement of blood pressure. Artery Res. 2020.
198. Olsen MH, Riberholt C, Capion T, Berg R, Møller K. Reliability of non-invasive arterial blood pressure measurement in patients with aneurysmal subarachnoid hemorrhage. Physiol Meas. 2022.
199. Gorbunov V, Fedorova E, Platonova E. Multiple modern methods of blood pressure measurement and the 2018 European Society of Hypertension guidelines. Ration Pharmacother Cardiol. 2020;16:126–32.
200. Nakagawa N, Hasebe N. Impact of the 2017 ACC/AHA hypertension guidelines on the next blood pressure guidelines in Asia. Curr Hypertens Rep. 2019;21:1–5.
201. Kamón T, Kaneko H, Itoh H, Kiriyama H, Mizuno Y, Morita H, Yamamichi N, Komuro I. Gender-specific association between blood pressure category and cardio-ankle vascular index: a community-based cohort study. J Cardiol. 2019.
202. Vischer A, Winterhalder C, Leonardi L, Eckstein J, Burkard T. Impact of American vs. Canadian style blood pressure measurement on blood pressure classification according to the 2017 ACC/AHA Task Force hypertension guidelines. J Hypertens. 2018;36:e6.
203. Bakris G. Similarities and differences between the ACC/AHA and ESH/ESC guidelines for high blood pressure. Circ Res. 2019.
204. Armstrong C. High blood pressure: ACC/AHA releases updated guideline. Am Fam Physician. 2018;97(6):413–5.
205. Aleyadeh W, Hutt-Centeno E, Ahmed HM, Shah NP. Hypertension guidelines: treat patients, not numbers. Cleve Clin J Med. 2019;86:47–56.
206. Schutte A. What are the financial implications of the 2017 AHA/ACC high blood pressure guideline? Eur J Prev Cardiol. 2018;25:1109–10.
207. Wilkins L. Correction to: 2017 ACC/AHA/AAPA/ABC/ACPM/AGS/APhA/ASH/ASPC/NMA/PCNA guideline for the prevention, detection, evaluation, and management of high blood pressure in adults. Hypertension. 2018;71(6):e140–4.
208. Hayer R, Kirley K, Tsipas S, Allen J, Hanson D, Johnson EL. Redesigning blood pressure measurement training in healthcare schools. Med Educ Online. 2022;27.
209. Wagner S. Blood pressure self-measurement. Adv Exp Med Biol. 2016;956:97–107.
210. Karvounis E, Vavva MG, Giannakeas N, Tzallas A, Smanis I, Tsipouras M. A hospital healthcare monitoring system using IoT technologies. In: Proc 6th SEEDA-CECNSM. IEEE; 2021. p. 1–6.
211. Salah W, Zneid BA. Evolution of microcontroller-based remote monitoring system applications. Int J Electr Comput Eng. 2019;9:2354.
212. Kumbhalwar SD, Badole TU, Mendhe P, Gadhave S. Health monitoring system. Int J Technol. 2015;5(1):50–6.
213. Luo S, Li Q, Liu H. Design of a multifunctional remote monitoring system for wards. Proc SPIE. 2022.
214. Naveena DA. IoT-based patient healthcare monitoring system. Int J Res Appl Sci Eng Technol. 2023; https://doi.org/10.22214/ijraset.2023.54653.
215. Liu K, Wang H, Xu Y. Enhancing ICU outcomes through intelligent monitoring systems: integration of AI and real-time analytics. Crit Care Technol J. 2024;58(1):12–21.
216. Poncette AS, Mosch L, Spies C, et al. Improvements in patient monitoring in the intensive care unit: survey of current and future technologies. JMIR Med Inform. 2020;8(7):e16204.
217. Li C, Zhang Y, Chen M. Uses of a real-time automatic nosocomial infection monitoring system in the ICU. J Biomed Inform. 2024;149:104393.

218. Pichaisnith V, Pichaisnith P, Tosuksa S, Srisornchat S, Shuapetcharasophon S, Kasitipradith N. The feasibility of applying microcomputer in community hospital management in Thailand. 2017.
219. Li L, Fang X, Yi W, Li T. Health monitoring system for medical staff based on STM32 MCU. Front Sci Eng. 2023.
220. Sudha MS, Selvakumar R. A hospital healthcare monitoring system using wireless sensor networks. In: International conference on emerging trends in engineering, science and sustainable technology (ICETSST-2017). SSRG; 2017.
221. Schmidt T, Bech C, Brabrand M, Wiil U, Lassen A. Factors related to monitoring during admission of acute patients. J Clin Monit Comput. 2016;31(4):641–9.
222. Bećirović F, Spahić L, Merdović N, Gurbeta-Pokvić L, Badnjević A. Advancement of post-market surveillance of medical devices leveraging artificial intelligence: patient monitors case study. Technol Health Care. 2025;33(2):974–80.
223. Zainuddin AA, Superamaniam S, Andrew AC, Muraleedharan R, Rakshys J, Miriam J, Bostomi MASM, Rais AMA, Khalidin Z, Mansor A, Taufik MSM. Patient monitoring system using computer vision for emotional recognition and vital signs detection. In Proc IEEE SCOReD. IEEE; 2020. p. 22–7.
224. European Parliament and Council of the European Union. Regulation (EU) 2017/745 on medical devices (MDR). Off J Eur Union. 2017.
225. Ghosh R. Use of artificial intelligence in medical devices for post-market safety surveillance: challenges and opportunities. Biomed Eng Lett. 2024;14(1):25–32.
226. Khinvasara S, Tzenios N, Junaid M. Post-market surveillance of medical devices using AI: emerging frameworks and global implications. J Healthc Inform Res. 2024;8(1):45–59.
227. Pearson S, Koyner J, Patel B. Management of respiratory failure. Clin J Am Soc Nephrol. 2022;17:572–80.
228. Barbas CSV, Nemer SN. Advanced modes of mechanical ventilation. Mechanical ventilation [Working Title]. 2021.
229. Janssens JP, Michel G, Rabec C. Long-term mechanical ventilation: recommendations of the Swiss Society for Pulmonology. Respiration. 2021;99(10).
230. Kharasch ED, Dumas TC, Johnson MA. Detecting ventilator-induced diaphragmatic dysfunction in long-term mechanical ventilation. 2020.
231. Maung AA, Kaplan LJ. Mechanical ventilation: advanced ventilation and adjuncts. DeckerMed Critical Care of the Surgical Patient. 2018.
232. Spahić L, Jeremić L, Lalatović I, Muratović T, Džuho A, Pokvić LG, Badnjević A. Machine learning for improved medical device management: a focus on defibrillator performance. Technol Health Care. 2024.
233. Ediboğlu O. Mechanical ventilation for patients with COPD. In: Chronic obstructive pulmonary disease – a current conspectus. IntechOpen; 2021.
234. Tahmid MT, Bappa MN. Advancing noninvasive mechanical ventilation. bioRxiv. 2024.
235. Dalamagka MI. COVID-19 and mechanical ventilation. GSC Adv Res Rev. 2024;19(02):204–7.
236. Kwak S. Home mechanical ventilation in children with chronic respiratory failure: a narrative review. J Yeungnam Med Sci. 2022.
237. Hu Y, Li X, Shi Y. Advances in clinical application of adaptive support ventilation. Chin J Appl Clin Pediatr. 2018.
238. Roberts H, Wallace T, Foster B. Design considerations for modern breathing circuits. Med Eng J. 2018;13(2):77–92.
239. Taylor R, Simmons L, Howard G. Dual-hose ventilation circuits: functionality and performance. J Intens Care Technol. 2022;27(4):98–110.
240. Lopez M, Reed J, Torres D. Humidification techniques in ventilatory support. Pulm Care J. 2023;22(1):98–112.
241. Davies M, Parker G, Wright H. Impact of gas humidification on airway health. Pulm Res J. 2019;18(6):212–28.

242. Evans S, Lopez J, Brooks K. Expiratory valve function in modern ventilators. Respir Ther Adv. 2021;25(3):144–57.
243. Nguyen P, Carter J. The role of PEEP in lung protection strategies. Pulm Crit Care Rev. 2018;20(4):85–99.
244. Haas R, Horton J. Aerosol therapy with inhalers during mechanical ventilation. Can J Health Technol. 2024;4.
245. Smith J, Black A, Weber C. Understanding intrapulmonary pressure changes during mechanical ventilation. Am J Respir Physiol. 2019;29(2):188–201.
246. Gonzalez E, Tran B, White C. Comparison of dual-hose and single-hose ventilator circuits. Respir Mech. 2018;11(5):201–14.
247. Miller C, Patel N. Patient-specific ventilatory settings and interface selection. Crit Care Med. 2023;41(2):202–15.
248. Brown D, White J, Green P. Electrical and gas supply requirements for ventilators. Eng Med. 2020;12(4):100–13.
249. Anderson R, Smith K, Taylor L. Portable ventilators and hospital transport solutions. J Respir Ther. 2021;19(3):78–91.
250. Lee K, Thompson J, Brown P. Compressed gas systems for medical ventilation. Eng Respir Care. 2019;9(3):64–77.
251. Garcia F, Patel M, Khan Z. Self-sustaining ventilators using ambient air technology. Biomed Eng Rev. 2022;16(2):178–92.
252. Williams D, Clark P. Power requirements for medical ventilators: an overview. J Clin Eng. 2018;16(2):55–70.
253. Davies R, Grant T, Hughes B. Optimizing gas mixers for ventilatory efficiency. Int J Respir Sci. 2023;21(2):88–104.
254. Harris T, Green R, Patel V. Advances in electronic gas mixing for ventilators. J Biomed Devices. 2020;14(3):129–40.
255. Wilson J, Torres B, Reed M. Ensuring accuracy in gas mixing systems for ventilators. J Respir Ther. 2022;24(1):187–203.
256. Young H, Marshall E, Bennett D. Pressure generators in mechanical ventilators: advances and challenges. Pulm Med Rev. 2021;19(2):113–26.
257. Parker D, Stevens M, Hall R. Manual ventilation devices and their applications. Emerg Med Technol. 2019;17(5):222–35.
258. Chen Y, Huang T, Zhou X. Anesthesia workstations and ventilator mechanics. J Clin Eng. 2023;30(1):45–57.
259. Sanchez L, Gordon F. Visualizing ventilator parameters: the impact of modern display systems. J Respir Technol. 2023;28(3):120–36.
260. Barnes M, Carter L, Kim S. Alarm systems in intensive care ventilators: a review. Crit Care Technol. 2022;28(5):220–35.
261. Bangaru S. Initiating mechanical ventilation in critically ill patients: a contemporary overview. 2024.
262. Goligher EC, Ferguson ND. Clinical challenges in mechanical ventilation: optimizing lung and diaphragm protection. 2016.
263. Vuković D, Šumar S, Dupovac S, Badnjević A. Cost effectiveness analysis of medical devices in legal metrology system. In: Badnjević A, Cifrek M, Magjarević R, Džemić Z, editors. Inspection of medical devices. Series in biomedical engineering. Cham: Springer; 2024.
264. Morgan S, Wright K, Diaz A. Touchscreen interface evolution in modern ventilators. J Med Technol. 2020;26(6):310–25.
265. Foster C, Wilson R, Sanchez P. Alarm fatigue in ICU ventilators: challenges and solutions. Healthc Technol. 2019;15(7):90–109.
266. Pokvić LG, Deumić A, Softić A, Badnjević A. Application of artificial intelligence for management of maintenance and prediction of performances. In: Badnjević A, Cifrek M, Magjarević R, Džemić Z, editors. Inspection of medical devices. Series in biomedical engineering. Cham: Springer; 2024.

267. Stewart R, Ford H. Monitoring oxygen saturation and $CO_2$ levels in ventilated patients. Crit Care Sci. 2018;14(6):305–19.
268. Spahić L, Bećirović F, Badnjević A, Gurbeta Pokvić L. Industry 4.0 & medical devices – application of artificial intelligence for surveillance and management. In: Application of Industry 4.0 – an opportunity for a new step forward in all industrial branches. 2022.
269. Mujkić A, Baralić E, Ombašić A, Bećirović LS, Pokvić LG, Badnjević A. Machine intelligence in biomedical data modeling, processing, and analysis. In: 2022 11th Mediterranean conference on embedded computing (MECO). IEEE; 2022. p. 1–10.
270. Zhang X, Aroulmozhi V, Prasad A. Reliability and safety testing of a ventilator with remote verification tools. J Biomed Eng Technol. 2024.
271. Eghbali S, Alhanai T, Ghassemi M. Distribution-free uncertainty quantification in reinforcement learning-based ventilator control. IEEE J Biomed Health Inform. 2024.
272. Miller RD, Eriksson LI, Fleisher LA, Wiener-Kronish JP, Cohen NH, Young WL. Miller's anesthesia. 9th ed. Elsevier; 2020.
273. Brown DL, Miller RD, Pardo MC, Miller TE. Miller's anesthesia review. 2nd ed. Elsevier; 2018.
274. Ehrenwerth J, Eisenkraft JB, Berry JM. Anesthesia equipment: principles and applications. 3rd ed. Elsevier; 2020.
275. Dorsch JA, Dorsch SE. Understanding anesthesia equipment. 6th ed. Lippincott Williams & Wilkins; 2017.
276. Begashvili I. Minimal fresh gas flow anesthesia. 2019.
277. Loeb RG, Eisenkraft JB. The anesthesia machine and workstation: developments in functionality, software integration, and monitoring. Curr Anesthesiol Rep. 2021;11(1):24–31.
278. Glenski TA, Levine L. The implementation of low-flow anesthesia at a tertiary pediatric center: a quality improvement initiative. Pediatr Anesth. 2020;30:1139–45.
279. Mitterlechner T, Paal P, Schroeder D, Wenzel V, Herff H. Safer employment of nitrous oxide in anesthesia machines—a technical simulation. Med Gas Res. 2018;8:54–6.
280. Jette CG. The anesthesia machine: managing exhaled and waste gases. DeckerMed Anesthesiol. 2019.
281. Shin H, Yu H, Bae G, Huh H, Park JY, Kim J. The effect of fresh gas flow rate and type of anesthesia machine on time to reach target sevoflurane concentration. BMC Anesthesiol. 2017;17:10.
282. Barash PG, Cullen BF, Stoelting RK, Cahalan MK, Stock MC. Clinical anesthesia. 8th ed. Wolters Kluwer; 2017.
283. Hashemi M, Yousefzadeh M, Yazdani A, Behmanesh H. Machine learning–guided anesthesiology: a review of recent applications and future directions. J Clin Anesth Monit. 2024;58(2):115–23.
284. Shah S. Safety features in modern anaesthetic machines: an update. J Anesth Crit Care Open Access. 2017;7.
285. Zahid M, Kumar V, Khan MU. Enhancing anesthesia precision: integration of BIS monitoring with automated feedback systems. J Clin Anesth Pain Manag. 2024;6(1):10–8.
286. Char DS, Burgart AM. Machine learning implementation in clinical anesthesia: opportunities and ethical challenges. Anesth Analg. 2020;131(4):1085–91.
287. Bottiroli G, Calini A, Castelli G, Bignami E, Bonfanti S. The repurposed use of anesthesia machines to ventilate critically ill patients with COVID-19: A physiologic comparison with ICU ventilators. J Clin Monit Comput. 2021;35(4):837–44.
288. Martinović M, Kosović M, Spahić L, Softić A, Pokvić LG, Badnjević A. Machine learning for improved medical device management: a focus on dialysis machines. Technol Health Care. 2025; https://doi.org/10.1177/09287329251328815.
289. Ramalingam H, Vinayagam S, Manivannan K. A hidden danger of delivering hypoxic gas mixture during low flow anaesthesia in modern anaesthesia machine. Indian J Anaesth. 2022;66:677–8.

290. Dill N. 'No volatile agent' as a standard alarm on anaesthetic workstations – a reply. Anaesthesia. 2019;74:252.
291. Jamil M, Shahzad S, Hussain S, Bukhari HA, Huda A. Comparison of manual mode with automatic gas control mode for sevoflurane consumption in Maquet Flow-I anesthesia machine. Pak J Med Health Sci. 2022.
292. Aytolign D, Wudineh K, Mekonnen T, Asres S, Tsegaye D, Yimam A. Assessment of pre-anesthesia machine check and airway equipment preparation among anesthesia providers in Ethiopia. Ann Med Surg. 2022;76:103556.
293. Faddy S, Jennings P. Biphasic versus monophasic waveforms for transthoracic defibrillation in out-of-hospital cardiac arrest. Cochrane Database Syst Rev. 2016;2:CD006762.
294. Hagihara A, Onozuka D, Ono J, Nagata T, Hasegawa M. Interaction of defibrillation waveform with time to defibrillation or number of attempts on survival from out-of-hospital cardiac arrest. Resuscitation. 2018;122:54–60.
295. Wankmüller C, Rohrer U, Fischer P, Nürnberger P, Kolesnik E. Potential and challenges in airborne automated external defibrillator delivery by drones in a mountainous region. Drones. 2024;8.
296. Ruiz J, Ruiz de Gauna S, González-Otero D, Sáiz P, Gutiérrez J, Veintemillas J, Bastida J, Alonso D. Circulation assessment by automated external defibrillators during cardiopulmonary resuscitation. Resuscitation. 2018.
297. Inácio J, dos Santos Gomes da Rosa M, Shah J, Rosário J, Vissoci J, Manica A, Rodrigues C. Monophasic and biphasic shock for transthoracic conversion of atrial fibrillation: systematic review and network meta-analysis. Resuscitation. 2016;100:66–75.
298. Gorbunov B, Nesterenko I, Telyshev D, Selishchev S. Areas of effectiveness of half-sine monophasic and biphasic depolarizing defibrillation pulses on the diagram of energy/phase of fibrillation cycle. Ural Radio Eng J. 2021.
299. Sahu P, Acharya S, Totade M. Evolution of pacemakers and implantable cardioverter defibrillators in cardiology. Cureus. 2023.
300. Rickard J, Wilkoff B. Advances in implantable cardioverter defibrillator therapy. Expert Rev Cardiovasc Ther. 2016;14:291–9.
301. Link MS, Myerburg R, Estes NAM. Eligibility and disqualification recommendations for competitive athletes with cardiovascular abnormalities. Circulation. 2015.
302. Nehme Z, Andrew E, Nair R, Bernard S, Smith K. Versus semiautomatic rhythm analysis and defibrillation for out-of-hospital cardiac arrest. 2017.
303. Zhang H, Li R, Zhao D, Liu Y. Effects of current pacing and electrical field on turbulence induced by voltage oscillations in hearts. In: Proc Int Conf Math Stat Appl Math (MSAM). Atlantis Press; 2015. p. 33–6.
304. Bun S, Squara F, Scarlatti D, Théodore G, Latcu D, Hasni K, Benaich FA, Allouche E, Saoudi N, Ferrari E. Technological advances in cardiac pacing and defibrillation. Heart Vessels Transpl. 2019;3:95–101.
305. Li Y, Wang K, Li Q, Bai X, Zhang H. Role of If (funny current) on biological pacemaker – insight from a ventricular model. Comput Cardiol Conf (CinC). 2018;45:1–4.
306. Bødtker H, Stærk M, Lauridsen K, Jæger A, Løfgren B. Automated external defibrillation: not that easy! Untrained laypeople place AED pads poorly. Circulation. 2015.
307. Wang R. Computational investigation of the mechanisms underlying the cardiac pacemaker and its dysfunction. Doctoral dissertation; 2016.
308. Ambesh P, Kapoor A. Biological pacemakers: concepts and techniques. Natl Med J India. 2017;30:324–6.
309. Korpas D, Barta P. Paced electrical field modeling within ischemic myocardium. In: IFMBE Proc. Springer; 2019.
310. Szigethy XJ, Willson CJ, Salcido DD, Defilippi DA, Menegazzi J. Automated external defibrillator shock advisement performance among multiple human electrocardiographic rhythms and devices. Circulation. 2019.

311. Ahmed S, Hilal-Alnaqbi A, Hemairy MA, Al Ahmad M. ECG abnormality detection algorithm. Int J Adv Comput Sci Appl. 2018.
312. Bhakta D, Foreman L. Progress in implantable cardioverter-defibrillator therapy: advancement beyond technology alone. Trends Cardiovasc Med. 2015;25(7):612–3.
313. Krasteva V, Ménétré S, Jekova I, Stoyanov T, Jost D, Frattini B, Lemoine S, Lemoine F, Thomas V, Didon J. Comparison of pediatric and adult ECG rhythm analysis by automated external defibrillators during out-of-hospital cardiac arrest. Comput Cardiol Conf (CinC). 2018.
314. Mitacchione G. Cardiac implantable electronic devices breakthrough: are we ready to face the future? J Clin Med. 2022;11.
315. Mattei E, Vivarelli C, Franci D, Pavoncello S, Aureli T, Calcagnini G, Censi F. Pacemakers, implantable defibrillators, and 5G technology: what we need to know. Health Phys. 2023;125:202–6.
316. Komosa ER, Wolfson DW, Bressan MC, Cho H, Ogle B. Implementing biological pacemakers: design criteria for successful transition from concept to clinic. Circ Arrhythm Electrophysiol. 2021.
317. Fitzgerald A, Johnson MD, Hirsch J, Rich MA, Fidler R. Inconsistent shock advisories for monomorphic VT and torsade de pointes: a prospective experimental study on AEDs and defibrillators. Resuscitation. 2015;92:137–40.
318. Ricci R. Cardiac pacing: basic concepts. In: The ESC textbook of cardiovascular medicine. 3rd ed. Oxford University Press; 2018. p. 1974–8.
319. Yakovleva L. Permanent electrical cardiac pacing in bradyarrhythmias. Med Ukr. 2021.
320. Leech C, Perkins G. Shockingly simple? Should you use manual or automated defibrillation in out-of-hospital cardiac arrest? Emerg Med J. 2022;39:344–5.
321. Medjedovic E, Stanojevic M, Jonuzovic-Prosic S, Ribic E, Begic Z, Cerovac A, Badnjevic A. Artificial intelligence as a new answer to old challenges in maternal-fetal medicine and obstetrics. Technol Health Care. 2024;32(3):1273–87.
322. Lin J, Zhang Q, Xu X. Development of an infant incubator intelligent control strategy. Med Eng Phys. 2022;108:103897.
323. Badnjevic A, Gurbeta L, Jimenez ER, Iadanza E. Testing of mechanical ventilators and infant incubators in healthcare institutions. Technol Health Care. 2017;25(2):237–50.
324. Ibrahim A, Chua M, Tan S. Design and development of an automated infant incubator for temperature control. Biomed Signal Process Control. 2022;76:103640.
325. Lopez M, Han S, Zhao X. Innovations in neonatal transport incubators: a review. Healthc Technol Lett. 2022;9(2):34–40.
326. Brown J, Smith L, Taylor K. Cybersecurity considerations in neonatal medical devices. J Neonatal Care. 2021;35(4):312–8.
327. Sousa R, Ferreira J. Advances in humidity control in neonatal incubators. J Med Devices. 2021;45(3):1256–63.
328. Spahić L, Gurbeta Pokvić L, Badnjević A. Machine learning techniques for performance prediction of medical devices: infant incubators. IFMBE Proc. 2019;73:483–90.
329. Watanabe T, Okuda T. Noise reduction strategies in neonatal incubators. Pediatr Int. 2023;65(5):456–63.
330. Park H, Kim S. Comparative study of neonatal incubator control systems. Med Eng Res. 2023;32(1):20–8.
331. Lee D, Chang Y. Regulation updates for neonatal life-support equipment. Med Devices Technol. 2020;8(1):7–12.
332. Tran P, Nguyen A. Humidity optimization for preterm infant care. J Pediatr Nurs. 2023;69(3):121–7.
333. Ahmad M, Jamal R. Clinical evaluation of incubator air quality on neonatal outcomes. Clin Neonatol. 2022;41(2):210–7.
334. Thomas L, White R. New approaches to neonatal incubator alarm management. Pediatr Crit Care Med. 2020;21(11):923–30.

335. Li Y, Deng J. Portable neonatal incubators: advances and challenges. Healthc Technol Innov. 2022;13(2):78–85.
336. Campbell K, McCarthy P. Long-term follow-up of premature infants: the role of early incubator care. Early Hum Dev. 2021;157:105357.
337. Mendes A, Oliveira T. Neonatal incubators: future trends in automation and control. Biomed Eng Adv. 2023;16:100092.
338. Silva R, Gonçalves P. Neonatal care innovation: from incubators to integrated systems. J Healthc Eng. 2022;2022:6238489.
339. Merdović N, Spahić L, Hundur M, Pokvić LG, Badnjević A. Advancement of post-market surveillance of medical devices leveraging artificial intelligence: infusion pumps case study. Technol Health Care. 2024;33(2):915–21.
340. Howe RD. Robotics for surgery. Annu Rev Biomed Eng. 1999;1:211–40.
341. Kazanzides P, Kapoor A, Kim YJ, Ferrier N, Iordachita I, Fischer GS, Taylor RH. An open-source research kit for the da Vinci® surgical system. In: Proceedings of the IEEE international conference on robotics and automation (ICRA). IEEE; 2014. p. 6434–9.
342. Dario P, Hannaford B, Menciassi A. Smart surgical tools and augmenting devices. IEEE Trans Robot Autom. 2003;19(5):782–92.
343. Liang W, et al. Current advancements in therapeutic approaches in orthopedic surgery: a review of recent trends. Front Bioeng Biotechnol. 2024;12:Article 9.
344. Schakir T, Chand M. Clinical applications of handheld robotic devices in general surgery: a mini-review. Int J Surg. 2024;176(4):1297–301.
345. Bottura B, et al. Surgeon experience, robotic perioperative outcomes, and complications in gynecology. Rev Assoc Med Bras. 2022;68(11):1514–8.
346. Shen Y, et al. Efficacy of computed tomography features in predicting stage III thymic tumors. Oncol Lett. 2017;13(1):29–36.
347. Wahlstedt ER, Wahlstedt JC, Rosenberg JS, de Vries CR. Life cycle of surgical devices: global, environmental, and regulatory considerations. World J Surg. 2023;48:1045–55.
348. Zhalechian M, Saghafian S, Robles O. Harmonizing safety and speed: a human-algorithm approach to enhance the FDA's medical device clearance policy. 2024. https://doi.org/10.2139/ssrn.4863134.
349. Camarillo DB, Krummel TM, Salisbury JK Jr. Robotic technology in surgery: past, present, and future. Am J Surg. 2004;188(2 Suppl):2S–15S.
350. Topol E. Deep medicine: how artificial intelligence can make healthcare human again. Basic Books; 2019.
351. Lupton D. The quantified self: a sociology of self-tracking. Polity Press; 2020.
352. Park S, Lee S, Shin S. Personalized digital health and artificial intelligence in medicine: a review. Annu Rev Med. 2021;72:255–68.
353. Bates DW, Saria S, Ohno-Machado L, Shah A, Escobar G. Big data in health care: using analytics to identify and manage high-risk and high-cost patients. Health Aff. 2018;33(7):1123–31.
354. Piwek L, Ellis DA, Andrews S, Joinson A. The rise of consumer health wearables: promises and barriers. PLoS Med. 2016;13(2):e1001953.
355. Steinhubl SR, Muse ED, Topol EJ. The emerging field of mobile health: using smartphones for health monitoring and diagnosis. Lancet Digit Health. 2017;1(3):e157–67.
356. Tison GH, Sanchez JM, Ballinger B, Singh A. Passive detection of atrial fibrillation using a commercially available smartwatch. JAMA Cardiol. 2018;3(5):409–16.
357. Sawan M. Miniaturized medical devices: innovation and application. Biomed Eng. 2018;4(1):22–39.
358. Darwish A, Hassanien AE. Wearable and implantable wireless sensor network solutions for healthcare monitoring. Sensors. 2020;10(5):5561–95.
359. Rosen HJ, Gorno-Tempini ML, Goldman WP, Kirsch HE. Advances in implantable medical devices: a review. Neurology. 2021;45(8):654–68.
360. Chen M, Hao Y, Hwang K, Wang L, Wang L. Disease prediction by machine learning over big data from healthcare communities. IEEE Access. 2019;5:8869–79.

361. He Y, Guo X, Qian H. The internet of medical things (IoMT) in smart healthcare: applications, challenges, and future trends. J Healthc Inform Res. 2021;5(4):287–308.
362. Rahmani AM, Liu X, Liljeberg P. Internet of things in health care: from medical devices to smart systems. Futur Gener Comput Syst. 2018;86:297–312.
363. Islam SMR, Kwak D, Kabir MH, Hossain M, Kwak KS. The internet of things for health care: a comprehensive survey. IEEE Access. 2019;3:678–708.
364. Jiang F, Jiang Y, Zhi H, Dong Y, Li H, Ma S, Wang Y. Artificial intelligence in healthcare: past, present, and future. Stroke Vasc Neurol. 2021;2(4):230–43.
365. Shin D, Hwang H, Kim J. Artificial intelligence in medicine: challenges and opportunities. Biomedical Informatics. 2020;39(6):785–99.
366. Troccaz J. Medical robotics: where we come from, where we are and where we could go. Ind Robot. 2008;35(4):289.
367. Brassetti A, Ragusa A, Tedesco F, Prata F, et al. Robotic surgery in urology: history from PROBOT® to HUGO™. Sensors (Basel). 2023;23(16):7104.
368. Dinger S, Dickens J, Pantanowitz A. Robotic arm for remote surgery. 2013. https://doi.org/10.48550/arXiv.1307.5641.
369. Schreiber DA, Shak DB, Norbash AM, Yip MC. An open-source 7-axis robotic platform to enable dexterous procedures within CT scanners. In: 2019 IEEE/RSJ international conference on intelligent robots and systems (IROS). IEEE; 2019.
370. Berger J, Unger M, Keller J, Reich CM, et al. Design and validation of a medical robotic device system to control two collaborative robots for ultrasound-guided needle insertions. Front Robot AI. 2022;9.
371. Unger M, Berger J, Melzer A. Robot-assisted image-guided interventions. Front Robot AI. 2021;8.
372. Poignant A, Jarrasse N, Morel G. Virtually turning robotic manipulators into worn devices: opening new horizons for wearable assistive robotics. arXiv:2211.08483v1. 2022.
373. Thai MT, Phan PT, Wong S, Lovell NH, et al. Advanced intelligent systems for surgical robotics. Adv Intell Syst. 2020.
374. Avgousti S, Christoforou EG, Panayides AS, Voskarides S, et al. Medical telerobotic systems: current status and future trends. BioMed Eng OnLine. 2016.
375. Okamura AM, Mataric MJ, Christensen HI. Medical and health-care robotics. IEEE Robot Autom Mag. 2010.
376. Denecke K, Baudoin CR. A review of artificial intelligence and robotics in transformed health ecosystems. Front Med. 2022;9.
377. Devanne M, Nguyen SM, Rémy-Néris O, Le Gales-Garnett B, et al. A co-design approach for a rehabilitation robot coach for physical rehabilitation based on the error classification of motion errors. In: IRC 2018: second IEEE international conference on robotic computing, Jan 2018, Laguna Hills, CA. IEEE; 2021.
378. Lim JH, He K, Yi Z, Hou C, et al. Adaptive learning-based upper-limb rehabilitation training system with collaborative robot. Annu Int Conf IEEE Eng Med Biol Soc. 2023; https://doi.org/10.1109/EMBC40787.2023.10340313.
379. Tsumura R, Koseki Y, Nitta N, Yoshinaka K. Toward fully automated robotic platform for remote auscultation. Int J Med Robot. 2023;19:e2461.
380. Lawrie L, Gillies K, Davies L, Torkington J, et al. Current issues and future considerations for the wider implementation of robotic-assisted surgery: a qualitative study. BMJ Open. 2022;12.
381. Lagomarsino M, Groenhuis V, Casadio M, Welleweerd MK, et al. Image-guided breast biopsy of MRI-visible lesions with a hand-mounted motorised needle steering tool. In: 2021 International symposium on medical robotics, ISMR 2021. IEEE; 2021.
382. Morone G, Pirrera A, Meli P, Giansanti D. Ethics and automated systems in the health domain: design and submission of a survey on rehabilitation and assistance robotics to collect insiders' opinions and perception. Healthcare. 2022;10.

383. Kleiner LW, Wright JC, Wang Y. Evolution of implantable and insertable drug delivery systems. J Control Release. 2014.
384. Rimon MTI, Hasan MW, Hassan MF, Cesmeci S. Advancements in insulin pumps: a comprehensive exploration of insulin pump systems, technologies, and future directions. Pharmaceutics. 2024;16.
385. Bally L, Thabit H, Hovorka R. Finding the right route for insulin delivery: an overview of implantable pump therapy. Expert Opin Drug Deliv. 2017;14:1103–11.
386. Barnard KD, Kropff J, Choudhary P, Neupane S, et al. Acceptability of implantable continuous glucose monitoring sensor. J Diabetes Sci Technol. 2018;12:634–8.
387. Sora ND, Shashpal F, Bond EA, Jenkins AJ. Insulin pumps: review of technological advancement in diabetes management. Am J Med Sci. 2019;358(5):326–31.
388. Haveman JW, Logtenberg SJJ, Kleefstra N, Groenier KH, et al. Erratum to: surgical aspects and complications of continuous intraperitoneal insulin infusion with an implantable pump. Langenbecks Arch Surg. 2019;404:21.
389. Meng E, Hoang T. MEMS-enabled implantable drug infusion pumps for laboratory animal research, preclinical, and clinical applications. Adv Drug Deliv Rev. 2012;64:1628–38.
390. Yan B, Li B, Kunecke F, Gu Z, Guo L. Polypyrrole-based implantable electroactive pump for controlled drug microinjection. ACS Appl Mater Interfaces. 2015;7:14563–8.
391. Payne M, Pooke F, Geoffrey Chase J, Jake C, Holder-Pearson L, Knopp J. The separation of insulin pump hardware and software – a novel and low-cost approach to insulin pump design. IFAC-PapersOnLine. 2021;54(15):502–7.
392. Schaeffer NE, Parks LJ, Verhoef ET, Morgan CA, Stal M. Insulin pumps and remote software updates: a new way forward. J Diabetes Sci Technol. 2015.
393. Ellis RJ, Angelos P, Jarnagin WR, Kemeny NE, Merkow RP. Abrupt discontinuation of the Codman hepatic artery infusion pump: considerations in the era of precision medicine. J Am Coll Surg. 2019;229:217–9.
394. Coutant T, Laniesse D, Sykes JM. Advances in therapeutics and delayed drug release. Vet Clin North Am Exotic Anim Pract. 2019;22:501–20.
395. McCrea DL. A primer on insulin pump therapy for health care providers. Nurs Clin North Am. 2017;52(4):553–64.
396. U.S. Food and Drug Administration (FDA). Software as a Medical Device (SaMD): Clinical Evaluation - Guidance for Industry and Food and Drug Administration Staff. 2017.
397. Litvinova O, Klager E, Tzvetkov NT, Kimberger O, et al. Digital pills with ingestible sensors: patent landscape analysis. Pharmaceuticals. 2022;15.
398. Byrne C, Lim CL. The ingestible telemetric body core temperature sensor: a review of validity and exercise applications. Br J Sports Med. 2006;41:126–33.
399. Chun HJ, Tanabe S, Choi M, Saurin J. Current status and future directions of capsule endoscopy. Gastroenterol Res Pract. 2016;2016.
400. Abramson A, Caffarel-Salvador E, Khang M, Dellal D, et al. An ingestible self-orienting system for oral delivery of macromolecules. Science. 2019;363:611–5.
401. Cummins G. Smart pills for gastrointestinal diagnostics and therapy. Adv Drug Deliv Rev. 2021;177.
402. Hoffmann SV, O'Shea JP, Galvin P, Jannin V, Griffin BT. State-of-the-art and future perspectives in ingestible remotely controlled smart capsules for drug delivery: a GENEGUT review. Eur J Pharm Sci. 2024;203:106911.
403. Cicha I, Priefer R, Severino P, Souto EB, Jain S. Biosensor-integrated drug delivery systems as new materials for biomedical applications. Biomolecules. 2022;12.
404. GiDoctor. SmartPill™ motility capsule. Motility test. GI Doctor; 2024.
405. Iddan G, Meron G, Glukhovsky A, Swain P. Wireless capsule endoscopy. Nature. 2000;405:417.
406. Kim G, Abbas A, Mahato K. Ingestible biosensors for personalized health. In: Biosensors for personalized healthcare. Springer; 2024. p. 393–418.

407. Gurbeta L, Badnjevic A, Maksimovic M, Omanovic-Miklicanin E, Sejdic E. A telehealth system for automated diagnosis of asthma and chronic obstructive pulmonary disease. J Am Med Inform Assoc. 2018;25(9):1213–7.
408. Islam SH, Kwak D, Kabir MH, Hossain MS, Kwak K-S. The internet of things for health care: a comprehensive survey. IEEE Access. 2015;3:678–708.
409. Gültekin M, Şahin M. The use of artificial intelligence in mental health services in Turkey: what do mental health professionals think? Cyberpsychol J Psychosoc Res Cyberspace. 2024;18(1).
410. Crnčević N, Hukić M, Deumić S, Selimagić A, Dozić A. Gastrointestinal tract microbiome effect and role in disease development. Diseases. 2022;10.
411. Klugman CM, Dunn LB, Schwartz J, Cohen IG. The ethics of smart pills and self-acting devices: autonomy, truth-telling, and trust at the dawn of digital medicine. Am J Bioeth. 2018.
412. Pokvić LG, Spahić L, Badnjević A. Implementation of Industry 4.0 in transformation of medical device maintenance systems. 2020.
413. Batra S, Baker R, Wang T, Forma F, et al. Digital health technology for use in patients with serious mental illness: a systematic review of the literature. Med Devices (Auckl). 2017.

# Chapter 3
# Clinical Engineering and Healthcare Technology Management

This section explores the principles, practices, and emerging trends in clinical engineering and healthcare technology management. It begins by introducing the foundations of the field, highlighting the role of clinical engineers in ensuring the safe, effective, and efficient use of medical technologies, and outlining the essential skills and competencies required for technical, regulatory, and interdisciplinary collaboration (Sect. 3.1). Building on this foundation, the section examines medical device management and safety, with a focus on post-market surveillance, regulatory compliance, risk management, and strategies to address deficiencies in device monitoring (Sect. 3.2). It then addresses quality, compliance, and sustainability, emphasizing the use of computerized maintenance management systems, environmentally responsible device management, and strategies to optimize performance while reducing ecological impact (Sect. 3.3). Together, these chapters demonstrate how clinical engineering integrates technical expertise, regulatory knowledge, and management practices to enhance patient safety, healthcare quality, and sustainable technology deployment.

## 3.1 Foundations of Clinical Engineering and Healthcare Technology Management

Clinical engineering is a specialized branch of biomedical engineering that focuses on applying engineering principles to healthcare [1]. It plays a crucial role in ensuring the safe, efficient, and effective use of medical technology in patient care. As healthcare continues to evolve with rapid technological advancements, integrating engineering expertise into medical environments has become indispensable.

Clinical engineering emerged as a distinct discipline in the mid-twentieth century when hospitals recognized the need for dedicated professionals to manage increasingly complex medical devices [2]. With the advent of electronic medical



A. Badnjević et al., *Biomedical Instrumentation*, Series in BioEngineering,
https://doi.org/10.1007/978-3-032-10978-1_3

equipment, the demand for engineers capable of maintaining, calibrating, and optimizing these technologies grew significantly. Over the years, the field has expanded to encompass device maintenance, healthcare technology management, regulatory compliance, risk assessment, and innovation in medical technology [3].

The role of a clinical engineer is inherently interdisciplinary. These professionals work at the intersection of medicine, engineering, and regulatory science, ensuring that medical devices meet the highest standards of functionality and safety [4]. Their contributions are crucial in hospital settings, where they support physicians, nurses, and technicians by ensuring that medical equipment functions properly, thereby contributing to improved patient outcomes [5, 6].

Moreover, clinical engineers are responsible for the strategic management of healthcare technology. This includes evaluating new medical devices before procurement, assessing their clinical benefits, and ensuring their integration into existing hospital systems [1]. The decisions they make can impact not only patient care but also healthcare costs and operational efficiency. Given the financial constraints in healthcare, clinical engineers must balance the need for advanced technology with cost-effectiveness, ensuring that hospitals invest in devices that provide the best value for patient care [7, 8].

As the healthcare industry embraces digital transformation, clinical engineering has expanded to include fields such as artificial intelligence in medicine, telehealth, and wearable health monitoring devices. These new technologies present opportunities and challenges, requiring clinical engineers to continuously update their skills and knowledge [3]. With a strong foundation in engineering and a deep understanding of medical applications, clinical engineers are poised to play a crucial role in shaping the future of healthcare technology.

Clinical engineers play a vital role in various aspects of healthcare operations. One of their primary responsibilities is ensuring that medical equipment functions reliably and safely. This involves overseeing the entire lifecycle of medical devices, from selection and acquisition to maintenance and eventual decommissioning. Proper equipment management reduces downtime, prevents malfunctions, and minimizes risks to patients and healthcare providers.

Clinical engineers are also key players in health technology assessment (HTA), where they evaluate the effectiveness, safety, and cost of medical devices before they are integrated into healthcare facilities. Through rigorous testing and analysis, they determine whether a particular device meets the required clinical and technical standards [4]. This process prevents hospitals from investing in ineffective or unsafe technologies.

Another critical role of clinical engineers is their contribution to patient safety. Medical devices, such as ventilators, infusion pumps, and imaging systems, are essential for diagnosing and treating patients; however, their improper use or malfunction can have severe consequences. Clinical engineers work closely with hospital staff to develop standard operating procedures (SOPs) for device usage, train medical personnel on proper operation, and establish protocols for regular maintenance. Beyond safety, clinical engineers play a fundamental role in regulatory compliance. Healthcare institutions must adhere to strict national and international regulations governing the use of medical technology. Compliance with standards set by organizations such as the International Organization for Standardization (ISO), the U.S. Food and Drug Administration (FDA), and the European Medicines Agency (EMA) is essential to maintaining operational approval [1, 9]. Clinical engineers ensure that hospitals and healthcare facilities meet these regulatory requirements by conducting audits, documenting compliance, and implementing necessary modifications. Additionally, as healthcare increasingly relies on interconnected medical devices, cybersecurity has become essential to clinical engineering. Many modern medical technologies, including patient monitoring systems and electronic health records, are connected to hospital networks, making them vulnerable to cyber threats. Clinical engineers work to secure these systems by implementing robust cybersecurity measures, monitoring for potential breaches, and ensuring compliance with data protection laws such as the Health Insurance Portability and Accountability Act (HIPAA) [4, 10].

Clinical engineers play a crucial role in disaster preparedness and emergency response within healthcare settings. During public health crises, such as the COVID-19 pandemic, their expertise was invaluable in managing medical equipment shortages, setting up emergency healthcare facilities, and ensuring the functionality of life-saving devices, including ventilators. Their ability to troubleshoot and adapt to rapidly changing circumstances makes them indispensable in emergencies. Ultimately, clinical engineers play a crucial role in supporting research and innovation in medical technology [7]. They collaborate with industry professionals, academic institutions, and healthcare providers to develop new medical devices and improve existing technologies. Their involvement in research and development (R&D) facilitates the translation of medical needs into engineering solutions, leading to advancements in diagnostic tools, therapeutic devices, and healthcare automation. With their unique combination of technical expertise and clinical insight, clinical engineers drive innovation and contribute to the ongoing evolution of modern medicine.

### 3.1.1 Skills and Competencies Required in Clinical Engineering

Clinical engineers must possess a diverse set of skills that combine technical proficiency, analytical thinking, and strong communication abilities to excel in their field. Their role requires a deep understanding of engineering principles, biomedical applications, and healthcare operations (Figs. 3.1 and 3.2).

One of the most critical competencies in clinical engineering is technical expertise. Clinical engineers must thoroughly understand the design, electronics, signal processing, and control systems of medical devices. They must be proficient in troubleshooting complex medical equipment, conducting performance evaluations, and ensuring devices meet regulatory standards. Knowledge of software

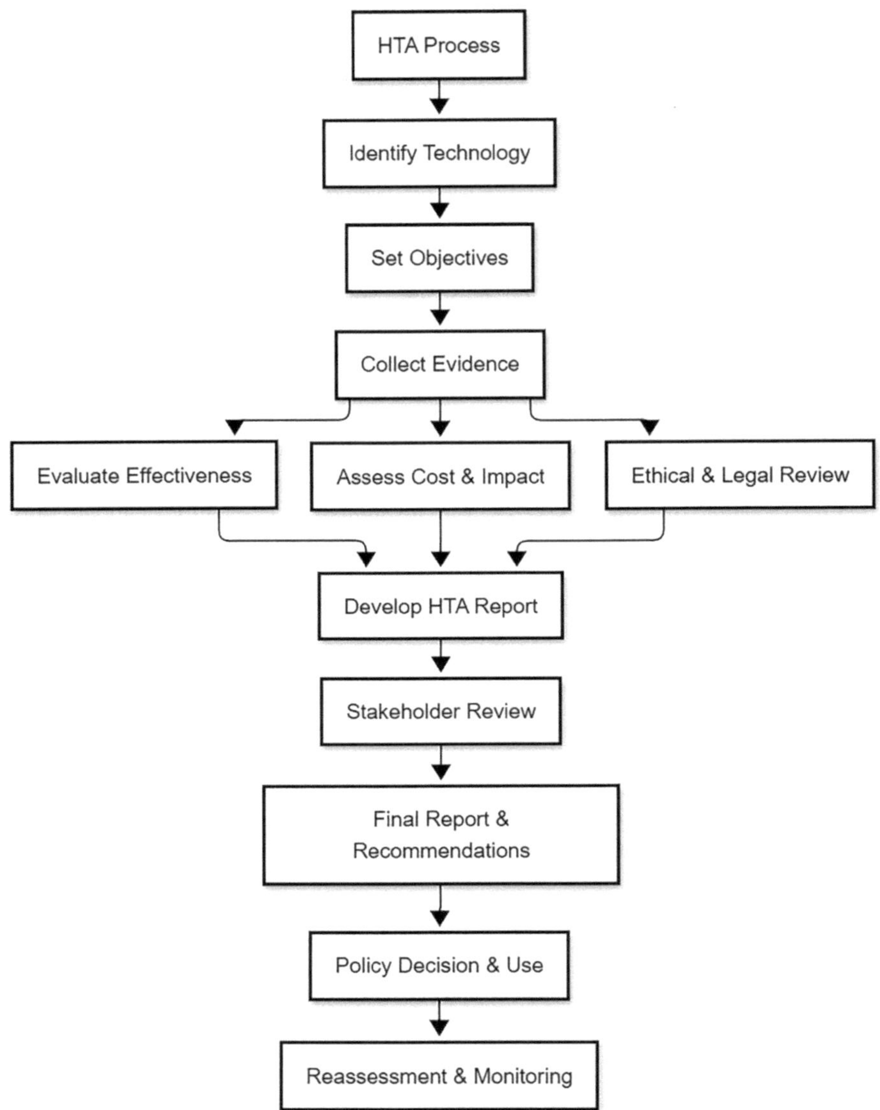


**Fig. 3.1** Health technology assessment (HTA) process

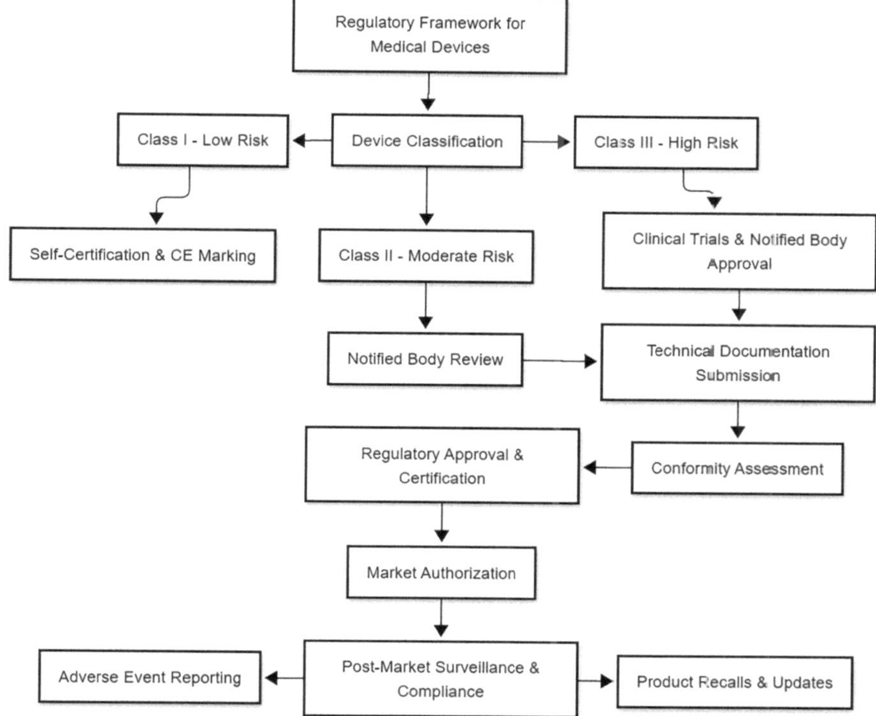


**Fig. 3.2** Regulatory framework for medical devices

development and programming languages such as Python or MATLAB is also beneficial, particularly as medical devices incorporate artificial intelligence and machine learning algorithms [5].

Beyond technical skills, clinical engineers must have analytical and problem-solving abilities [1]. They are often tasked with diagnosing equipment malfunctions, optimizing device performance, and identifying potential risks associated with medical technology. This requires critical thinking and the application of engineering principles to real-world clinical challenges.

Regulatory knowledge is another vital skill for clinical engineers. They must be well-versed in international medical device regulations, including ISO 13485 (Quality Management Systems for Medical Devices) and FDA guidelines. Understanding these regulations ensures that healthcare institutions remain compliant and that medical devices meet the safety and efficacy standards set by the FDA [11] and the WHO [12].

Additionally, clinical engineers must have strong interpersonal and communication skills. They frequently collaborate with physicians, nurses, hospital administrators, and regulatory bodies, translating technical information into practical applications for healthcare providers. Effective communication is essential for training medical personnel on device usage, writing technical reports, and advising hospital management on procurement decisions [13, 14].

As healthcare technology evolves, clinical engineers must develop expertise in emerging fields, including artificial intelligence, telemedicine, and cybersecurity. Integrating AI-powered diagnostic tools, wearable health monitors, and remote patient monitoring systems requires clinical engineers to stay updated with the latest advancements in medical technology. Continuous learning through professional development programs, industry conferences, and certification courses is essential to keeping pace with these innovations [15, 16].

In addition to technical and regulatory knowledge, project management skills are increasingly valuable in clinical engineering. Managing medical device procurement, installation, and maintenance requires careful planning, budgeting, and coordination with multiple stakeholders. Clinical engineers must be adept at managing complex projects, ensuring that technology is implemented efficiently while meeting clinical and financial constraints [17].

## 3.2 Medical Device Management and Safety

Medical devices (MDs) form the backbone of modern healthcare, playing a crucial role in disease prevention, diagnosis, treatment, and patient monitoring. These devices range from simple tools, such as thermometers and blood pressure cuffs, to highly complex systems, including MRI scanners, pacemakers, and robotic surgical instruments. Given their direct impact on patient health and clinical outcomes, ensuring their safety, reliability, and effectiveness is paramount for healthcare providers, regulatory bodies, and manufacturers alike.

The lifecycle of a medical device does not end once it receives regulatory approval and enters the market. Instead, it must undergo continuous scrutiny to ensure it continues to perform as intended, while identifying any previously undetected risks or malfunctions. This ongoing monitoring process is known as post-market surveillance (PMS), a crucial regulatory function designed to track the performance of medical devices in real-world conditions and mitigate emerging risks. PMS is an essential complement to pre-market testing, which, despite rigorous clinical trials and laboratory testing, cannot fully predict a device's behavior across diverse patient populations, settings, and use cases [14]. Regulatory authorities worldwide, including the U.S. Food and Drug Administration (FDA), the European Medicines Agency (EMA), and the World Health Organization (WHO), have developed detailed guidelines and regulations to govern PMS. The European Union's Medical Device Regulation (MDR) and the FDA's Quality System Regulation (QSR) outline strict requirements for manufacturers to monitor and report safety concerns, conduct post-market clinical follow-ups, and take corrective actions when necessary [11, 18]. Similar frameworks exist in other regions, including China, Canada, Japan, and Australia, each with specific regulatory nuances that govern PMS operations [12].

However, despite structured PMS protocols, challenges remain in their implementation. Many regulatory frameworks rely heavily on manufacturers for self-reporting adverse events, which introduces potential biases and gaps in data collection. Additionally, inconsistencies in regulatory approaches across different regions can lead to discrepancies in device performance, safety monitoring, and recall procedures. The lack of harmonized global reporting systems and standardized methodologies further complicates the surveillance process, creating a fragmented landscape that may compromise patient safety [19]. Moreover, advancements in medical technology introduce new complexities in PMS. The increasing integration of artificial intelligence (AI), software-driven diagnostics, and interconnected medical devices through the Internet of Things (IoT) necessitates new approaches to safety monitoring. Traditional PMS methods, which primarily focus on mechanical failures and adverse event reporting, may not be sufficient to track algorithmic biases, cybersecurity threats, or software updates that can alter device performance after market release. This highlights the need for innovative surveillance mechanisms, including AI-driven analytics, real-time data collection, and predictive risk modeling to enhance the effectiveness of PMS strategies [15].

This chapter aims to provide a comprehensive review of PMS, examining its regulatory landscape, challenges, real-world case studies of PMS deficiencies, and strategies for improvement. By examining the intricacies of post-market surveillance, this review highlights opportunities for enhancing PMS frameworks and ensuring a safer, more effective healthcare environment for patients worldwide (Fig. 3.3).

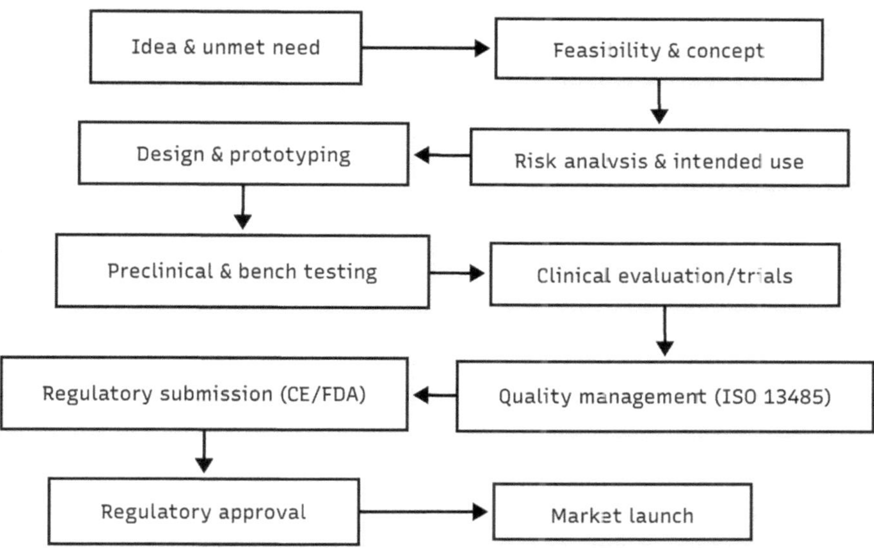


**Fig. 3.3** Medical device process—from idea to market (pre-market process)

### 3.2.1 The Regulatory Landscape of Post-Market Surveillance

The regulatory landscape for PMS is diverse, with countries implementing varying oversight and reporting requirements for medical devices. Regulations are primarily focused on ensuring that MDs continue to meet safety, performance, and efficacy standards after they have been placed on the market. Key regulatory frameworks governing PMS include those implemented by the European Union, the United States, China, Canada, Australia, and Japan [14].

**European Union (EU)**

The EU has one of the most stringent regulatory frameworks for medical devices. The MDR [20], which replaced the Medical Device Directive (MDD), introduced stricter requirements for PMS. Under MDR, manufacturers must establish and maintain a PMS system to actively and systematically collect, record, and analyze relevant data on MDs' quality, performance, and safety throughout their lifecycle. Key requirements under the EU MDR include:

- Post-Market Clinical Follow-up (PMCF): Manufacturers must conduct ongoing clinical evaluations to assess device performance and detect potential safety issues.
- Periodic Safety Update Reports (PSUR): Class IIa, IIb, and III devices are required to report periodically on safety and performance.
- Vigilance and Incident Reporting: Manufacturers must report serious incidents and field safety corrective actions (FSCA) within strict timelines (15 days for serious incidents, 2 days for public health threats).
- European Databank on Medical Devices (EUDAMED): A centralized platform for storing information on device registration, clinical investigations, PMS, and market surveillance activities.

**United States (FDA)**

In the United States, the FDA regulates PMS under the Federal Food, Drug, and Cosmetic Act (FDCA) and the QSR. The FDA's PMS mechanisms include:

- MDR: Manufacturers, device user facilities, and importers must report adverse events, malfunctions, and device-related deaths or serious injuries.
- Post-Approval Studies (PAS): FDA may require manufacturers to conduct additional studies after a device is approved to gather further safety and effectiveness data.
- MedSun Program: A voluntary surveillance system where hospitals and healthcare institutions report MD-related issues.
- Recall and Safety Alerts: The FDA has the authority to issue recalls and safety communications to protect public health.

#### China

China's National Medical Products Administration (NMPA) enforces PMS through State Council Order No. 739. This regulation strengthens PMS by:

- Mandatory adverse event reporting for manufacturers and healthcare institutions.
- Stricter PMS data collection requirements.
- Increased inspections at manufacturing and distribution sites.

#### Japan

Japan's Pharmaceuticals and Medical Devices Agency (PMDA) enforces PMS through:

- GVP Ordinance (Good Vigilance Practice): Mandates periodic safety reports.
- Sentinel Medical Networks: AI-driven risk detection systems.
- Field Inspections: Ensuring compliance with PMS regulations.

#### Canada and Australia

Canada's Health Canada and Australia's Therapeutic Goods Administration (TGA) require PMS through:

- Mandatory reporting of adverse events and recalls.
- Market authorization renewals based on PMS data.
- Integration of real-world evidence (RWE) in regulatory decisions.

### *3.2.2 Challenges in PMS Implementation*

Despite the clear regulatory frameworks established for PMS, several challenges hinder its effective implementation. These challenges range from inconsistencies in reporting mechanisms and underreporting of adverse events to a lack of harmonized methodologies and difficulties in tracking device performance in diverse clinical settings.

#### Inconsistent Reporting Mechanisms

One of the significant obstacles to effective PMS is the inconsistency in adverse event reporting mechanisms across different regulatory jurisdictions. In the EU, serious incidents must be reported within 15 days, whereas in the US, medical device-related deaths and serious injuries must be reported to the FDA within

30 days [11, 18]. These variations create discrepancies in reporting practices, making it challenging to track device safety on a global scale [21]. Furthermore, some countries have voluntary reporting systems, which can significantly underreport safety concerns [19].

#### Underreporting of Adverse Events

Adverse event underreporting remains a critical issue in PMS. Studies have shown that healthcare professionals, including physicians and nurses, often fail to report device-related complications due to a lack of awareness, time constraints, or fear of legal repercussions [13]. Manufacturers dominate the reporting process, contributing over 96% of all adverse event reports, while healthcare professionals and patients contribute significantly less [21]. This reliance on manufacturers for data collection introduces potential biases, as companies may downplay issues to avoid regulatory scrutiny [22].

#### Lack of Global Harmonization in PMS Standards

The absence of standardized PMS protocols across different regulatory agencies poses another challenge. While organizations like the International Medical Device Regulators Forum (IMDRF) have recommended harmonized reporting frameworks, global adoption remains limited. Countries such as China and Japan enforce stricter PMS requirements than the US and EU, leading to regulatory fragmentation that makes global data comparison and device performance tracking challenging [15].

#### Challenges in Post-Market Clinical Follow-Up (PMCF)

PMCF is a crucial component of PMS, requiring manufacturers to collect real-world clinical data on device performance. However, many manufacturers do not conduct PMCF studies unless explicitly required by regulators [13]. This results in a lack of long-term safety data, making it challenging to evaluate a device's performance over time and across diverse patient populations [19].

#### Limited Real-World Evidence Integration

Real-world evidence (RWE) can enhance patient management systems (PMS) by leveraging patient data from electronic health records (EHRs), registries, and wearable devices. However, the integration of RWE into PMS frameworks remains limited due to concerns over data privacy, challenges in standardization, and difficulties in aggregating data across healthcare institutions. Regulatory bodies, such as the

FDA, have launched initiatives to incorporate real-world evidence (RWE) in decision-making; however, widespread adoption is still in progress [11].

#### Difficulties in Tracking Device Performance Across Healthcare Institutions

Medical devices are used in various healthcare settings, from large hospitals to small outpatient clinics. Tracking their performance across these diverse environments is challenging due to differences in maintenance practices, calibration protocols, and user expertise [6]. A lack of centralized databases linking device performance data across healthcare institutions further exacerbates this issue, limiting the ability to conduct comprehensive safety assessments [22].

These challenges underscore the need for enhanced PMS strategies, including improved reporting mechanisms, global harmonization of PMS regulations, and the integration of AI-driven monitoring systems to detect and predict device failures more effectively. By addressing these limitations, regulatory bodies, manufacturers, and healthcare institutions can collaborate to develop a more robust PMS framework that ensures patient safety and enhances the overall reliability of medical devices in clinical practice.

### *3.2.3 Case Studies of PMS Deficiencies*

Several real-world cases highlight the consequences of inadequate PMS. During the COVID-19 pandemic, many emergency-use ventilators were deployed without sufficient clinical testing, leading to device malfunctions and patient harm [23]. Furthermore, retrospective analyses of device recalls indicate that software failures are among the most common causes of MD safety issues [24].

An independent inspection of mechanical ventilators and incubators revealed that nearly 30% of these devices failed to meet performance standards, necessitating recalibration or removal from clinical use [6]. Similar studies on anesthesia machines and defibrillators found failure rates exceeding 13%, raising concerns about the adequacy of PMS frameworks in ensuring device reliability [22].

### *3.2.4 Strategies for Improving PMS*

To address the challenges in PMS implementation, it is crucial to develop harmonized, evidence-based methodologies that ensure consistency, transparency, and efficiency in post-market monitoring. Several strategic approaches have been proposed to enhance the effectiveness of PMS, including standardized global reporting, third-party performance verification, integration of AI and big data, and expansion of medical device registries.

### Standardized Global Reporting Systems

A significant challenge in PMS is the lack of standardized adverse event reporting systems across regulatory bodies. The International Medical Device Regulators Forum (IMDRF) has proposed guidelines for a globally harmonized adverse event reporting system, but adoption remains inconsistent across different regions.

Establishing uniform reporting criteria for medical device failures and adverse events would enhance data comparability and improve the accuracy of risk assessments. For example, EUDAMED in the EU and MAUDE in the US serve as adverse event databases but operate under different criteria and timelines, making cross-jurisdictional data analysis difficult [14]. A unified, internationally recognized reporting structure could mitigate these discrepancies and improve regulatory decision-making.

### Third-Party Performance Verification

Relying solely on manufacturers for PMS introduces potential biases and conflicts of interest, as self-reported data may not always present an accurate picture of device performance. Independent third-party performance assessments, conducted by accredited inspection bodies, would increase accountability and ensure unbiased evaluations [17].

Countries incorporating medical devices into legal metrology frameworks have demonstrated improved compliance and safety outcomes. For example, legal metrology frameworks in Bosnia, Herzegovina, and Serbia mandate independent inspections of critical medical devices such as ventilators and defibrillators, leading to more transparent PMS data [22]. Expanding this approach globally would standardize performance verification and reinforce public trust in medical devices.

### Integration of AI and Big Data in PMS

Artificial intelligence (AI) and big data analytics present significant opportunities for improving PMS by automating the detection of device failures and predicting potential risks. AI algorithms can process large volumes of real-world data from electronic health records (EHRs), adverse event reports, and device telemetry to identify patterns that may indicate emerging safety concerns [15, 16].

Japan has already begun leveraging AI-based monitoring tools and sentinel networks to streamline PMS activities. These AI-driven surveillance systems analyze device performance in real-time, allowing regulators to take proactive measures before issues escalate [15, 25]. Implementing similar AI-driven strategies in other regions would improve PMS efficiency and enhance patient safety.

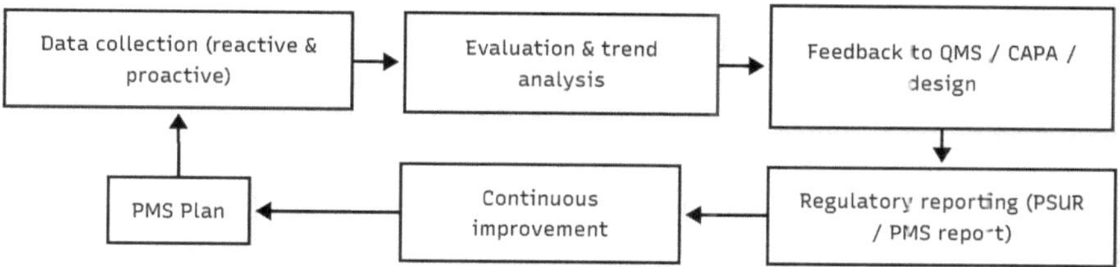


**Fig. 3.4** Suggested methodology for post-market surveillance of medical devices

**Expansion of Medical Device Registries**

Transitioning from static administrative registries to dynamic databases incorporating real-world performance data would significantly improve PMS. Medical device registries should be linked with patient registries to provide comprehensive safety assessments and facilitate long-term tracking of device performance [26].

Countries with well-established registry systems, such as Germany and Sweden, have successfully utilized registry data to monitor the long-term performance of implants and other high-risk devices, facilitating the faster identification of faulty products [14]. Expanding the scope of these registries and integrating real-world evidence (RWE) into PMS frameworks would provide a more holistic view of device safety and efficacy (Fig. 3.4).

### 3.2.5 *Future Research*

Post-market surveillance of medical devices is a critical component of healthcare safety and regulatory oversight. The need for effective, harmonized, and evidence-based product management systems (PMS) mechanisms grows as medical devices become increasingly sophisticated and interconnected. This paper has identified key challenges in PMS implementation, including inconsistent reporting mechanisms, underreporting of adverse events, lack of global harmonization in regulatory frameworks, and difficulty tracking device performance across healthcare settings. These challenges underscore the necessity for strategic improvements to ensure patient safety and enhance device reliability.

One of the most pressing concerns in PMS is the inconsistency in reporting adverse events. While some countries enforce mandatory reporting requirements, others operate under voluntary disclosure models, resulting in discrepancies in data quality and availability. Strengthening global PMS frameworks through standardized reporting systems, such as those proposed by the International Medical Device Regulators Forum (IMDRF), would significantly enhance transparency and comparability of safety data across jurisdictions [8]. Moreover, centralizing PMS data within shared international databases, similar to EUDAMED in the EU, would improve collaboration between regulators and healthcare institutions [14].

Relying on the manufacturer's self-reported data introduces potential bias and limits the effectiveness of PMS. Implementing third-party performance verification, as seen in countries with legal metrology frameworks, such as Bosnia and Herzegovina and Serbia, could provide a more objective assessment of device safety and functionality [22]. Expanding such independent oversight mechanisms worldwide would reinforce accountability and improve public confidence in medical devices.

Integrating artificial intelligence (AI) and big data analytics presents a transformative opportunity for PMS. AI-driven tools can analyze vast amounts of real-world evidence (RWE) from electronic health records (EHRs), wearable devices, and patient registries to detect patterns that may indicate emerging safety risks. Countries like Japan are pioneering AI-based PMS approaches, demonstrating the potential of these technologies to enhance real-time surveillance and proactive risk management [15]. Adopting AI-driven PMS strategies across regulatory bodies would optimize device monitoring and facilitate faster responses to safety concerns.

Additionally, expanding the scope of medical device registries to incorporate real-world performance data would significantly improve PMS efficiency. Linking patient registries with device registries would provide a more comprehensive understanding of long-term safety and efficacy. Countries with well-established registry systems, such as Germany and Sweden, have successfully utilized these databases to track the performance of implants and high-risk devices, enabling more effective recall and remediation processes [14]. Future PMS frameworks should prioritize the expansion and interconnectivity of such registries to facilitate global collaboration and data sharing.

As medical technologies evolve, PMS frameworks must also adapt to address new risks associated with AI-driven diagnostics, cybersecurity threats, and remote medical devices. Future PMS strategies should consider developing robust monitoring mechanisms for software-driven medical devices, including automated alerts for software vulnerabilities and periodic performance assessments of AI algorithms. The growing use of telemedicine and remote patient monitoring further emphasizes the need for PMS systems to track device functionality in non-traditional healthcare settings.

Improving PMS requires coordinated efforts from regulators, manufacturers, healthcare institutions, and technology providers. Regulatory bodies can create a more effective and transparent PMS framework by embracing standardized reporting systems, independent performance verification, AI-driven analytics, and enhanced medical device registries. These improvements will enhance patient safety and contribute to the overall trust and reliability of medical devices in modern healthcare.

Future research should focus on evaluating the effectiveness of AI-based PMS strategies, assessing the impact of global PMS harmonization efforts, and exploring novel regulatory approaches to address emerging challenges in medical device safety. As the healthcare landscape evolves, ensuring a dynamic and responsive PMS system will be essential to safeguarding patient well-being and supporting the continued advancement of medical technology.

## 3.3 Quality, Compliance, and Sustainability in Clinical Engineering

Clinical engineering is responsible for the safe and effective use of medical devices within healthcare institutions [27]. As technological advancements in medical devices continue to evolve, clinical engineers face increasing challenges related to the maintenance, compliance, and sustainability of these devices. This chapter examines the intersection of quality, compliance, and sustainability in clinical engineering, focusing on the utilization of Computerized Maintenance Management Systems (CMMS), strategies for reducing environmental impacts, and fostering sustainable practices in medical device procurement, maintenance, and waste management [28].

At the heart of clinical engineering is the imperative to ensure that medical devices operate safely and effectively, meeting regulatory standards and the operational needs of healthcare providers. This task has become increasingly complex as the healthcare industry has evolved with technological advancements and the expanding role of clinical engineering in the oversight and management of medical devices [29]. Clinical engineers oversee the lifecycle of medical equipment, from installation and calibration to regular maintenance, repair, and disposal. Ensuring the safety and functionality of medical devices is crucial, as these devices have a direct impact on patient health and outcomes. As a result, the management of medical devices and their maintenance processes has evolved into a highly sophisticated practice that requires technical expertise, an understanding of regulatory frameworks, operational efficiency, and sustainability considerations [30].

A key tool in this process is the Computerized Maintenance Management System (CMMS), which tracks, manages, and schedules maintenance for medical devices. The advent of CMMS has revolutionized clinical engineering by providing a centralized digital platform that allows for the monitoring and control of all aspects of medical device maintenance. This includes preventive maintenance (PM), corrective maintenance (CM), inventory management, and compliance reporting. Through CMMS, clinical engineers are empowered to streamline maintenance operations, reduce the risk of human error, and ensure that medical devices are maintained according to the highest safety and efficacy standards. By automating various processes, CMMS significantly reduces the administrative burden on clinical engineers, enabling them to focus more on technical and clinical tasks, ultimately enhancing the efficiency of healthcare delivery [31].

One of the central tenets of clinical engineering is optimizing the utilization of healthcare resources. Medical devices, a significant capital investment for healthcare institutions, must be managed effectively to maximize their lifespan and functionality. CMMS plays a vital role in this process by allowing clinical engineers to manage device inventories and track the lifecycle of each device. Through real-time tracking, CMMS ensures that medical devices are maintained according to their manufacturer-recommended schedules, helping to prevent premature wear and tear or breakdowns that could result in costly repairs or replacements. This automation of maintenance scheduling reduces the administrative burden on staff, decreases the likelihood of human error, and improves the overall operational efficiency of the healthcare institution [1].

Preventive maintenance (PM) is a crucial aspect of clinical engineering, as it aims to identify and address potential problems before they result in equipment failure. CMMS streamlines scheduling and tracking of these maintenance tasks, ensuring they are completed promptly. Medical devices are often heavily relied upon for critical patient care, and any unexpected downtime can have serious consequences. By automating preventive maintenance scheduling, CMMS helps minimize the risk of equipment failure and ensures that devices are performing optimally. Additionally, it allows clinical engineers to track maintenance history and identify trends that could indicate recurring issues or underlying problems with specific devices or equipment models. Through data-driven insights, CMMS can help clinical engineers make informed decisions about whether devices must be repaired, replaced, or upgraded [5].

Corrective maintenance (CM), which involves repairing or replacing equipment that is broken or malfunctioning, is another crucial function of a CMMS. CMMS provides an organized system for tracking repair requests, dispatching technicians, and documenting the status of repairs. By maintaining detailed records of each repair, CMMS enables clinical engineers to track the history of issues and identify recurring patterns that may indicate more systemic problems with specific devices or equipment categories. By streamlining corrective maintenance workflows, CMMS helps reduce downtime and ensures that repairs are completed promptly, thus improving the availability of medical devices for patient care [8] (Figs. 3.5 and 3.6).

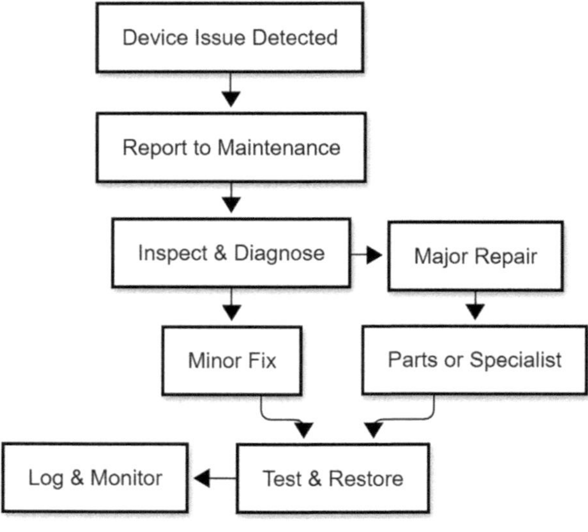


**Fig. 3.5** Corrective maintenance workflows

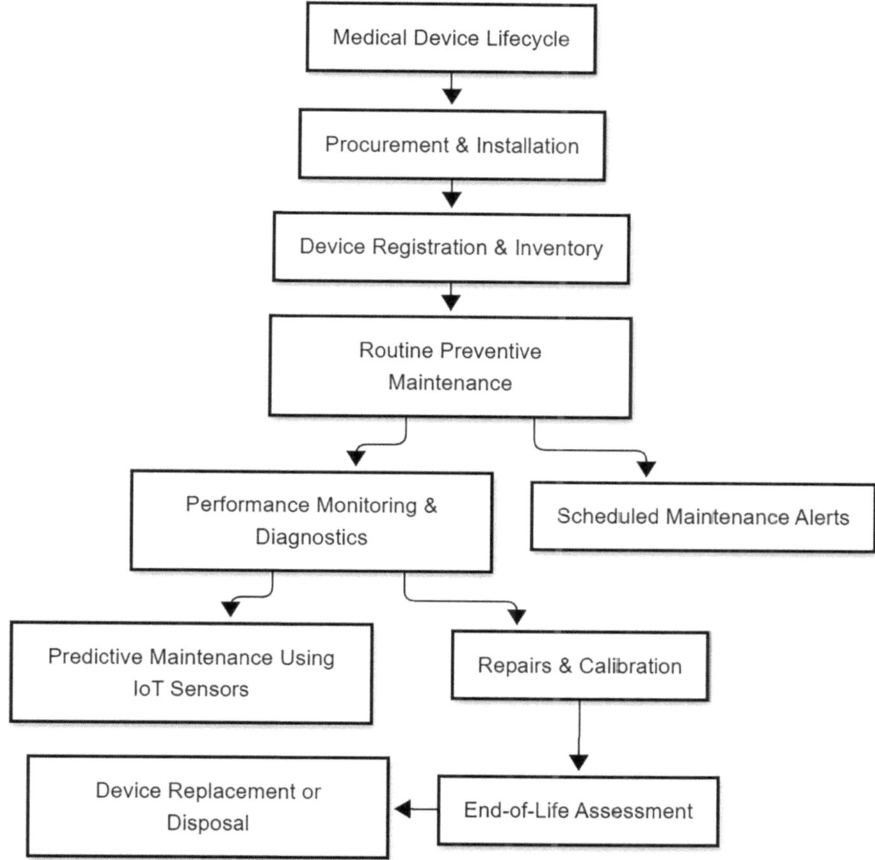


**Fig. 3.6** Preventive maintenance scheduling and device lifecycle tracking

The application of CMMS extends beyond simple tracking of maintenance schedules. Advanced CMMS platforms now incorporate features that allow clinical engineers to move from a reactive maintenance approach to a more proactive one. One of the key innovations in CMMS is the integration of predictive maintenance capabilities. Predictive maintenance relies on real-time data collection, performance analytics, and machine learning algorithms to predict when a medical device is likely to fail or require service [32]. By analyzing historical data, including usage patterns, environmental conditions, and device-specific performance data, predictive maintenance algorithms can forecast potential failures before they occur.

This predictive approach enables clinical engineers to take preemptive action, addressing maintenance issues before they escalate into significant problems that result in equipment downtime or patient safety concerns. For example, a predictive maintenance system might identify a particular device experiencing increased wear on one of its components, suggesting that a replacement part is needed before the device fails. By addressing issues proactively, predictive maintenance helps to reduce unplanned downtime, minimize the costs associated with emergency repairs, and ensure that devices remain in good working order. Furthermore, predictive maintenance allows clinical engineers to optimize the lifespan of medical devices, as they can address problems at the early stages of wear and tear, thus avoiding more expensive repairs or replacements down the line.

Predictive maintenance relies on various data inputs, including sensor readings, usage data, and historical repair information. Many modern medical devices feature sensors that provide real-time data on their operational status, including temperature, pressure, and vibration. This data can be fed into the CMMS platform, where it is analyzed and used to generate predictive insights. For example, a diagnostic imaging system might utilize data from its cooling system to predict when the cooling unit is likely to fail, enabling clinical engineers to replace the part before it causes a system shutdown. Healthcare institutions can achieve significant cost savings and improve patient care by integrating predictive maintenance into the overall maintenance strategy.

### 3.3.1 CMMS and Regulatory Compliance

In addition to improving operational efficiency, CMMS also plays a critical role in maintaining regulatory compliance. Healthcare institutions are subject to a wide range of regulations and standards aimed at ensuring patient safety, including those set by bodies such as the U.S. Food and Drug Administration (FDA), the European Medicines Agency (EMA), and international standards like ISO 13485 [33]. These regulations require that medical devices be maintained, calibrated, and tested regularly to ensure their safety and efficacy. Non-compliance with these standards can result in legal liabilities, regulatory sanctions, and, most importantly, risks to patient safety.

A robust CMMS allows clinical engineers to maintain detailed records of maintenance activities, repairs, and inspections, providing an audit trail that can be reviewed in the event of an inspection by regulatory agencies. This documentation demonstrates that healthcare institutions comply with regulatory requirements and adhere to established maintenance protocols. For example, suppose a regulatory body inspects a healthcare facility. In that case, the CMMS can provide an audit trail that documents when each medical device was last serviced, the nature of the service performed, and the results of any testing or calibration activities [14, 34]. This ability to provide comprehensive, accessible records of all maintenance activities is a key factor in ensuring compliance with regulatory requirements.

Maintaining accurate and up-to-date records also supports the continuous improvement of maintenance processes. CMMS platforms can help identify recurring issues with specific devices or equipment categories, informing decision-making about repairs, replacements, or upgrades. For example, if a specific device requires frequent repairs, clinical engineers can analyze the data to identify potential root causes, such as poor quality components or inadequate maintenance protocols. This information can then improve maintenance procedures and prevent future failures (Fig. 3.7).

In this way, CMMS helps maintain compliance and fosters a culture of continuous improvement, driving better outcomes for both healthcare providers and patients. As medical devices become increasingly interconnected, the need for interoperability between devices and healthcare information systems has become more critical. Interoperability refers to the ability of different systems and devices to communicate and exchange data seamlessly, which is essential for coordinating patient care, improving diagnostic accuracy, and ensuring patient safety. CMMS platforms play a key role in facilitating interoperability, as they often integrate with other healthcare information systems, such as electronic health records (EHRs), laboratory information systems (LIS), and hospital information systems (HIS). By enabling data to flow seamlessly between devices and systems, CMMS facilitates the creation of a more integrated and efficient healthcare environment [27, 35].

For example, when a clinical engineer schedules preventive maintenance on a medical device, this information can be communicated to the relevant clinical staff, ensuring they are aware of potential device unavailability. Similarly, CMMS can track device usage data and integrate with EHRs to ensure that devices are properly calibrated for the specific needs of each patient.

This interoperability is critical in complex healthcare settings where multiple systems and devices are used simultaneously. CMMS helps improve operational

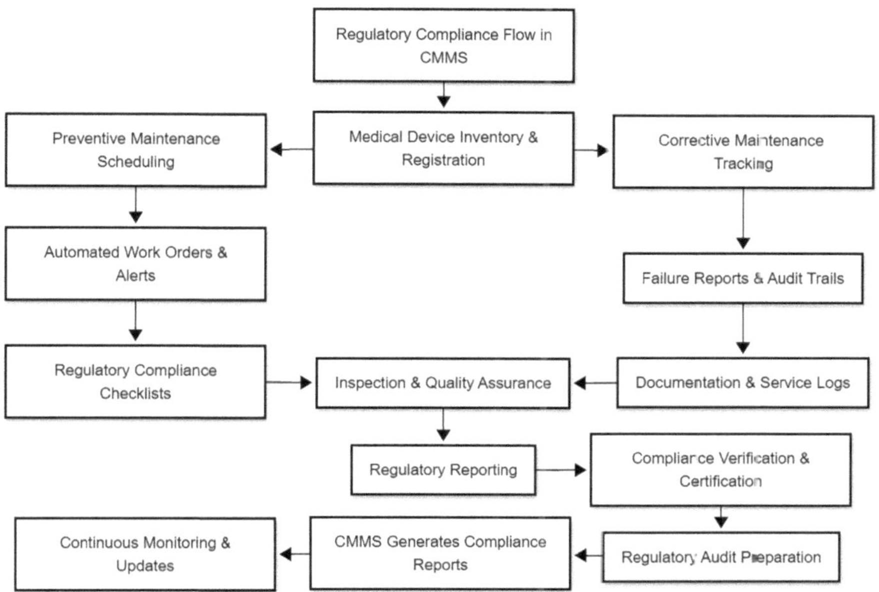


**Fig. 3.7** Regulatory compliance flow through CMMS

efficiency, reduce errors, and enhance patient care by supporting data sharing and communication between devices. Using CMMS, clinical engineers can automate key processes, reduce downtime, enhance predictive maintenance capabilities, and maintain compliance with regulatory requirements. Furthermore, CMMS supports interoperability and integration between medical devices and healthcare information systems, fostering a more efficient and coordinated healthcare environment. As healthcare systems evolve and the complexity of medical devices increases, CMMS will remain a critical component of clinical engineering, enabling healthcare institutions to deliver high-quality care while minimizing costs and risks. As healthcare's future increasingly relies on technology and data, CMMS will play a crucial role in ensuring that medical devices are safe, effective, and sustainable, contributing to improved patient outcomes and enhanced healthcare delivery.

## 3.3.2 *Sustainability in Clinical Engineering*

As sustainability becomes an increasingly important consideration in healthcare, clinical engineers must adopt practices that reduce the environmental impact of medical devices throughout their life cycles. This includes the entire process, from procurement and installation to operation, maintenance, and disposal. The healthcare sector is a significant consumer of resources, and medical devices contribute to environmental challenges such as energy consumption, material waste, and hazardous chemical use. Clinical engineers, therefore, must take a comprehensive approach to sustainability that aligns with global efforts to reduce environmental impacts [28] (Fig. 3.8).

Energy consumption is one of the' most significant environmental impacts of medical devices in many healthcare settings. Medical devices are often used

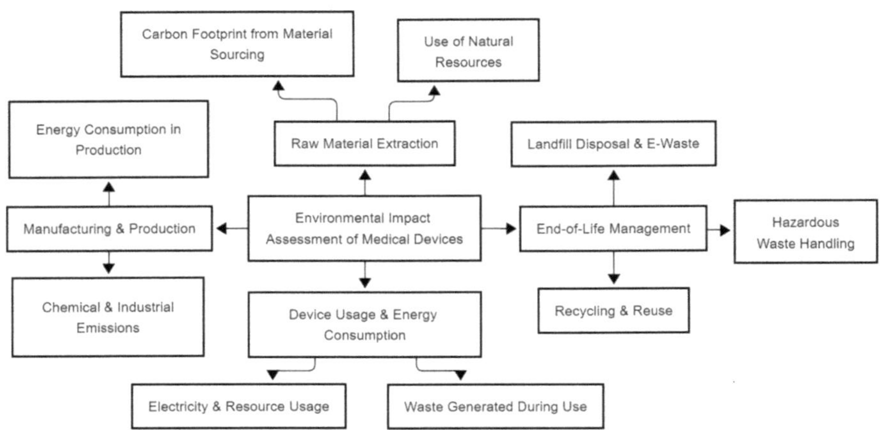


**Fig. 3.8** Environmental impact assessment of medical devices

continuously, or for long periods, throughout the day, particularly in intensive care units or diagnostic imaging departments. Devices such as MRI machines, X-ray systems, and ventilators require significant energy, adding to the overall energy demand of healthcare institutions [29]. As such, clinical engineers are increasingly focusing on selecting and implementing energy-efficient devices that help reduce the operational costs of healthcare facilities while lowering their carbon footprint [36].

Energy-efficient medical devices are designed to consume less power during use, contributing to financial savings and environmental sustainability. A prime example is the shift from traditional incandescent light bulbs to LED lighting in healthcare settings. Similarly, when not in active use, modern diagnostic equipment often comes equipped with energy-saving features, such as automatic shut-off functions or low-power modes. By adopting energy-efficient devices, healthcare providers can achieve notable reductions in energy consumption, leading to lower utility bills and a reduced environmental impact from their operations (Fig. 3.9).

Adopting energy-efficient medical devices is not just about reducing the direct energy consumption of equipment but also about designing and selecting devices optimized for performance with minimal resource use. For example, devices engineered to be more durable and long-lasting require fewer replacements, which reduces the overall demand for raw materials and energy needed for production. This extends to integrating devices equipped with energy-saving sensors or automatic diagnostics that improve operational efficiency over time [37]. Another key aspect of sustainability in clinical engineering is the responsible management of materials and resources used in medical devices. Many medical devices contain hazardous materials, such as mercury in thermometers or lead in specific diagnostic equipment, which require careful handling and disposal. Clinical engineers are crucial in properly managing these devices, minimizing the risk of harmful environmental contamination. For instance, older diagnostic devices may contain materials that, when improperly disposed of, can leach into the environment and pose significant risks to public health. By selecting medical devices designed with safer, more sustainable materials, clinical engineers can help reduce the healthcare sector's environmental footprint. This includes opting for devices made from recyclable

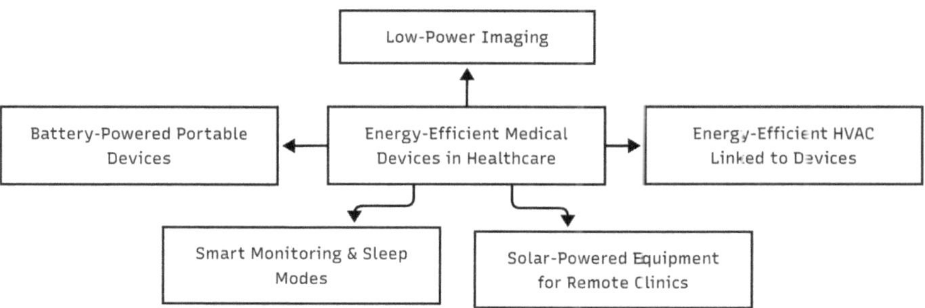


**Fig. 3.9** Energy-efficient medical devices in healthcare settings

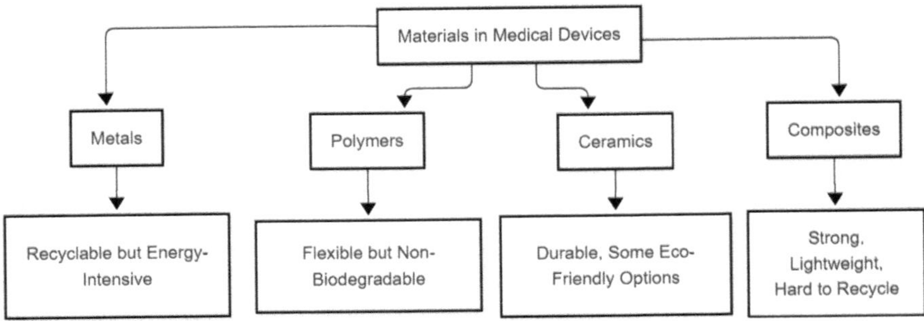


**Fig. 3.10** Materials used in medical devices and their sustainability impact

materials or those free from toxic substances like mercury or lead. Additionally, clinical engineers can work with manufacturers to encourage the design and production of more sustainable devices that are easier to recycle or dispose of safely at the end of their life. The goal is to reduce the environmental impact of medical device waste, ensuring that devices are disposed of in a manner that minimizes their effect on ecosystems and human health (Fig. 3.10).

In practice, sustainability can also be achieved through initiatives like remanufacturing and refurbishment. Medical devices that are no longer in use can be remanufactured to meet modern standards, thereby reducing the need for new devices and, consequently, the consumption of raw materials and energy. Refurbishing devices allows them to be reused, saving hospitals the cost of purchasing brand-new equipment and extending the lifespan of existing devices. Clinical engineers can collaborate with manufacturers and healthcare institutions to develop protocols for refurbishing devices that are still serviceable but may require updated components or technologies (Fig. 3.11).

In addition to energy and material management, clinical engineers are also focused on reducing the carbon footprint associated with the transportation and logistics of medical devices. The global supply chain for medical devices frequently involves substantial travel and transportation, thereby contributing to the healthcare industry's overall environmental footprint. By sourcing medical devices locally or regionally, clinical engineers can help minimize transportation-related emissions [33, 38]. Additionally, optimizing the supply chain to reduce the need for frequent shipments and packaging can further contribute to reducing environmental harm.

At the end of a medical device's life, its disposal presents another opportunity for clinical engineers to promote sustainability. Devices that are improperly discarded can contribute to landfill waste and environmental contamination. However, responsible disposal practices, such as recycling and handling hazardous materials safely, can significantly reduce this impact. Clinical engineers can play a crucial role by ensuring that devices are properly decommissioned and their components are either recycled or disposed of safely, by local environmental standards. Furthermore,

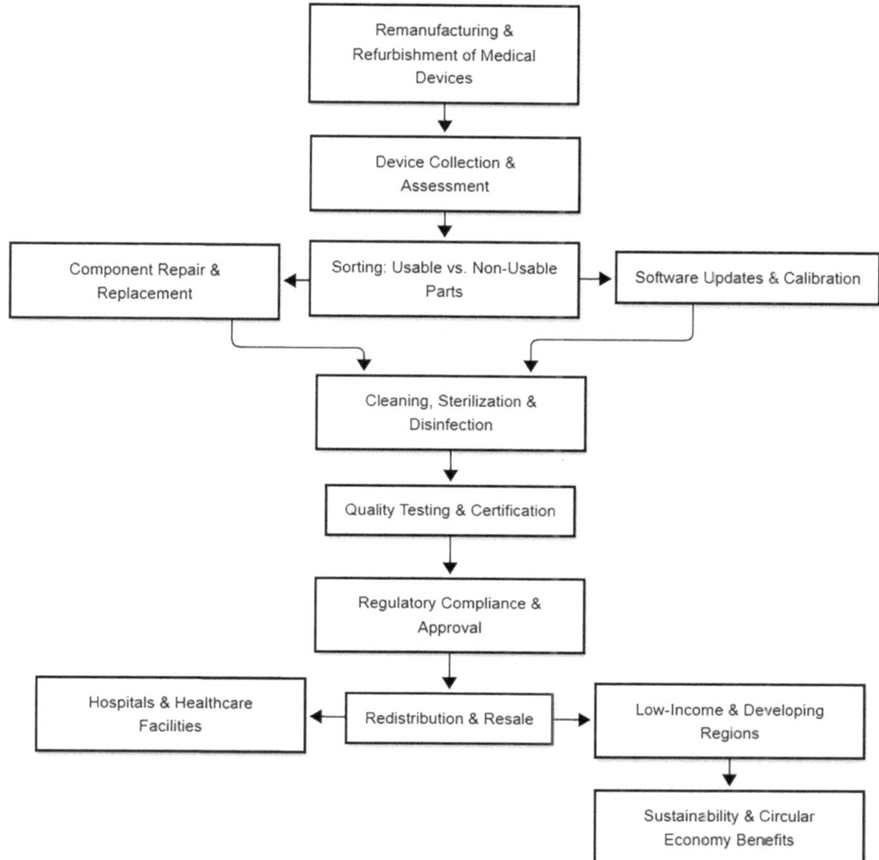


**Fig. 3.11** Remanufacturing and refurbishment of medical devices

clinical engineers can advocate for the adoption of take-back programs or partnerships with manufacturers that provide recycling services for medical devices at the end of their life cycles.

By adopting energy-efficient devices, prioritizing sustainable materials, implementing refurbishment programs, and ensuring proper disposal, clinical engineers contribute to the larger global effort to reduce environmental impacts and promote sustainability in healthcare. The integration of these sustainable practices not only benefits the environment but also leads to operational cost savings and enhanced long-term resource management. As healthcare institutions continue to embrace sustainability, clinical engineers will ensure that medical devices support patient health and the planet's well-being (Fig. 3.12).

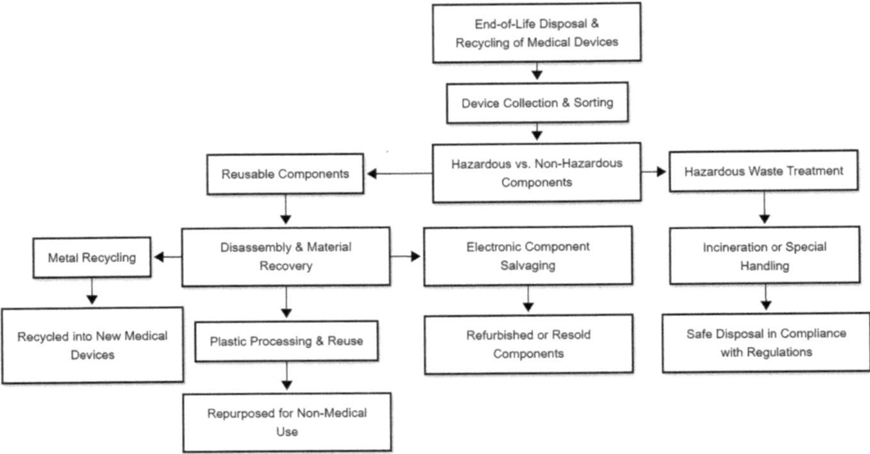


**Fig. 3.12** End-of-life disposal and recycling of medical devices

## 3.3.3 *Reducing the Environmental Impact of Medical Devices*

The environmental impact of medical devices is a growing concern as the healthcare sector seeks to minimize its carbon footprint and waste generation. While essential for patient care, medical devices contribute to environmental degradation in several ways, including energy consumption, emissions, the use of hazardous materials, and the generation of electronic waste (e-waste). As healthcare institutions strive for sustainability, clinical engineers are uniquely positioned to influence the environmental performance of medical devices by implementing strategies to reduce their impact on the environment [31]. Their role is crucial in addressing the environmental challenges posed by the widespread use of medical technologies, particularly as the healthcare sector increasingly moves toward sustainability goals (Fig. 3.13).

Energy consumption is one of the primary environmental concerns associated with medical devices. Many medical devices, such as MRI machines, X-ray machines, diagnostic imaging equipment, and laboratory instruments, require significant energy. The energy demand can be substantial in healthcare facilities, where numerous devices are used continuously or for extended periods. The high energy requirements of medical devices contribute not only to operational costs but also to the carbon footprint of healthcare institutions [27]. In light of this, clinical engineers play an essential role in mitigating the environmental impact of energy consumption by selecting energy-efficient devices and implementing strategies that optimize energy usage. One strategy to reduce energy consumption is to adopt energy-efficient medical devices that meet established energy performance standards. Devices with certifications like the Energy Star label indicate they meet high energy-efficiency standards, helping healthcare institutions reduce energy usage and operational costs. Clinical engineers can work with procurement teams to prioritize energy-efficient models when selecting or upgrading new devices. For example, advanced imaging

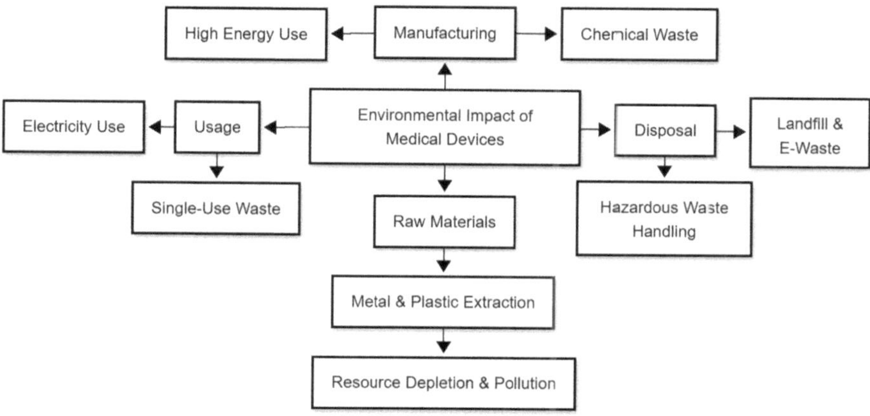


**Fig. 3.13** Environmental impact of medical devices

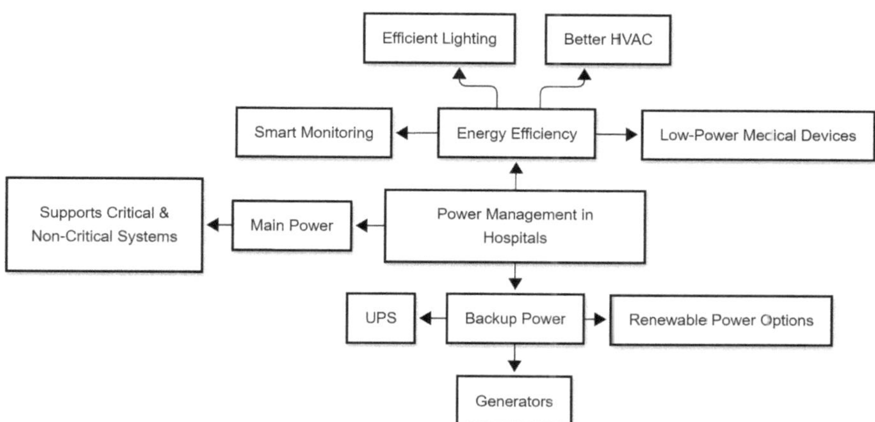


**Fig. 3.14** Power management in healthcare facilities

technologies like MRI machines and CT scanners can be chosen based on their energy consumption ratings, which can vary significantly between models.

In addition to selecting energy-efficient devices, healthcare institutions can implement strategies to optimize energy usage. One such strategy is using power management systems that automatically power down devices when not in use, helping to reduce standby energy consumption. Furthermore, clinical engineers can advocate for the installation of energy-saving technologies, such as motion sensors that control lighting or temperature, ensuring that energy is used only when necessary. Ensuring that devices are powered off at the end of the day or during periods of inactivity can further reduce energy consumption. These small but impactful changes can add up over time, significantly reducing the overall environmental footprint of healthcare facilities (Fig. 3.14).

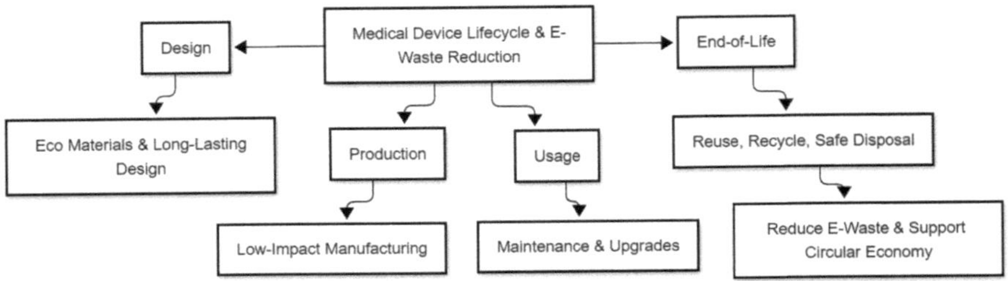


**Fig. 3.15** Lifecycle of medical devices and e-waste reduction

Medical devices also generate electronic waste (e-waste), one of the fastest-growing categories of waste worldwide. E-waste consists of discarded electronic devices that contain both valuable materials, such as gold and copper, and hazardous substances, such as lead, mercury, and cadmium. Improper e-waste disposal can lead to environmental contamination and pose significant health risks to the environment and individuals working in the recycling industry. Therefore, managing e-waste is a crucial aspect of reducing the environmental impact of medical devices.

Clinical engineers play a key role in reducing e-waste by selecting medical devices with longer life cycles. Devices built to last not only reduce the frequency of replacements but also minimize the resources required for manufacturing new ones. Healthcare institutions can also prioritize modular and easily upgradeable devices, allowing for the replacement of only specific components rather than the entire device. This can extend the life of medical devices and reduce their need for disposal (Fig. 3.15).

Another approach to reducing e-waste is through the repair and refurbishment of medical devices, rather than their complete replacement. Many medical devices, costly ones such as diagnostic imaging machines or surgical equipment, can be refurbished to meet modern standards and reused in healthcare settings. Clinical engineers can collaborate with manufacturers and third-party service providers to develop and implement refurbishment programs, extending the life of old devices and diverting them from landfills. Additionally, clinical engineers must ensure that devices are properly recycled at the end of their useful life [33]. This involves working with certified e-waste recycling companies that can safely dismantle and recycle the components of medical devices. Devices containing valuable materials, such as metals and plastics, should be sent to recycling facilities that specialize in extracting these materials, which can be reused to produce new devices. Proper recycling reduces e-waste and conserves valuable resources, contributing to a more sustainable healthcare system [39].

One of the most significant contributors to the environmental impact of medical devices is the use of hazardous materials. Many medical devices, particularly older models, contain toxic substances such as mercury, lead, and certain chemicals, which can pose serious environmental and health risks if not properly managed. For example, thermometers, blood pressure cuffs, and some diagnostic equipment may contain mercury, which can contaminate the environment if not disposed of

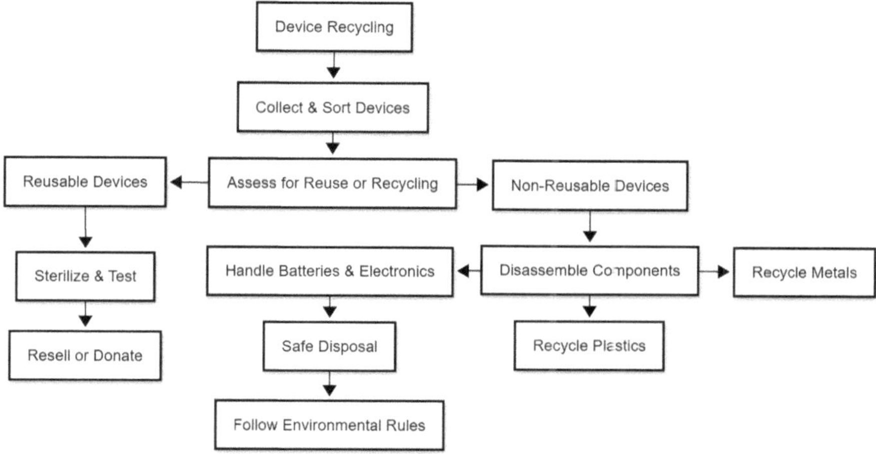


**Fig. 3.16** Medical device recycling process

correctly. Lead is commonly found in older radiation therapy equipment, while specific medical devices may use harmful chemicals in their components (Fig. 3.16).

Medical devices containing hazardous materials are disposed of safely, by local, national, and international environmental regulations. Proper disposal involves identifying materials that require careful handling and ensuring they are sent to facilities that can safely manage hazardous waste. Furthermore, clinical engineers can play a proactive role in advocating for the use of safer, non-toxic alternatives in the design of new medical devices. By encouraging manufacturers to use materials free from harmful substances like mercury or lead, clinical engineers can significantly reduce the environmental impact of medical devices [36] (Fig. 3.17).

As part of their sustainability efforts, clinical engineers can also work with manufacturers and policymakers to promote the use of safer, non-toxic materials in the design and manufacturing of medical devices. For example, non-mercury thermometers, lead-free radiation shielding, and devices made from biocompatible and recyclable materials can significantly reduce the environmental footprint of healthcare technologies. This advocacy can extend to supporting manufacturers committed to using environmentally friendly materials and adopting more sustainable production methods. Furthermore, clinical engineers can encourage the integration of life cycle assessments (LCAs) when selecting medical devices. LCAs are comprehensive evaluations that consider the environmental impacts of a product across its entire life cycle, from raw material extraction to disposal. Using LCA as a decision-making tool, clinical engineers can help ensure that medical devices are selected based on their overall sustainability performance, including energy efficiency, material use, recyclability, and the potential for harmful emissions [16].

The environmental impact of medical devices is an important consideration that clinical engineers must address to contribute to a more sustainable healthcare system. Clinical engineers can play a crucial role in minimizing the environmental

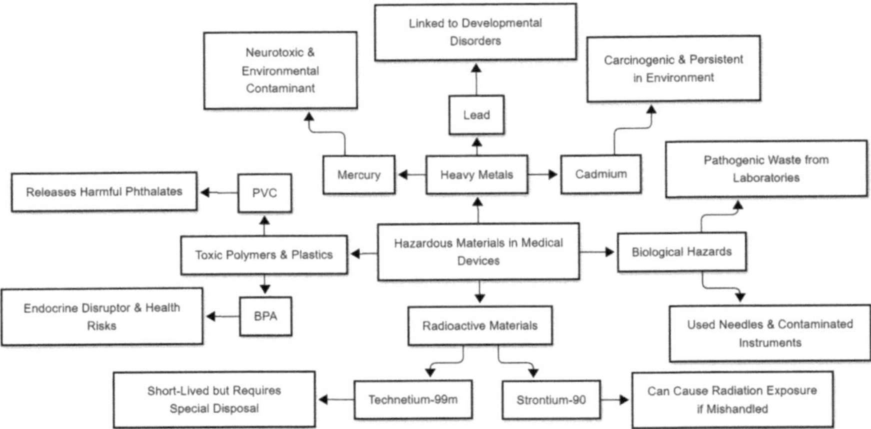


**Fig. 3.17** Hazardous materials in medical devices

footprint of healthcare technologies by focusing on energy consumption, e-waste reduction, and the safe management of hazardous materials. Adopting energy-efficient devices, promoting repair and refurbishment programs, and advocating for safer, non-toxic materials all represent key strategies in this ongoing effort. As healthcare institutions continue to adopt sustainability practices, clinical engineers will be at the forefront of ensuring that medical devices contribute to both patient health and the health of the planet.

Sustainable procurement is a critical aspect of reducing the environmental impact of medical devices. The procurement process involves selecting and purchasing devices from manufacturers, and this decision has significant implications for the sustainability of healthcare operations. Clinical engineers must work closely with procurement teams to select devices that meet sustainability criteria, including energy efficiency, recyclability, and the use of environmentally friendly materials. This requires a thorough understanding of the life cycle of medical devices, from manufacturing to disposal, and the ability to assess the environmental performance of different products [4, 10]. In addition to selecting sustainable products, clinical engineers should also consider the environmental performance of suppliers and manufacturers. This includes evaluating their commitment to sustainability, such as whether they adhere to environmental standards, implement green manufacturing practices, or engage in product take-back programs. Healthcare institutions can reduce their overall environmental impact by working with suppliers that prioritize sustainability (Fig. 3.18).

Waste management is another critical aspect of sustainability in clinical engineering. The healthcare sector generates significant waste, including medical device packaging, used parts, and obsolete equipment. Clinical engineers must develop and implement waste management strategies that minimize the amount of waste sent to landfills and promote recycling and reuse. This may involve working with waste management providers to ensure that medical device waste is properly sorted and

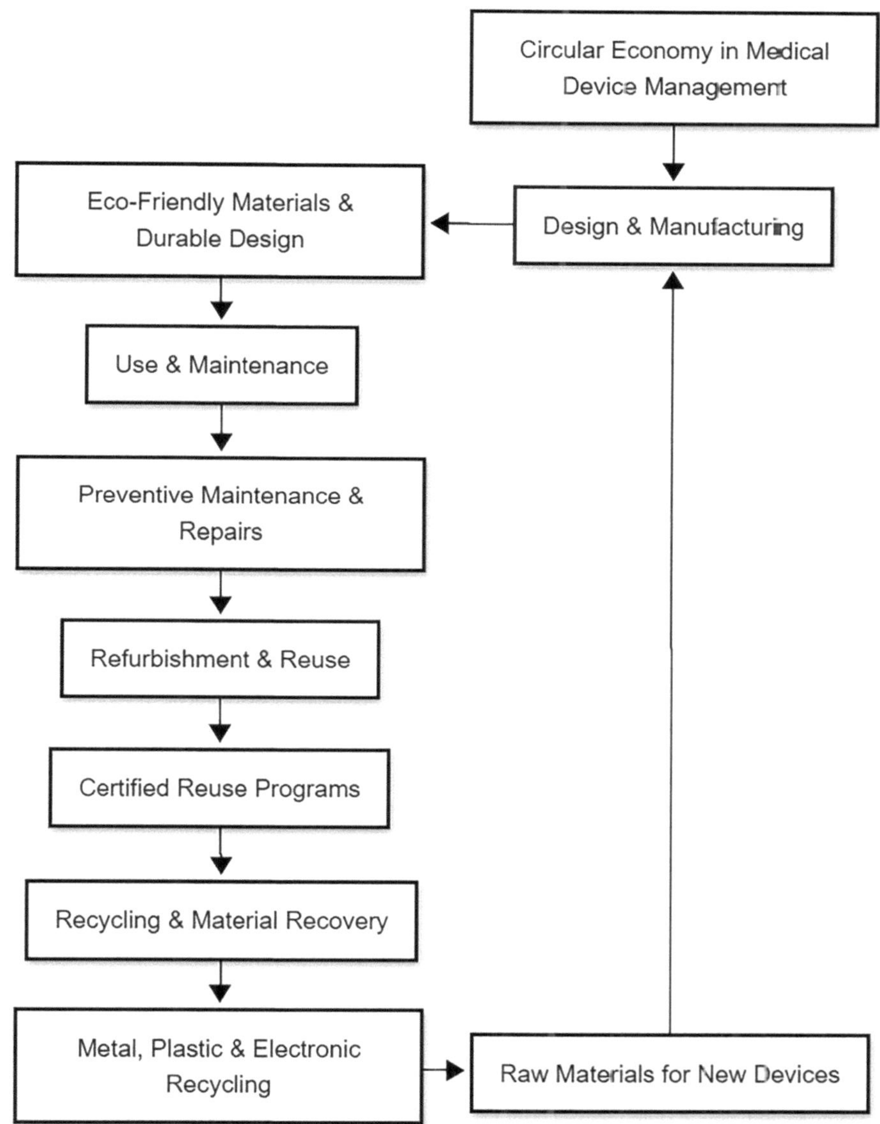


**Fig. 3.18** Diagram of a circular economy model applied to medical device management

recycled, as well as educating staff on best practices for waste reduction. To further enhance sustainability, healthcare institutions can adopt circular economy principles, focusing on extending the lifecycle of medical devices through repair, refurbishment, and reuse. By embracing circular economy models, clinical engineers can reduce the demand for new devices, conserve resources, and lower the environmental impact of healthcare operations.

## References

1. Kelvin-Agwu MC, Adelodun MO, Igwama GT, Anyanwu EC. The role of biomedical engineers in enhancing patient care through efficient equipment management. Int J Front Med Surg Res. 2024;6(1):11–8.
2. Iadanza E. Clinical engineering handbook. Elsevier; 2019;2.
3. Frize M. Health Care Engineering Part I: Clinical Engineering and Technology Management. Springer Nature. 2022;1:27–49.
4. Darrow JJ, Avorn J, Kesselheim AS. FDA regulation and approval of medical devices: 1976–2020. JAMA. 2021;326(5):420–32.
5. Sun L, Yin C, Xu Q, Zhao W. Artificial intelligence for healthcare and medical education: a systematic review. Am J Transl Res. 2023;15(7):4820.
6. Badnjević A, Gurbeta L, Jimenez ER, Iadanza E. Testing of mechanical ventilators and infant incubators in healthcare institutions. Technol Health Care. 2017;25:237.
7. Abbaszada Y. Digital transformation in healthcare systems: challenges and opportunities. AGORA Int'l J Jurid Sci. 2025;19:147.
8. Badnjević A, Pokvić LG, Hasičić M, Bandić L, Mašetić Z, Kovačević Ž. Evidence-based clinical engineering: machine learning algorithms for prediction of defibrillator performance. Biomed Signal Process Control. 2019;54:101629.
9. Badnjević A, Avdihodžić H, Pokvić LG. Artificial intelligence in medical devices: past, present and future. Psychiatr Danub. 2021;33:101–6.
10. Pokvic LG, Spahic L, Badnjevic A. Implementation of industry 4.0 in transformation of medical device maintenance systems. Handbook of Research on Integrating Industry 4.0 in Business and Manufacturing. 2020;512–32.
11. U.S. Food and Drug Administration. Medical Device Regulation: Overview of Device Regulation. FDA; 2021.
12. World Health Organization. Global report on health technology assessment. WHO; 2020.
13. Johnson JA. FDA regulation of medical devices. Congressional Research Service; 2012.
14. Badnjević A, Pokvić LG, Deumić A, Bećirović LS. Post-market surveillance of medical devices: a review. Technol Health Care. 2022;30:1315–29.
15. Pharmaceuticals and Medical Devices Agency (PMDA). Initiatives for medical device innovation and emerging technology. PMDA; 2021.
16. Kovačević Ž, Pokvić LG, Spahić L, Badnjević A. Prediction of medical device performance using machine learning techniques: infant incubator case study. Health Technol. 2020;10:151–5.
17. David Y, Judd T. Evidence-based impact by clinical engineers on global patient outcomes. Health Technol. 2020;10(2):517–35.
18. European Union. Regulation (EU) 2017/745 on medical devices (MDR). Official Journal of the European Union; 2017.
19. Fraser AG, Butchart EG, Szymański P, Caiani EG, Crosby S, Kearney P, Van de Werf F. The need for transparency of clinical evidence for medical devices in Europe. Lancet. 2018;392(10146):521–30.
20. European Commission. Guidance on Post-Market Surveillance (PMS) for Medical Devices. EU Commission; 2020.
21. Yadav AR, Pawar AR, Shete AS, Jadhav NR, Kumbhar AR, Jadhav NM, Gejage SM. Comparative analysis of medical device adverse event reporting forms for patients and industries across various countries, and the introduction of a unified generic form for harmonization. Expert Rev Med Devices. 2025;22(1):49–62.
22. Badnjević A, Pokvić LG. Legal metrology framework for medical devices. Clinical Engineering Handbook. 2020;774–79.

23. Arabi YM, Azoulay E, Al-Dorzi HM, Phua J, Salluh J, Binnie A, Citerio G. How the COVID-19 pandemic will change the future of critical care. Intensive Care Med. 2021;47(3):282–91.
24. Kramer DB, Xu S, Kesselheim AS. Regulation of medical devices in the United States and European Union. N Engl J Med. 2012;366:848–55.
25. Bećirović F, Spahić L, Merdović N, Gurbeta Pokvić L, Badnjević A. Advancement of post-market surveillance of medical devices leveraging artificial intelligence: patient monitors case study. Technol Health Care. 2025;33:974–80.
26. Spahić L, Sredović U, Kurpejović Z, Mrdanović E, Pokvić G, Badnjević A. Machine learning for improved medical device management: a focus on infant incubators. Technol Health Care. 2025;33:2034–40.
27. Li Y, Pan X, Han Y, Taylor JE. Sustainable healthcare facilities: a scoping review. J Constr Eng Manag. 2021;147(12):03121007.
28. Hoveling T, Nijdam AS, Monincx M, Faludi J, Bakker C. Circular economy for medical devices: barriers, opportunities and best practices from a design perspective. Resour Conserv Recycl. 2024;208:107719.
29. Khider MO, Hamza AO. Medical equipment maintenance management system: review and analysis. J Clin Eng. 2022;47(3):151–9.
30. Shankar L, Singh CD, Singh R. AI and CMMS: a powerful duo for enhanced maintenance in manufacturing. Educ Adm Theory Pract. 2024;30(5):8647–54.
31. Manchadi O, Ben-Bouazza FE, Jioudi B. Predictive maintenance in healthcare system: a survey. IEEE Access. 2023;11:61313–30.
32. Judd T, David Y. The growing role of clinical engineering: merging technology at the point of care. Glob Clin Eng J. 2022;5(1):29–32.
33. Amaral C, Paiva M, Rodrigues AR, Veiga F, Bell V. Global regulatory challenges for medical devices: impact on innovation and market access. Appl Sci. 2024;14(20):9304
34. Lin Z, Kang J, Wei Y, Zou B. Maintenance management strategies for medical equipment in healthcare institutions: a review. BME Horiz. 2024;2:2024135.
35. Hrvat F, Spahić L, Pokvić LG, Badnjević A. Artificial neural networks for prediction of medical device performance based on conformity assessment data: infusion and perfusor pumps case study. 2020 9th Mediterranean Conference on Embedded Computing (MECO). 2020;1–4.
36. Badnjevic A. Evidence-based maintenance of medical devices: current shortage and pathway towards solution. Technol Health Care. 2023;31:293–305.
37. Montesinos L, Checa Rifá P, Rifá Fabregat M, Maldonado-Romo J, Capacci S, Maccaro A, Piaggio D. Sustainability across the medical device lifecycle: a scoping review. Sustainability. 2024;16(4):1433.
38. Spahić L, Jeremić L, Lalatović I, Muratović T, Džuho A, Pokvić LG, Badnjević ASAIG. Machine learning for improved medical device management: a focus on defibrillator performance. Technol Health Care. 2025;33(2):737–43.
39. Spahić L, Pokvić LG, Badnjević A. Inspection and testing of infusion pumps. Inspection of Medical Devices: For Regulatory Purposes. Springer Nature. 2023;377–98.

# Chapter 4
# Laboratory Devices

This section provides a comprehensive overview of key laboratory devices that underpin modern clinical diagnostics. It begins with biochemical analyzers, tracing their historical development, technical characteristics, and diverse applications in patient monitoring and diagnostic decision-making (Sect. 4.1). The section then examines polymerase chain reaction (PCR) devices, detailing their mechanisms, types, and role in molecular diagnostics and pathogen detection (Sect. 4.2). Sequencing machines are presented next, highlighting their evolution from early methods to next-generation platforms, their technical features, and clinical applications in genomics and personalized medicine (Sect. 4.3). Finally, from genomes to molecules, mass spectrometry devices are explored, emphasizing their analytical capabilities, types, and contributions to biomarker discovery, proteomics, metabolomics, and therapeutic drug monitoring (Sect. 4.4). Across all chapters, regulatory considerations and compliance standards are addressed, and future perspectives highlight emerging innovations that enhance accuracy, efficiency, and integration in laboratory diagnostics.

## 4.1 Biochemical Analyzers

Biochemistry analyzers play a pivotal role in modern clinical laboratories by enabling rapid, precise quantification of biochemical constituents in bodily fluids such as blood and urine. These instruments are essential for diagnosing diseases, monitoring patient health, and guiding therapeutic decisions [1]. In response to growing demands for high-throughput, reliable, and automated diagnostics, the technological capabilities of these analyzers have advanced considerably.

Recent innovations include the integration of microfluidic platforms and lab-on-a-chip technologies, which facilitate faster analysis with minimal reagent



A. Badnjević et al., *Biomedical Instrumentation*, Series in BioEngineering,
https://doi.org/10.1007/978-3-032-10978-1_4

consumption and reduced sample volumes [2]. Additionally, the incorporation of artificial intelligence (AI) and machine learning (ML) has significantly enhanced data interpretation, contributing to improved diagnostic accuracy and more timely clinical decision-making. Despite these advancements, critical challenges remain, particularly in standardization, calibration, and quality control. Variability across platforms can affect the comparability and reliability of test results, underscoring the need for stringent validation and regulatory oversight [3].

### *4.1.1 History*

The emergence of biochemical analyzers marked a transformative milestone in the evolution of diagnostic methodologies within clinical laboratories, significantly enhancing daily operational workflows. Initially, biochemical testing was conducted manually, requiring intensive labor from laboratory personnel and relying primarily on early twentieth-century colorimetric techniques. While these methods laid the foundation for technological advancement in clinical chemistry, they were inherently prone to human error, limiting their reliability and restricting widespread clinical use. A significant shift occurred in the 1950s with the advent of automated biochemical analyzers, which revolutionized laboratory diagnostics by enabling high-throughput and more consistent analyses. One of the earliest breakthroughs was the Technicon AutoAnalyzer, which introduced continuous flow analysis for enzymes and metabolites, significantly improving accuracy and throughput.

Technological advancements throughout the twentieth century led to the development of discrete analyzers, which enabled the individual testing of multiple analytes with reduced sample and reagent volumes. These systems also integrated computer-based data processing, elevating both the precision and efficiency of biochemical testing while reducing manual errors [4]. These developments expanded the clinical utility of biochemical tests, accelerating both diagnostic workflows and therapeutic monitoring. In recent years, the convergence of microfluidics, nanotechnology, and artificial intelligence has further advanced the capabilities of biochemical analyzers. These innovations have not only improved sensitivity and specificity but also enabled point-of-care testing and personalized diagnostics, aligning with the broader movement toward precision medicine [2].

### *4.1.2 Technical Characteristics*

#### Hardware

The hardware infrastructure of biochemical analyzers is designed to facilitate rapid, precise, and reliable analysis of biological samples. At the core of these systems lies the optical detection module, which typically includes interference filters for wavelength selection—usually within the 340–670 nm range—and a stable light source, most often a halogen lamp. These filters are essential for isolating specific wavelengths, ensuring that only the desired light reaches the sample for accurate photometric measurements.

A critical component in this system is the reaction cuvette, which serves as the vessel where the biochemical reaction between the reagent and the sample occurs. Made from high-grade optical glass or transparent polymers, these cuvettes must maintain strict dimensional and optical consistency to minimize measurement variability. Within the reaction chamber, Peltier elements are commonly employed to provide thermal regulation, a key factor for enzymatic reactions that are highly sensitive to temperature fluctuations. Modern analyzers also incorporate robotic arms, precision pipetting systems, and automated reagent dispensers. These mechanisms enhance efficiency, reduce human error, and standardize operations across high-throughput workflows. Fluid management systems, including waste disposal units and rinse stations, are integrated to prevent cross-contamination and maintain system hygiene (Fig. 4.1).

Additionally, electronic control modules manage a wide range of operational tasks, including the timing of optical pulses, signal amplification, and data transmission. These systems play a central role in synchronizing the hardware functions and ensuring accurate real-time analysis and data display.

## Software

The software embedded within biochemical analyzers serves as the backbone for automation, data processing, and system integration. It transforms the analyzer into an intelligent diagnostic platform, capable of real-time monitoring, quality control, and seamless communication with external healthcare systems. Software functionalities span several core domains:

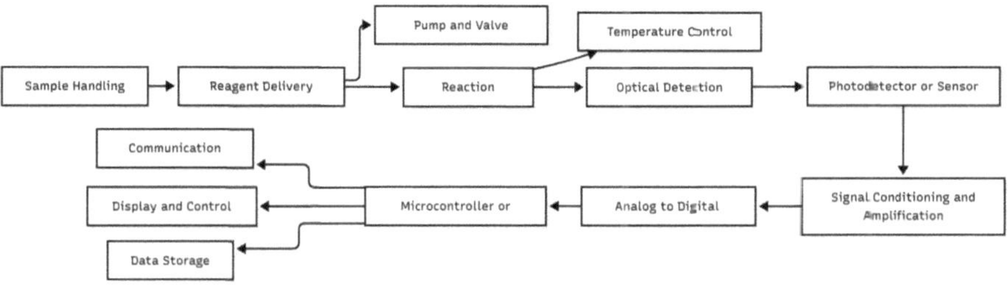


**Fig. 4.1** Block diagram of the hardware components of a biochemical analyzer

#### Sample Identification

Advanced biochemical analyzers are equipped with software that ensures precise sample tracking through the use of barcodes or QR codes. When a sample tube is loaded into the analyzer, the code is automatically read and linked to the patient's electronic health record. This functionality minimizes identification errors and enables traceability throughout the entire analytical process, which is crucial for validating results and resolving discrepancies [5].

#### Reagent Handling and Inventory Management

The software manages reagent selection, tracking, and inventory control. It monitors expiration dates and usage levels, and automatically assigns reagents to tests. For instance, Roche's cobas analyzers utilize software that alerts users to low reagent levels or calibration requirements, thereby enhancing operational continuity and reducing the risk of contamination or test failure.

#### Analysis, Timing, and Workflow Automation

Precise timing of dosing, incubation, and photometric measurement is critical to the accuracy of test results. The software coordinates these steps with exact timing algorithms. Incubation parameters and mixing protocols are tailored per assay requirements, and several samples can be processed in parallel, thereby increasing analyzer throughput [6]. Moreover, the software automates test repetition in cases of out-of-range results, issues maintenance alerts, and logs instrument performance for traceability. It can also execute self-diagnostic routines and error correction mechanisms to prevent system downtime.

#### Data Management and System Integration

The software architecture is designed to handle large volumes of data securely and efficiently. It supports bi-directional communication with Laboratory Information Systems (LIS) and Hospital Information Systems (HIS), ensuring that test results are rapidly and accurately incorporated into clinical records [6]. Advanced analyzers use real-time quality control algorithms to compare internal control samples against reference standards. Some platforms enable dynamic calibration curve adjustments based on historical trends or environmental conditions, thereby enhancing the accuracy of results [7].

Regulatory Compliance and Cybersecurity

Modern systems incorporate user authentication, activity logging, and encrypted data storage to comply with regulatory frameworks such as ISO 15189 and GDPR. Given the increasing relevance of data security in healthcare, the software must provide audit trails, restricted access, and protection against unauthorized data breaches [8].

### *4.1.3 Types of Devices*

Biochemical analyzers can be broadly categorized based on their degree of automation, portability, and clinical application. The primary classifications include manual, semi-automated, fully automated, and point-of-care (POC) analyzers. Each category serves a distinct role in clinical diagnostics, offering specific advantages and limitations depending on laboratory capacity, testing volume, and clinical urgency.

**Manual Analyzers**

Manual biochemical analyzers represent the earliest generation of diagnostic technology. Initially introduced in the early twentieth century, these systems required significant manual labor and were based on fundamental techniques such as colorimetry. Although they laid the groundwork for biochemical testing, their susceptibility to human error and lengthy processing times limited their widespread clinical adoption.

The introduction of the AutoAnalyzer in the 1950s revolutionized biochemical testing by automating colorimetric reactions through a continuous flow system. This innovation enabled faster and more consistent analyses, reducing the workload on laboratory personnel. By the late twentieth century, further advancements led to discrete analyzers, which supported multiple simultaneous tests using smaller reagent volumes, greater precision, and early computer integration [4]. These innovations transformed laboratory workflows and enhanced the reliability of clinical diagnostics. Modern developments—such as the integration of microfluidics, nanotechnology, and artificial intelligence—have further refined analyzer capabilities, extending their use to decentralized environments including outpatient clinics and emergency settings [2]. This progress is central to the emergence of personalized medicine and point-of-care diagnostics.

## Semi-Automated Analyzers

Semi-automated biochemical analyzers bridge the gap between manual and fully automated systems. These devices automate analytical measurement and data processing while still requiring manual steps for sample preparation and reagent loading. Their cost-effectiveness, compact footprint, and operational simplicity make them well-suited for small to medium-sized laboratories and healthcare settings with limited infrastructure (Fig. 4.2).

Semi-automated analyzers demonstrated a strong correlation with fully automated systems across key biochemical parameters, including cholesterol, urea, SGOT, and SGPT. However, results indicated that triglyceride measurements exhibited higher variability in semi-automated formats, emphasizing that some assays may be more sensitive to manual processing steps. Despite these limitations, semi-automated analyzers continue to serve as reliable diagnostic platforms, particularly in areas where fully automated systems are not accessible. Their hybrid design maintains analytical robustness while offering affordability and adaptability in diverse clinical environments.

## Fully Automated Analyzers

Fully automated biochemical analyzers have dramatically improved the speed, accuracy, and reproducibility of laboratory diagnostics. These systems integrate every stage of testing—including sample loading, reagent dispensing, incubation,

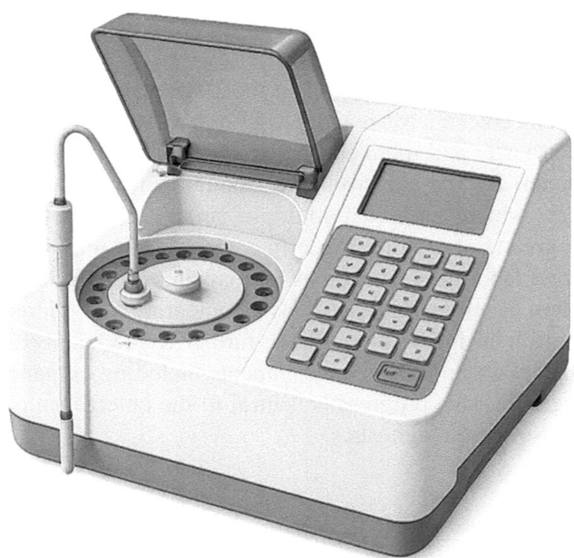

**Fig. 4.2** Semi automated analyzer

optical measurement, and result interpretation—into a seamless automated workflow [9]. This comprehensive automation minimizes human error, enhances throughput, and significantly reduces turnaround times, making these analyzers ideal for high-volume clinical laboratories. Advanced models are equipped with real-time quality control systems, automated maintenance alerts, and full integration with Laboratory Information Systems (LIS), which facilitates data traceability and streamlines laboratory operations [10].

Although the initial investment for fully automated analyzers is high, the long-term benefits in terms of efficiency, scalability, and analytical consistency often outweigh the cost [11]. Their widespread adoption has become a cornerstone of modern clinical laboratory infrastructure.

**Point-of-Care (POC) Analyzers**

Point-of-care biochemical analyzers have redefined diagnostic accessibility by enabling immediate testing at or near the patient's location. These portable, user-friendly devices are especially valuable in emergency departments, ambulatory clinics, rural health settings, and during home-based care [12]. Recent innovations in biosensor design and microfluidics have enhanced the analytical performance of point-of-care (POC) systems, enabling the conduct of complex biochemical assays with minimal sample volumes and short processing times [13]. Integration with mobile apps, cloud storage, and wireless data transmission enables real-time patient monitoring and remote clinical oversight, further enhancing the capabilities of these systems.

Despite their advantages, POC analyzers must still overcome challenges related to standardization, quality control, and regulatory compliance [14]. Nevertheless, as technology advances, these systems are expected to expand their roles in chronic disease management, telemedicine, and personalized therapy planning [15].

### *4.1.4 Clinical Applications*

Biochemistry analyzers play a critical role in modern medicine by enabling the rapid and precise quantification of biochemical markers in bodily fluids. Their diagnostic and monitoring capabilities are essential across a wide range of medical specialties, including cardiology, endocrinology, nephrology, and infectious disease management [1].

In cardiology, these analyzers are used to measure cardiac biomarkers such as troponins and natriuretic peptides, which are pivotal for the early detection and management of myocardial infarction and heart failure [16]. In endocrinology, biochemical analyzers assess hormone levels—including insulin, thyroid hormones, and cortisol—supporting the diagnosis and treatment of conditions such as diabetes mellitus, thyroid dysfunctions, and adrenal disorders [17]. In the context of nephrology, analytes such as creatinine, urea, and electrolytes are routinely measured to assess kidney function and guide therapeutic interventions in patients with renal impairment [18]. In infectious diseases, biochemistry analyzers enable the rapid detection of inflammatory markers and pathogen-associated antigens, facilitating prompt diagnosis and targeted antimicrobial therapy [19].

Emerging innovations have further expanded their utility into the realm of personalized medicine, allowing clinicians to tailor treatments based on individual biochemical profiles [15]. Additionally, integration with hospital information systems (HIS) supports streamlined data handling, enhances clinical decision-making, and improves continuity of care [20].

### *4.1.5 Regulatory Considerations*

Biochemical analyzers employed in clinical laboratories are subject to rigorous regulatory oversight to ensure diagnostic accuracy, operational reliability, and patient safety. These instruments must comply with established standards and certification requirements set forth by regulatory bodies such as the U.S. Food and Drug Administration (FDA), the European Medicines Agency (EMA), and the International Organization for Standardization (ISO).

In the United States, the FDA regulates in vitro diagnostic (IVD) devices under the Medical Device Amendments to the Federal Food, Drug, and Cosmetic Act (FD&C Act). Biochemical analyzers are generally classified as Class II medical devices, necessitating either a premarket notification (510(k)) or a premarket approval (PMA), depending on their risk profile and intended use [21]. Additionally, laboratories utilizing these analyzers must adhere to the Clinical Laboratory Improvement Amendments (CLIA), which enforce stringent quality control measures and proficiency testing standards.

In the European Union, biochemical analyzers are regulated under the In Vitro Diagnostic Regulation (IVDR) (EU) 2017/746, which imposes comprehensive requirements for device safety, performance evaluation, clinical evidence, and post-market surveillance. The regulation aims to enhance transparency and traceability across the diagnostic device lifecycle, ultimately improving clinical outcomes and patient protection [22].

Globally, ISO 13485 defines the requirements for quality management systems specific to medical device design and manufacturing. This standard ensures consistent product development, regulatory conformity, and risk mitigation across international markets [23]. Moreover, the Clinical and Laboratory Standards Institute (CLSI) provides detailed procedural guidelines and performance benchmarks that support standardization in biochemical testing workflows.

### 4.1.6 Future Perspectives

The incorporation of cutting-edge technologies is poised to redefine the functionality and clinical impact of biochemical analyzers fundamentally. Among the most transformative developments is the integration of artificial intelligence (AI) and machine learning (ML) algorithms, which significantly elevate analytical precision, data processing efficiency, and interpretative accuracy. These technologies empower analysts to decode complex biochemical datasets with enhanced reliability, thereby supporting more informed and timely clinical decisions [24].

AI and ML algorithms also facilitate the interrogation of large-scale laboratory datasets to identify diagnostic patterns and subtle anomalies that conventional analysis may overlook. For example, ML models have demonstrated success in predicting mortality risk among patients with rheumatoid arthritis by processing diverse clinical and serological markers, enabling clinicians to tailor therapies with greater precision. In laboratory diagnostics, AI-driven clinical decision support systems (CDSS) are becoming increasingly common. These systems assist in interpreting test results, flagging inconsistencies, and minimizing errors across all stages of laboratory workflows. The resulting increase in diagnostic speed and accuracy strengthens the utility and reliability of biochemical analyzers in diverse clinical contexts.

Moreover, AI contributes to the development of personalized reference intervals, dynamically adjusted based on individual variables such as age, sex, and comorbidities. This individualized approach enhances diagnostic specificity and reduces false interpretations in heterogeneous patient populations. Another significant advancement lies in the field of biochemical sensors, particularly in the design of flexible, skin-adherent systems capable of continuously monitoring biomarkers through noninvasive fluids such as sweat. These wearable sensors transmit physiological data in real time, offering new opportunities for chronic disease management and remote patient monitoring [25].

Microfluidic "lab-on-a-chip" systems represent a parallel innovation, enabling rapid and low-cost biochemical analyses at the point of care. The incorporation of nanomaterials, particularly graphene and its derivatives, has significantly enhanced the sensitivity, specificity, and operational robustness of these platforms. Graphene's superior electrical conductivity and mechanical flexibility make it an ideal substrate for next-generation biosensors embedded within microfluidic devices [26]. Looking ahead, the convergence of AI, wearable technology, and microfluidics is expected to yield highly advanced diagnostic platforms that support real-time health tracking, early disease detection, and precision-guided treatment strategies. These integrated systems hold the potential to redefine patient care models by enabling proactive, personalized, and scalable healthcare delivery [24–26].

## 4.2 PCR Devices

Polymerase chain reaction (PCR) amplification techniques have revolutionized pathogen detection by offering rapid, sensitive, and specific identification of microbial targets. The scope of PCR-based applications continues to expand, with an increasing number of amplification methods now utilized in FDA field laboratories for the detection of pathogens, including Salmonella, Escherichia coli, Shigella, Vibrio spp., hepatitis A virus (HAV), and noroviruses (NoV).

However, one of the principal challenges associated with PCR is its extreme sensitivity, which also renders it highly susceptible to contamination. Even trace amounts of previously amplified DNA (amplicons) or target nucleic acids introduced via aerosols, surfaces, or laboratory equipment can lead to false-positive results. This poses significant issues in regulatory and clinical settings, where diagnostic accuracy is paramount. To mitigate PCR carryover contamination, rigorous preventive strategies must be implemented [27]. The primary line of defense involves the mechanical separation of laboratory spaces, with dedicated rooms or segregated workstations for sample preparation, amplification, and post-PCR analysis.

Additionally, chemical, ultraviolet (UV), and enzymatic decontamination approaches are employed to degrade residual amplicons. For example, UV irradiation of work surfaces, use of dUTP/UNG (uracil-DNA glycosylase) systems, and application of DNA-degrading reagents can substantially reduce the risk of residual DNA contaminating new assays. Prompt detection and source tracking of contaminants are also critical. To support this, a rapid method for identifying carryover contamination through DNA sequencing of suspected amplicons has been developed. This allows laboratories to distinguish between accurate pathogen-specific amplification and inadvertent contamination. When combined with stringent workflow practices, decontamination protocols, and rapid detection tools for contamination, these strategies can effectively eliminate carryover contamination. This ensures that PCR assays maintain their high sensitivity and specificity, enabling their reliable use in regulatory and diagnostic applications.

### *4.2.1 History*

Few scientific innovations in the past century have had as profound an impact on biology and genetics as the polymerase chain reaction (PCR) [28]. Its development revolutionized molecular research by enabling rapid, specific, and exponential amplification of DNA sequences from minimal starting material.

The journey began with challenges in DNA sequencing using the Sanger method, which produced weak signals when analyzing single-copy genes due to low DNA concentrations. Kary Mullis addressed this by introducing a denaturation step to separate double-stranded DNA (dsDNA) into single strands (ssDNA), and by adding a reverse primer to define the length of the amplicon. This allowed the amplification of two DNA copies per cycle [29]. However, each high-temperature denaturation step destroyed the DNA polymerase, requiring manual addition for every cycle—a process that proved labor-intensive. This limitation was overcome by using Taq polymerase, an enzyme derived from the thermophilic bacterium Thermus aquaticus, which retains activity even at 94 °C. The introduction of Taq polymerase enabled fully automated thermal cycling without the need for polymerase replenishment [30]. Early thermal cyclers, such as the 'Baby Blue' prototype, facilitated time-domain temperature cycling, where the sample remained stationary as temperatures changed. An alternative, the spatial-domain cycler, moved the sample through three zones with fixed temperatures, though time-domain systems are now more widely used.

The foundation for PCR was laid much earlier. In 1957, Arthur Kornberg discovered the first DNA polymerase, demonstrating that DNA synthesis requires a primer and proceeds in a single direction. In the 1970s, Gobind Khorana and his team advanced the concept of DNA replication using synthetic primers and templates. Although these techniques used DNA polymerase repeatedly, they lacked exponential amplification. Notably, Kjell Kleppe, working in Khorana's lab, proposed a two-primer system—an idea that prefigured the basic principle of PCR. In parallel, the biotechnology company Cetus Corporation, founded in 1971, became a hub for molecular biology innovation. Kary Mullis, working at Cetus, was involved in oligonucleotide synthesis and later revisited the concept of using two primers to flank a DNA target sequence [31, 32]. In 1983, he realized that repeated cycles of denaturation, annealing, and extension could trigger a chain reaction of DNA amplification—a breakthrough that led to the birth of PCR [33].

Initial trials used Sanger sequencing as a framework, and though early amplification products were not visible on agarose gels, Southern blotting confirmed the presence of increased DNA. Refinements in primer and probe design gradually improved specificity and yield, making PCR products eventually visible by gel electrophoresis. The technique was formally patented in 1987 after the successful cloning and sequencing of the amplified DNA. In 1985, Perkin-Elmer and Cetus entered a joint venture to commercialize PCR instruments and reagents. This led to the development of the first Taq-based thermal cyclers, and the commercial release of AmpliTaq DNA polymerase in 1987 marked the beginning of widespread adoption.

By assembling existing components—primers, polymerase, nucleotide precursors, and thermal cyclers—PCR emerged as a transformative tool in diagnostics, forensics, genomics, and biotechnology. Its invention remains a landmark achievement in molecular biology, catalyzing a new era of scientific inquiry and medical innovation.

## *4.2.2 Technical Characteristics*

### Hardware

Real-time PCR (qPCR) systems comprise several integrated hardware components designed to facilitate thermal cycling and real-time fluorescence detection of nucleic acid amplification. The core components include:

Thermal Cycling Module

This unit precisely controls temperature changes required for DNA denaturation, primer annealing, and extension. Most modern systems utilize Peltier elements, solid-state thermoelectric devices that can rapidly heat and cool. These modules can establish thermal gradients, which are particularly useful for optimizing annealing temperatures within a single run. Some systems alternatively use heated or cooled air chambers, in which samples are suspended and exposed to temperature-controlled airflow for each cycle.

Optical Detection System

The detection unit monitors fluorescence intensity during each cycle, enabling quantification of DNA amplification in real-time. Fluorescent signals originate from intercalating dyes or sequence-specific probes. Light sources commonly include:

- Light Emitting Diodes (LEDs): Arranged either above each well or in stationary arrays, LEDs can excite multiple wells simultaneously.
- Halogen Lamps: Emit broad-spectrum light, filtered to excite specific fluorophores.
- Lasers: Emit narrow-bandwidth, high-intensity light for precise excitation of select dyes; however, their utility in multiplexing is limited due to spectral restrictions.

Detection devices convert emitted light into measurable signals:

- Photodiodes: Compact and reliable, these sensors convert light into electrical current with a broad spectral range.
- Charge-Coupled Devices (CCDs): Capture digital images of entire reaction plates; software interprets the fluorescence intensity across all wells.
- Photomultiplier Tubes (PMTs): Extremely sensitive detectors that amplify the light signal, often used in high-performance systems.

Reaction Formats

Thermal blocks are most commonly designed in 96-well plate format, accommodating reaction volumes between 1 and 125 μL. High-throughput platforms may utilize 384-well or microfluidic formats, where reaction volumes can be as low as nanoliters or even picoliters.

Integrated Control Interface

While most systems require a computer for full functionality, specific instruments (e.g., Bio-Rad's CFX96 and CFX384 Touch) include onboard interfaces allowing independent operation. However, external computers are typically used for comprehensive data analysis and long-term data storage.

**Software**

Real-time PCR software is essential for managing instrument operations and performing data analysis. It integrates four primary functional components:

Protocol Configuration

Users define temperature profiles, including denaturation, annealing, and extension steps, as well as the number of cycles. Parameters for fluorescence data acquisition (e.g., which steps and channels to monitor) are also specified in this section.

Plate Setup

The software interface allows for detailed mapping of each well, including the sample ID, target, and reference genes. This setup ensures accurate data interpretation and traceability across runs.

Data Collection

During the amplification process, fluorescence intensity is recorded in real time. These values are plotted against cycle number to visualize the accumulation of amplified product. A characteristic exponential increase in fluorescence indicates the presence of a target sequence.

Data Analysis

Post-run, the software calculates a baseline fluorescence level, either automatically or manually defined, to standardize comparison between wells. The quantification cycle (Cq)—formerly known as Ct—is determined based on a fluorescence threshold or through regression analysis (QIAGEN 2024). Two primary analysis methods are supported:

- Absolute Quantification: Compares Cq values from experimental samples to a standard curve derived from known concentrations. Results are expressed as nucleic acid amount (e.g., copies/μL, μg/sample).
- Relative Quantification: Assesses fold changes in gene expression by comparing the target gene's Cq value to that of a reference gene across different samples (e.g., treated vs. control), providing insights into differential gene expression.

Advanced software suites also support:

- Quality control alerts (e.g., melt curve analysis).
- Real-time monitoring of amplification efficiency.
- Exportable data formats for integration with LIMS and statistical tools.

### *4.2.3 Types of Devices*

**Standard PCR Workflow**

Polymerase Chain Reaction (PCR) is a powerful molecular technique used to amplify a specific DNA sequence exponentially. It operates on a cyclical temperature-driven process consisting of three main steps:

1. Denaturation (94–98 °C): During this step, the double-stranded DNA is heated to a high temperature, which disrupts the hydrogen bonds between complementary bases, resulting in the separation of the DNA into two single strands. This prepares the template for primer annealing.
2. Annealing (50–65 °C): The reaction mixture is cooled to a temperature suitable for primer hybridization. Primers, short single-stranded DNA sequences complementary to the target region's flanking areas, bind to each DNA template strand. The optimal annealing temperature depends on the primer sequence and GC content.
3. Extension (72 °C): The temperature is raised to the optimal working temperature for Taq DNA polymerase (a thermostable enzyme derived from Thermus aquaticus). The enzyme extends the primers by adding nucleotides that are complementary to the template strand, thereby synthesizing a new strand of DNA.

This cycle is repeated typically 25–40 times, doubling the amount of target DNA with each cycle and resulting in exponential amplification [31, 32].

### Hot-Start PCR

Hot-Start PCR is an enhanced version of traditional PCR designed to increase specificity and reduce non-specific amplification and primer-dimer formation. This method prevents premature enzymatic activity by inactivating DNA polymerase until the initial denaturation step. Several strategies are used:

- Antibody-mediated inhibition: An antibody binds to the polymerase, inhibiting its activity until high temperatures denature the antibody.
- Chemical modification: The polymerase is chemically altered to remain inactive until the denaturation temperature removes the modification.
- Encapsulation or physical separation: Enzymes and other reagents are physically separated until the reaction mixture is heated.

Hot-Start PCR is particularly useful for amplifying complex genomic DNA or low-abundance templates where specificity is critical [34] (Fig. 4.3).

### High-Fidelity Polymerases

Standard Taq polymerase lacks proofreading ability, making it prone to errors during DNA synthesis. High-fidelity polymerases, such as Pfu from Pyrococcus furiosus, have 3′–5′ exonuclease activity, which allows them to remove incorrectly incorporated nucleotides and replace them with the correct ones. This proofreading function significantly reduces the error rate. Applications requiring high accuracy, such as cloning, mutagenesis, or sequencing, benefit from the use of high-fidelity enzymes. Modern engineered variants (e.g., Phusion, Q5) combine high processivity with low error rates [32].

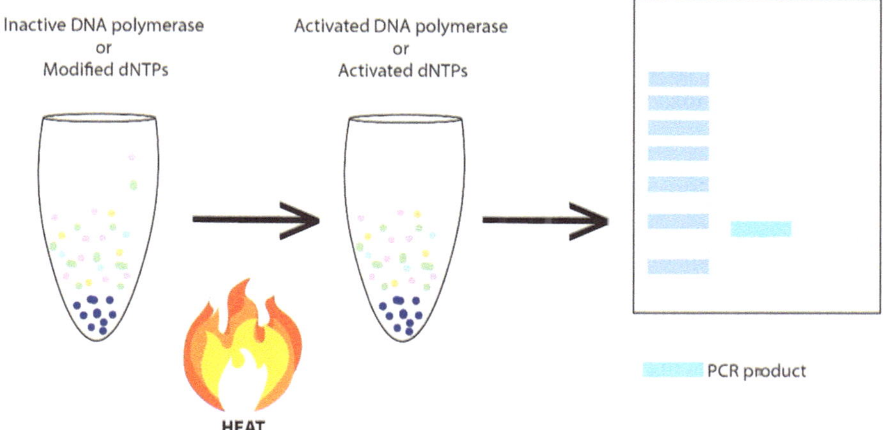


**Fig. 4.3** Hot-start PCR using antibody-linked Taq DNA polymerase (https://upload.wikimedia.org/wikipedia/commons/1/11/HSPCR.jpg)

### Reverse Transcription PCR (RT-PCR)

RT-PCR is used to study RNA by converting it into complementary DNA (cDNA) using the enzyme reverse transcriptase. This cDNA then serves as a template for PCR amplification [35, 36]. Steps include:

- RNA extraction: Isolating high-quality RNA from the biological sample.
- Reverse transcription: Using reverse transcriptase to synthesize cDNA from the RNA template.
- PCR amplification: Amplifying specific regions of the cDNA to analyze gene expression or detect RNA viruses.

RT-PCR is essential for transcriptome profiling, studying gene regulation, and diagnosing RNA-based pathogens such as SARS-CoV-2.

### Quantitative PCR (qPCR) and RT-qPCR

Quantitative PCR (qPCR), also known as real-time PCR, enables the quantification of nucleic acids in real-time by using fluorescent dyes or probes.

- Dye-based qPCR: Utilizes DNA-binding dyes like SYBR Green. As double-stranded DNA accumulates, fluorescence increases proportionally. While cost-effective and straightforward, this method lacks specificity and can amplify non-target products.
- Probe-based qPCR: Employs sequence-specific probes (e.g., TaqMan probes) labeled with a fluorophore and quencher. During amplification, the probe is degraded by polymerase, which separates the fluorophore and quencher, resulting in the emission of a fluorescence signal. This allows multiplexing and greater specificity.

RT-qPCR combines reverse transcription and quantitative PCR (qPCR) for dynamic quantification of RNA. It is widely used in clinical diagnostics, particularly for monitoring viral load [37–39].

### Isothermal Amplification

Isothermal amplification eliminates the need for thermal cycling by conducting amplification at a constant temperature [40]. Techniques include:

- LAMP (Loop-mediated Isothermal Amplification): Utilizes multiple primers and a strand-displacing DNA polymerase to amplify DNA at ~65 °C. The method produces a large amount of DNA in a short time and is detectable via fluorescence or colorimetric indicators.

- NASBA (Nucleic Acid Sequence-Based Amplification): Targets RNA amplification through the simultaneous activity of reverse transcriptase, RNase H, and T7 RNA polymerase.

These methods are ideal for point-of-care testing and resource-limited settings due to their simplicity and minimal equipment requirements.

**Digital PCR (dPCR)**

Digital PCR partitions the PCR reaction into thousands or millions of nanoliter-sized reactions. Each partition contains either zero or one (or a few) copies of the target DNA. Following amplification, partitions are scored as positive or negative for target amplification [33, 41].

- Absolute quantification: The ratio of positive to total partitions allows calculation of the precise number of target molecules, independent of standard curves.
- High sensitivity: Enables detection of rare alleles or mutations, low-copy-number targets, and subtle expression changes.

dPCR is increasingly used in precision oncology, infectious disease diagnostics, and copy number variation analysis.

### *4.2.4 Clinical Applications*

**Applications of PCR in Infectious Diseases**

Polymerase Chain Reaction (PCR) has become a cornerstone in the clinical diagnosis and surveillance of infectious diseases. Its ability to detect and amplify minute quantities of pathogen-specific nucleic acids makes it especially valuable for early and precise diagnosis. PCR is routinely used to detect a broad spectrum of pathogens, including bacteria, viruses, and protozoa. Applications include confirming the presence of specific infectious agents, identifying asymptomatic carriers, evaluating the spread of emerging infections, and detecting antimicrobial resistance genes [35].

Traditional diagnostic methods, such as bacterial or viral culture, serological assays, and enzyme-linked immunosorbent assays (ELISA), have limitations: they are labor-intensive, time-consuming, and expensive, and often lack sensitivity or specificity. For example, serological tests may yield false positives due to cross-reactivity. In contrast, PCR-based diagnostics offer high sensitivity and specificity, overcoming the "window period" of immunological detection by identifying pathogens during the early stages of infection or even in latent forms. Since the onset of the COVID-19 pandemic, PCR has been the primary diagnostic tool for SARS-CoV-2, providing rapid and reliable detection of the virus [42]. Emerging platforms, such as multiplex PCR, quantitative multiplex PCR, and microfluidic PCR, enable the simultaneous detection of multiple pathogens from a single sample, thereby optimizing diagnostic workflows.

PCR is also employed in pathogen genotyping. For instance, in human papillomavirus (HPV) diagnostics, PCR enables not only the detection of the virus but also the identification of specific oncogenic subtypes. This stratification is critical, as certain HPV genotypes pose a higher risk of cervical cancer. Quantitative PCR (qPCR) can monitor pathogen load, which is crucial in diseases such as HIV and hepatitis B (HBV), where viral load informs treatment decisions. Moreover, PCR facilitates rapid detection of antimicrobial resistance (AMR) genes in pathogens such as Klebsiella pneumoniae, which can harbor genes for extended-spectrum beta-lactamases (ESBLs), AmpC enzymes, and aminoglycoside-modifying enzymes (AMEs).

Digital PCR (dPCR), the third-generation PCR technology, further enhances sensitivity. It partitions the reaction into thousands of microdroplets, allowing for precise quantification and detection of low-frequency mutations. For example, dPCR has demonstrated superior detection of the H275Y mutation in oseltamivir-resistant H1N1 influenza virus and specific hepatitis C virus (HCV) mutations, outperforming conventional qPCR in sensitivity by up to 200-fold [38].

### Applications of PCR in Hereditary Diseases

PCR has revolutionized genetic diagnostics, particularly in prenatal and neonatal contexts. Traditional methods, such as Southern blotting and RFLP, while informative, are time-consuming, technically demanding, and less suited to high-throughput clinical workflows.

In prenatal testing, PCR is routinely used to detect chromosomal abnormalities and single-gene disorders. For instance, in the diagnosis of Down syndrome (Trisomy 21), dPCR-based non-invasive prenatal testing (NIPT) offers improved sensitivity and specificity compared to traditional serum biochemical testing (SBT), with a lower cost compared to next-generation sequencing (NGS)-based NIPT. For monogenic disorders such as thalassemia, Gap-PCR and NGS are used in tandem for effective mutation detection. The advent of droplet digital PCR (ddPCR) has further advanced non-invasive prenatal diagnostics (NIPD). Studies show that ddPCR can reliably detect mutations, such as IVS1-110 and beta +039 thalassemia, with high sensitivity and specificity, facilitating early diagnosis and management without the risks associated with invasive procedures [33]. Neonatal genetic screening is another vital area, enabling diagnosis and intervention within days of birth to prevent severe outcomes. qPCR is commonly used to screen for conditions such as hereditary deafness and metabolic disorders. Techniques like ARMS-PCR have been adapted for the rapid and accurate detection of mutations in diseases such as Wilson's disease.

### Applications of PCR in Cancer and Other Diseases

PCR plays a vital role in oncology, enabling early detection, molecular classification, and treatment monitoring. It is used to identify chromosomal translocations, oncogene activations, tumor suppressor gene inactivations, and mutations conferring drug resistance. For example, the Bcr-Abl fusion gene—a hallmark of chronic myeloid leukemia (CML)—can be detected and quantified via PCR before clinical symptoms arise, guiding early therapeutic intervention. PCR also facilitates the detection of tumor-associated microRNAs (miRNAs) such as miR-122 and miR-1258, which are implicated in hepatocellular carcinoma, breast cancer, and other malignancies. Changes in miRNA expression levels can serve as prognostic markers or indicators of therapeutic response.

In ovarian cancer, PCR-based detection of elevated HE4 mRNA levels offers a means for early diagnosis and monitoring of disease recurrence months before clinical symptoms appear. Similarly, in colorectal cancer (CRC), PCR is used to analyze gene expression profiles and microbiome alterations, supporting early diagnosis and personalized therapy. Liquid biopsies using PCR enable the real-time tracking of tumor gene expression from blood samples, providing a non-invasive alternative for disease monitoring and therapy optimization, particularly for patients with hematologic malignancies and those undergoing post-surgical cancer treatment. Together, these applications underline PCR's transformative impact across clinical diagnostics, particularly in infectious diseases, hereditary conditions, and oncology. As technologies like digital PCR and microfluidics mature, the scope and precision of PCR-based diagnostics will continue to expand.

## *4.2.5 Regulatory Considerations*

The use of Polymerase Chain Reaction (PCR) and its advanced derivatives in clinical diagnostics and public health mandates strict adherence to regulatory standards to ensure safety, accuracy, reproducibility, and clinical relevance. As PCR-based assays increasingly move from centralized laboratories to decentralized, point-of-care (POC) and even at-home settings, regulatory frameworks must evolve to address both established and emerging risks.

### Regulatory Frameworks and Approval Pathways

In the United States, PCR assays used for diagnostic purposes are classified as in vitro diagnostic (IVD) medical devices and regulated by the Food and Drug Administration (FDA) under the Federal Food, Drug, and Cosmetic Act (FD&C Act). Depending on the level of risk associated with the assay, these devices may require:

- Premarket Notification [510(k)] for moderate-risk devices.
- Premarket Approval (PMA) for high-risk diagnostics.
- Emergency Use Authorization (EUA) in cases of urgent public health needs (e.g., COVID-19 diagnostics).

PCR-based tests must demonstrate analytical validity (sensitivity, specificity, limit of detection), clinical validity (association with disease state), and clinical utility (impact on health outcomes). For multiplex or syndromic panels, cross-reactivity and interference studies are essential [43, 44].

In the European Union, IVDs are governed by the In Vitro Diagnostic Regulation, which came into full effect in May 2022. The IVDR mandates:

- Risk-based classification of IVDs (Class A to D).
- Performance evaluation and clinical evidence for all tests.
- Stricter oversight by notified bodies.
- Post-market surveillance and traceability.

PCR assays for detecting pathogens, such as HIV, HBV, or oncogenic mutations, fall into Class D, requiring independent review, batch verification, and possibly the involvement of a reference laboratory. IVDR also requires lab-developed tests (LDTs) to comply if they are marketed outside the facility in which they are developed. Globally, regulatory harmonization is supported by organizations such as the International Medical Device Regulators Forum (IMDRF) and guidance documents from the World Health Organization (WHO) for PCR-based diagnostics in low-resource settings [42, 45].

### Laboratory and Quality Standards

Clinical laboratories performing PCR-based diagnostics must adhere to national laboratory standards:

- In the U.S., laboratories must be CLIA-certified (Clinical Laboratory Improvement Amendments), which ensures competency in test validation, proficiency testing, and quality management.
- The College of American Pathologists (CAP) provides additional accreditation that emphasizes result accuracy and documentation in molecular diagnostics labs.
- Internationally, compliance with ISO 15189 (Medical laboratories—Requirements for quality and competence) is often required or recommended for molecular testing facilities.

Manufacturers of PCR reagents, consumables, and devices must also comply with ISO 13485, which governs quality management systems for medical devices, including design controls, risk management, and traceability [46].

### Regulatory Considerations for Emerging Platforms

The development of microfluidic PCR, digital PCR, isothermal amplification systems, and CRISPR-based diagnostics introduces novel challenges:

- These platforms often blur the lines between traditional IVDs and laboratory-developed tests (LDTs).
- Regulatory agencies now require validation of entire workflows, including sample preparation, nucleic acid extraction, amplification, and data interpretation.
- For point-of-care systems, human factor studies and usability testing are critical to ensure that non-specialist users (e.g., patients or field workers) can operate devices reliably.
- Cybersecurity and data privacy regulations, particularly for smartphone-based and IoT-enabled PCR systems, are becoming increasingly essential as diagnostic data is being increasingly digitized and transmitted via wireless networks.

### Ethical and Legal Considerations

PCR's ability to detect minute quantities of genetic material raises bioethical concerns related to:

- Privacy and consent, particularly in hereditary disease screening and newborn testing.
- Data governance for genomic information.
- Equitable access to high-sensitivity diagnostic tools across socioeconomic and geographical barriers.

National and international frameworks, including the General Data Protection Regulation (GDPR) in the European Union and HIPAA in the United States, govern the use of patient data generated through molecular diagnostics.

### Post-market Surveillance and Risk Management

Ongoing monitoring of PCR assay performance is crucial, particularly in dynamic settings such as infectious disease surveillance and oncology. Regulatory bodies increasingly require:

- Periodic performance re-evaluation.
- Adverse event reporting for diagnostic failures or misdiagnoses.
- Lot-to-lot verification for critical reagents.
- Environmental monitoring to prevent contamination in high-throughput laboratories.

In addition, performance requirements must be reevaluated as pathogen genomes evolve, particularly in the case of RNA viruses like SARS-CoV-2 or influenza, where mutations may affect primer or probe binding.

### *4.2.6 Future Perspectives*

PCR remains a foundational technology in molecular diagnostics, and its influence is set to expand with the integration of next-generation technologies. Techniques such as next-generation sequencing (NGS) heavily rely on PCR for target enrichment and library preparation, and this dependence is likely to grow stronger as sequencing technologies continue to evolve. Shortly, PCR will be central to advanced molecular diagnostics through innovations in microfluidics. These platforms are expected to enable parallel analysis of multiple samples in miniaturized, handheld point-of-care (POC) systems. One promising direction is the use of microfluidic devices to perform real-time RT-PCR on immunomagnetically isolated exosomal RNA, which could provide high-resolution insights into diseases such as cancer.

Droplet-based qPCR platforms are also gaining momentum, particularly for the purification of single-cell mRNA and gene expression profiling. These systems partition individual cells or nucleic acid targets into nanoliter droplets, enabling precise analysis of transcriptional heterogeneity. Similarly, digital RT-PCR on-chip-based platforms are becoming a standard for the absolute quantification of mRNA in single cells, which is essential for studying rare transcripts or low-copy-number targets, such as microRNAs (miRNAs). Another transformative advance is the use of emulsion PCR, which enables barcoding and amplification of nucleic acids within individual droplets. This technology has enabled the performance of single-cell RNA or DNA sequencing on complex tissue samples or heterogeneous cell populations. Currently, Oxford Nanopore Technologies offers the only commercial sequencing system that bypasses PCR entirely, using nanopore-based direct nucleic acid sequencing [41].

Paper-based PCR and LAMP (loop-mediated isothermal amplification) platforms are expected to see increasing adoption in low-resource and field settings. These systems promise rapid, affordable, and equipment-free molecular diagnostics, ideal for infectious disease detection, agricultural testing, and forensic applications. In forensic science, for instance, on-site DNA profiling chips could replace traditional lab-based workflows, enabling immediate identification at crime scenes. Commercially available systems such as BioFire FilmArray have already demonstrated the viability of on-chip pathogen detection, covering a wide range of bacterial and viral targets in clinical diagnostics [47]. The success of these platforms points toward a future where microfluidic PCR devices are routinely commercialized, tailored for diverse applications from hospitals to environmental monitoring stations.

The miniaturization of PCR technology will also continue, with integrated systems capable of performing sample preparation, nucleic acid extraction, amplification, and detection in a single unit. This trend is moving diagnostics closer to a sample-to-answer format for point-of-care (POC) applications. The COVID-19 pandemic accelerated this progress, with platforms like the ID NOW (initially designed for influenza detection via LAMP) being rapidly adapted for SARS-CoV-2 diagnostics. As of May 2020, 81 diagnostic kits had been granted Emergency Use Authorization (EUA) by the FDA, with the majority utilizing real-time reverse transcription-polymerase chain reaction (RT-PCR) technology. New frontiers also include CRISPR-based diagnostics, which are poised to complement or even replace traditional detection methods by enhancing specificity and multiplexing capacity. CRISPR-mediated identification of amplified sequences enables visual or lateral-flow readouts and can be integrated with PCR or isothermal methods [48].

Looking ahead, these detection platforms may become part of a broader Internet of Medical Things (IoMT). Smartphone-based systems—already capable of integrating cameras, sensors, and Bluetooth-enabled thermal control—may soon be adapted to operate entire diagnostic workflows. Android-based interfaces can control image capture, perform local data processing, and wirelessly transmit results to cloud-based servers or remote clinical centers for review. Alternative DNA amplification technologies, such as recombinase polymerase amplification (RPA) and loop-mediated isothermal amplification (LAMP), offer energy-efficient alternatives to traditional polymerase chain reaction (PCR), which is crucial for field-deployable diagnostics and battery-powered devices. Ultimately, portable digital PCR (dPCR) platforms are likely to become indispensable tools in clinical diagnostics, environmental surveillance, and forensic science, offering rapid, high-precision nucleic acid quantification without the need to transport samples to centralized laboratories, thereby preserving sample integrity and enabling real-time decision-making.

## 4.3 Sequencing Machines

Sequencing machines—also known as DNA and RNA sequencers—are sophisticated biomedical instruments engineered to decode the precise order of nucleotides in genetic material. For DNA, this sequence comprises adenine (A), thymine (T), cytosine (C), and guanine (G); in RNA, uracil (U) replaces thymine. These platforms have fundamentally transformed genomics by enabling rapid, high-throughput sequencing of entire genomes with exceptional accuracy and scalability. The adoption of sequencing technologies in medical, pharmaceutical, and research domains has dramatically accelerated genetic discovery and clinical diagnostics.

The evolution of sequencing technology can be categorized into three major generations. The first generation, Sanger sequencing, once the gold standard for DNA analysis, remains in niche use today due to its high fidelity but is limited by low throughput and cost inefficiency. Next-generation sequencing (NGS) technologies—pioneered by companies such as Illumina and Thermo Fisher (Ion

Torrent)—represent the second generation. These platforms enable the simultaneous sequencing of millions of DNA fragments, offering a balance between cost, speed, and accuracy that has catalyzed their widespread use in research and diagnostics. Emerging third-generation sequencing technologies, including Pacific Biosciences' Single Molecule Real-Time (SMRT) sequencing and Oxford Nanopore Technologies' nanopore-based systems, further extend sequencing capabilities by enabling real-time analysis and ultra-long read lengths. These advancements facilitate improved detection of structural variants, more comprehensive transcriptomics, and sequencing in low-resource or point-of-care settings.

Sequencing platforms are now integral across both clinical and research environments. In healthcare, they enable early and precise diagnosis of genetic disorders, detection of somatic mutations in oncology, and real-time tracking of pathogens during infectious disease outbreaks. In the realm of pharmacogenomics, sequencing enables the identification of genetic polymorphisms that influence drug metabolism, efficacy, and the risk of adverse reactions. This convergence of sequencing technology and personalized medicine is supported by pharmacy informatics, a field at the intersection of pharmaceutical sciences and health information systems. The integration of sequencing data into electronic health records (EHRs) enables clinical decision support systems (CDSS) to guide drug selection and dosage based on a patient's genomic profile. Such integration enhances therapeutic precision, minimizes adverse drug events, and improves overall clinical outcomes.

Furthermore, informatics tools are indispensable for the interpretation, storage, and secure management of the massive datasets generated by sequencing. As genomics continues to expand its footprint in clinical practice, pharmacy informatics will play a pivotal role in translating genetic data into actionable, patient-specific therapeutic strategies.

## *4.3.1 History*

The evolution of DNA sequencing technologies can be categorized into three transformative generations, each characterized by substantial improvements in throughput, cost-efficiency, accuracy, and clinical utility. These technological milestones have underpinned breakthroughs in genomics, enabling a wide range of applications, from large-scale genome mapping to personalized medicine and point-of-care diagnostics [49].

### First Generation: Sanger Sequencing and Early Automation

The first generation of DNA sequencing began with the landmark development of the Sanger method in 1977 by Frederick Sanger and colleagues. This technique, based on chain-termination chemistry, became the standard method for DNA sequencing for nearly three decades due to its reliability and precision. In 1986, the introduction of automated DNA sequencers by Applied Biosystems marked a pivotal advancement, enabling higher-throughput sequencing and reducing human error [50]. These innovations culminated in the launch of the Human Genome Project (1990–2003), a multinational effort that successfully sequenced the entire human genome. The project served as a technological and conceptual springboard, catalyzing further advancements in sequencing methodologies and bioinformatics infrastructure.

#### Second Generation: Next-Generation Sequencing (NGS)

The advent of next-generation sequencing (NGS) technologies in the early 2000s revolutionized genomics by introducing massively parallel sequencing. Companies like 454 Life Sciences (acquired by Roche), Illumina, and Thermo Fisher (Ion Torrent) developed platforms that could simultaneously sequence millions of DNA fragments in a single run. These platforms dramatically reduced the time and cost required for whole-genome and targeted sequencing, transforming research and clinical diagnostics. NGS technologies have since become integral to oncology (for somatic mutation profiling), infectious disease surveillance, rare disease diagnostics, and pharmacogenomics, where sequencing data guide the selection and dosing of therapeutic agents.

#### Third Generation: Real-Time and Single-Molecule Sequencing

The third generation of sequencing focuses on the real-time analysis of single DNA molecules, eliminating the need for PCR amplification. Technologies such as Pacific Biosciences' Single Molecule Real-Time (SMRT) sequencing and Oxford Nanopore Technologies' nanopore-based platforms offer significantly longer read lengths, direct epigenetic analysis, and rapid turnaround. Unlike earlier platforms, some third-generation sequencers are portable and field-deployable, enabling point-of-care testing, outbreak response, and environmental monitoring [51]. These capabilities have advanced applications in clinical metagenomics, genome assembly, and personalized medicine, particularly in contexts where speed, mobility, and read length are critical (Fig. 4.4).

### 4.3.2 Technical Characteristics

Modern sequencing platforms represent a convergence of advanced engineering and computational biology, designed to convert biological samples into meaningful genetic information with clinical and research applications. Their effectiveness depends on technical specifications, including sequencing accuracy, throughput, runtime, and data integration [52]. These characteristics vary by platform generation and impact both performance and usability in diagnostic settings.

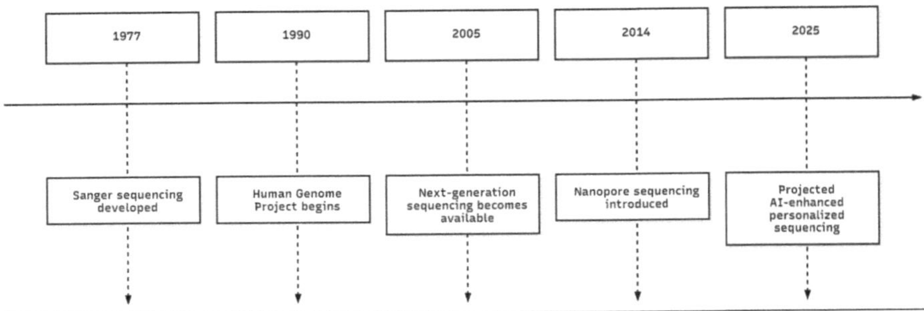


**Fig. 4.4** Timeline of DNA sequencing technologies

## Hardware

Sequencing systems comprise several key hardware components, including sample preparation units, sequencing reactors, detection modules, and environmental control systems. While the architecture differs across generations, these components are designed to work in concert to ensure accuracy, scalability, and operational robustness.

### Automated Library Preparation

Platforms such as Illumina's NeoPrep automate key preparatory steps—DNA fragmentation, end-repair, and adapter ligation—using robotic liquid handling systems. Automation reduces human error, enhances reproducibility, and minimizes contamination, making it essential for clinical and high-throughput environments [53].

### Sequencing Reactors

The core of any sequencer is its reactor unit, where sequencing chemistry is performed [51]:

- NGS systems like those from Illumina use flow cells embedded with optically transparent nanowells where bridge amplification occurs.
- Ion Torrent platforms utilize microfluidic chips and perform clonal amplification through emulsion polymerase chain reaction (emulsion PCR).
- Third-generation systems adopt amplification-free strategies: Pacific Biosciences uses Zero-Mode Waveguides (ZMWs) to observe real-time synthesis by single polymerases, whereas Oxford Nanopore embeds protein nanopores into membranes laid across microelectrode arrays for direct strand sequencing.

### Detection Technologies

Detection mechanisms differ based on sequencing chemistry [51]:

- Optical fluorescence detection (e.g., Illumina NovaSeq) uses multiple lasers to excite dye-labeled nucleotides, capturing images for each base incorporation.
- Semiconductor detection (Ion Torrent Genexus) uses CMOS sensors to detect pH shifts following nucleotide incorporation.
- Electrochemical detection in Oxford Nanopore systems monitors disruptions in ionic current as DNA strands pass through nanopores, interpreted via application-specific integrated circuits (ASICs).

### Environmental Control and Portability

High-end sequencing instruments incorporate advanced thermal control for precise reaction cycling, alongside integrated reagent dispensing and waste handling systems. Portable sequencers, such as the Nanopore MinION, feature built-in environmental safeguards, including vibration damping, which facilitates real-time surveillance in field settings—proven effective during outbreaks like Ebola and COVID-19 [54].

## Software

Sequencing workflows are driven by layered bioinformatics systems, which manage the acquisition, processing, analysis of variants, and clinical interpretation of raw data [55]. These pipelines determine how efficiently and accurately genetic data is translated into clinically actionable insights.

### Primary Analysis

The initial phase involves basecalling, converting raw signal data into nucleotide sequences [56, 57]:

- Illumina's Real-Time Analysis (RTA) software transforms fluorescence images into FASTQ files.
- Oxford Nanopore's MinKNOW software interprets changes in ionic current to derive sequences in real-time. Key output metrics, such as Phred quality scores (Q-scores), read lengths, and total data yield, are generated during this stage.

Secondary Analysis

In this phase, raw reads are mapped to reference genomes and analyzed for sequence variation [58, 59]:

- BWA-MEM is a widely used algorithm for aligning reads to genomes like GRCh38.
- GATK (Genome Analysis Toolkit) identifies variants (SNPs, indels) with clinical-grade accuracy.
- Emerging approaches leverage machine learning, with tools like DeepVariant using deep neural networks to improve variant calling precision and sensitivity.

Tertiary Analysis and Clinical Interpretation

This stage translates genomic findings into clinical relevance. Annotation platforms match genetic variants to known functional or therapeutic implications [48, 51]:

- PharmCAT (Pharmacogenomic Clinical Annotation Tool) assesses genotypes for pharmacogenes such as CYP2C9, CYP2D6, and TPMT to guide medication dosing.
- In oncology, databases such as CIViC (Clinical Interpretation of Variants in Cancer) link somatic mutations to evidence-based treatments.
- Clinical platforms, such as Apollo and Translational Software, interface with electronic health records (EHRs), embedding decision support into the pharmacy and clinical workflow. For example, alerts regarding the warfarin-VKORC1 interaction allow pharmacists to adjust anticoagulant dosing safely based on patient-specific genotypes.

### *4.3.3 Types of Devices*

Sequencing instruments differ substantially in their underlying principles, throughput capacity, and clinical relevance. These technologies are commonly categorized into three generational tiers—first, second, and third—each representing a leap in sequencing methodology, speed, and clinical utility. Understanding the technical distinctions between these generations is crucial for selecting the most suitable platform based on diagnostic, research, or therapeutic needs.

#### **First-Generation Sequencers: Capillary Electrophoresis Systems**

The first generation of sequencing devices was built upon the Sanger method, a technique that dominated molecular biology for decades due to its accuracy. Devices such as the ABI 3730 DNA Analyzer employed capillary electrophoresis to determine nucleotide sequences with high fidelity. Despite their limited throughput and time-intensive workflows, these instruments remain in use for targeted applications such as single-gene testing, confirmatory analysis, and small-scale diagnostics [49]. Their enduring value lies in their precision, reproducibility, and established role in regulatory-compliant workflows.

### Second-Generation Sequencers: High-Throughput NGS Platforms

The advent of next-generation sequencing (NGS), often referred to as second-generation sequencing, has transformed genomics by enabling the parallel sequencing of millions of DNA fragments. This dramatically lowered the cost per base and shortened turnaround times.

- Illumina platforms (e.g., MiSeq, NextSeq, NovaSeq) dominate the NGS landscape. These systems employ a sequencing-by-synthesis method using fluorescently labeled nucleotides, which delivers high accuracy, scalability, and efficient data generation. They are widely used in oncology, pharmacogenomics, infectious disease diagnostics, and population genomics.
- Ion Torrent systems (e.g., Ion PGM, Ion S5) offer a semiconductor-based alternative, detecting pH changes during nucleotide incorporation. These platforms offer moderate throughput and fast runtime, making them suitable for smaller labs and time-sensitive applications.

The flexibility and precision of NGS platforms support clinical workflows ranging from panel-based testing (e.g., pharmacogenetic markers like CYP2C19 or TPMT) to whole-exome or whole-genome sequencing in complex diagnostic cases.

### Third-Generation Sequencers: Long-Read and Real-Time Technologies

Third-generation sequencing platforms introduced significant innovations by enabling the direct sequencing of native DNA or RNA molecules, often without the need for amplification [51, 60]. This improves the detection of structural variants, epigenetic modifications, and repetitive regions of the genome.

- Pacific Biosciences (PacBio) offers SMRT (Single Molecule Real-Time) sequencing, known for its long, highly accurate reads (HiFi reads), which are essential for genome assembly, isoform identification, and the analysis of repeat-rich regions.
- Oxford Nanopore Technologies developed highly portable and scalable platforms like MinION, GridION, and PromethION. These devices detect nucleotide sequences based on disruptions in electrical current as DNA or RNA strands pass through biological nanopores. They support real-time sequencing and are ideal for field diagnostics, outbreak surveillance, and metagenomic profiling.

These third-generation devices are rapidly advancing clinical research and are increasingly integrated into translational workflows due to their portability, adaptability, and minimal infrastructure requirements.

**Emerging and Compact Platforms**

New entrants into the sequencing market are designing systems with clinical efficiency and decentralized accessibility in mind. Companies such as GenapSys and Singular Genomics are developing benchtop and ultra-rapid sequencers designed for point-of-care use, small laboratories, and focused diagnostic applications [54]. These innovations reflect a broader movement toward democratizing sequencing, making it as ubiquitous as other routine diagnostic tools in clinical laboratories.

**Clinical Implications in Pharmacy Practice**

For pharmacy and clinical genomics, the expanding range of sequencing devices supports both targeted and comprehensive testing strategies:

- Pharmacogenetic applications: Next-generation sequencing (NGS) or capillary systems can be used to detect variants in genes such as VKORC1, CYP2C9, or SLCO1B1, informing drug dosing.
- Comprehensive genomic profiling: Long-read platforms can be utilized for assessing complex diseases, including the detection of oncogenic fusions or whole transcriptome analysis.

Selecting the most suitable sequencing platform, based on the clinical question, sample type, and turnaround time, is crucial for translating genomic data into actionable, patient-specific treatment plans [51]. The convergence of speed, accuracy, and adaptability ensures that sequencing will continue to be a central pillar of personalized medicine and pharmacy informatics.

## *4.3.4 Clinical Applications*

Over the past two decades, sequencing technologies have fundamentally reshaped clinical practice by enabling the use of genetic information in routine medical decision-making. Their clinical scope encompasses diagnostics, therapeutic guidance, disease surveillance, and public health interventions—roles that are increasingly central to modern healthcare and pharmacy practice [61]. In particular, sequencing data supports the advancement of personalized medicine and data-driven pharmacological strategies.

### Pharmacogenomics and Drug Response

One of the most transformative applications of sequencing lies in pharmacogenomics, where genomic information is used to predict an individual's response to specific medications. Variants in genes encoding drug-metabolizing enzymes—most notably the cytochrome P450 family (e.g., CYP2D6, CYP2C19, CYP2C9)—can significantly influence the absorption, metabolism, and elimination of drugs. By identifying such variants, sequencing enables clinicians to tailor drug selection and dosing for improved efficacy and minimized adverse reactions [62].

This is particularly critical for medications with narrow therapeutic windows—such as warfarin, clopidogrel, and tricyclic antidepressants—where slight variations in drug metabolism can result in significant clinical consequences. Incorporating pharmacogenomic data into prescribing practices enhances drug safety and therapeutic precision, thereby reducing the need for trial-and-error approaches in medication management.

### Oncology and Tumor Profiling

In oncology, next-generation sequencing (NGS) has become a cornerstone of precision medicine. Sequencing tumor DNA enables the identification of oncogenic drivers, including mutations, gene fusions, and copy number alterations that guide the selection of targeted therapies [63]. For example:

- EGFR mutations in non-small cell lung cancer predict sensitivity to tyrosine kinase inhibitors.
- BRAF V600E mutations in melanoma inform the use of BRAF-targeted treatments.

Sequencing also reveals biomarkers of resistance and provides prognostic information, enabling oncologists and clinical pharmacists to make informed therapeutic decisions, optimize treatment regimens, and monitor disease progression in real-time.

### Infectious Disease and Pathogen Surveillance

Sequencing plays a pivotal role in the diagnosis and monitoring of infectious diseases, particularly in identifying drug resistance genes and characterizing emerging variants. For instance:

- Whole genome sequencing of Mycobacterium tuberculosis allows rapid detection of resistance to first- and second-line antibiotics.
- During the COVID-19 pandemic, real-time genomic surveillance of SARS-CoV-2 variants informed public health policies, vaccine formulation, and transmission control strategies.

These capabilities support precision antimicrobial stewardship and outbreak management, enabling early detection of resistance patterns and informed intervention [64, 65].

#### Rare and Undiagnosed Genetic Disorders

In the diagnosis of rare diseases, particularly in pediatric and neonatal care, whole-exome sequencing (WES) and whole-genome sequencing (WGS) have become indispensable tools. When conventional diagnostics fail, these methods enable the identification of de novo mutations, complex structural variants, and multigenic syndromes that may otherwise go undetected. Early genetic diagnosis can significantly impact clinical outcomes by guiding appropriate treatment, reducing unnecessary testing, informing reproductive counseling, and enhancing the quality of life for patients and their families [66].

#### Integration with Pharmacy Informatics

From a pharmaceutical perspective, sequencing data is increasingly integrated into electronic health records (EHRs) and clinical decision support systems (CDSSs). These platforms:

- Automatically flag gene–drug interactions (e.g., SLCO1B1 and statins).
- Provide dose adjustment recommendations.
- Alert clinicians to contraindications based on individual genetic risk.

This integration enhances the pharmacist's ability to intervene proactively in medication management, thereby reducing the likelihood of adverse drug events [67]. However, it also requires careful consideration of data privacy, standardization, and interoperability, emphasizing the multidisciplinary nature of genomic medicine.

### *4.3.5 Regulatory Considerations*

The clinical implementation of sequencing technologies is governed by a complex and evolving regulatory landscape that ensures accuracy, patient safety, adherence to ethical standards, and data protection. As these technologies increasingly influence diagnostic and therapeutic decision-making, particularly in pharmacy and personalized medicine, adherence to regulatory requirements is crucial for maintaining clinical validity and public trust.

### Regulatory Oversight in the United States

In the United States, the Food and Drug Administration (FDA) oversees sequencing technologies used in clinical settings. Devices must be classified and approved either as medical devices or, when developed and used within a single certified laboratory, as laboratory-developed tests (LDTs). The FDA evaluates sequencing systems and associated assays based on:

- Analytical validity: The test's ability to accurately detect genetic variants.
- Clinical validity: The association between detected variants and specific health conditions or drug responses.
- Clinical utility: The test's potential to improve clinical outcomes and guide patient care.

Notable examples of FDA-approved next-generation sequencing (NGS) platforms include the FoundationOne CDx assay for oncology applications and Oncomine Dx by Thermo Fisher Scientific, both of which serve as companion diagnostics for targeted therapies. Additionally, laboratories conducting sequencing for clinical purposes must meet the Clinical Laboratory Improvement Amendments (CLIA) requirements, which establish quality standards for laboratory testing. CLIA compliance ensures reproducibility and reliability in test results, which is critical for informing therapeutic decisions. Furthermore, accreditation bodies such as the College of American Pathologists (CAP) enforce rigorous quality assurance through proficiency testing, personnel qualifications, and facility audits.

### Regulatory Framework in the European Union

In the European Union, sequencing devices and diagnostic assays are regulated under the In Vitro Diagnostic Regulation (IVDR), which replaced the previous In Vitro Diagnostic Medical Device Directive (IVDD) as of May 2022. IVDR mandates stricter classification of genetic tests based on risk stratification, requiring:

- Demonstration of scientific validity, analytical performance, and clinical performance
- Independent review of high-risk tests by Notified Bodies
- Implementation of post-market surveillance and robust quality management systems

IVDR aims to harmonize standards across EU member states and increase transparency in genetic diagnostics, especially in the context of cross-border healthcare and pan-European research collaborations.

### Data Privacy and Ethical Use

Sequencing technologies generate vast amounts of sensitive genomic data, not only identifying individuals but also implicating familial and ancestral relationships [62]. To safeguard personal and family genetic information:

- The General Data Protection Regulation (GDPR) in the EU establishes stringent guidelines for obtaining informed consent, minimizing data collection, anonymizing data, and limiting secondary use of genomic data.
- In the U.S., the Health Insurance Portability and Accountability Act (HIPAA) governs how genomic and health-related data are stored, transmitted, and accessed within healthcare institutions.

Both frameworks aim to protect individual privacy while supporting responsible data sharing for public health, research, and clinical development.

### Direct-to-Consumer (DTC) Genetic Testing

The proliferation of direct-to-consumer (DTC) genetic testing services, offered by companies such as 23andMe and AncestryDNA, has introduced new regulatory challenges. Although accessible, these tests often lack the clinical validation and interpretive oversight required for medical decision-making. Concerns include:

- Variable test accuracy and reproducibility
- Misinterpretation of genetic risk without healthcare guidance
- Inadequate data protection and unclear ownership of genomic information

Regulatory bodies are now working to define clear boundaries between consumer and clinical testing, ensuring that individuals receive accurate and medically actionable results when sequencing is used for health-related purposes.

### Clinical Decision Support and Software Regulation

As genomic data becomes embedded in clinical decision support systems (CDSSs)—including those used in pharmacy practice—these software tools are increasingly subject to regulation as Software as a Medical Device (SaMD). Under FDA and EU MDR/IVDR guidance, such platforms must:

- Demonstrate algorithmic transparency and clinical reliability
- Undergo validation studies for their intended use
- Be designed with robust cybersecurity and data integrity measures

For pharmacists who depend on CDSSs to evaluate drug–gene interactions, suggest dosing adjustments, and manage complex regimens, regulatory compliance ensures both legal accountability and clinical efficacy [45, 58].

### 4.3.6 *Future Perspectives*

The landscape of genomic sequencing is undergoing rapid evolution, with advances that point toward faster processing times, lower costs, broader clinical integration, and increased accessibility. As the cost of whole genome sequencing (WGS) continues to decline—approaching the widely anticipated $100 threshold—its incorporation into routine clinical care is no longer speculative but increasingly practical. This trajectory holds significant implications for the field of pharmacy, particularly in advancing data-driven, patient-specific therapeutic strategies.

#### Next-Generation Portability and Point-of-Care Use

Emerging ultra-portable sequencing platforms, such as Oxford Nanopore's MinION, are redefining the traditional confines of genomics. These compact devices enable real-time sequencing outside centralized laboratories, facilitating deployment in community pharmacies, rural clinics, emergency settings, and field-based public health operations. This shift toward point-of-care (POC) genomics enhances diagnostic speed and precision, particularly during infectious disease outbreaks or for on-the-spot pharmacogenetic testing [54]. The potential to rapidly profile patient genotypes on-site enables pharmacists to tailor drug regimens in real-time, significantly reducing therapeutic delays and adverse outcomes.

#### Integration of Artificial Intelligence in Genomic Interpretation

As sequencing technologies generate exponentially increasing volumes of data, artificial intelligence (AI) and machine learning (ML) are emerging as indispensable tools for interpretation. AI-driven platforms can detect complex patterns across genomic variants that may correlate with drug efficacy, toxicity risk, or disease predisposition—patterns often imperceptible to traditional bioinformatics pipelines. When integrated with electronic health records (EHRs) and clinical decision support systems (CDSSs), these algorithms can generate personalized medication recommendations, thereby enhancing the pharmacist's ability to deliver targeted therapies efficiently and safely [68].

#### Proactive Pharmacogenomics

The future of pharmacogenomics is poised to shift from a reactive model—applied after treatment failure or adverse events—to a proactive paradigm. Comprehensive preemptive genetic profiling may become part of standard health assessments, embedded in patients' digital health records. This would empower prescribers and pharmacists to select medications based on a patient's pharmacogenetic profile before treatment begins, optimizing therapy from the outset. As this becomes routine, pharmacists will play an increasingly central role in interpreting genomic information, counseling patients, and refining individualized drug regimens.

### Addressing Challenges: Data Privacy, Training, and Regulatory Convergence

The expansion of sequencing in clinical practice hinges on resolving several key challenges:

- Data privacy and security: Genomic data is profoundly personal and must be protected under stringent frameworks. Cross-platform data sharing necessitates encryption, access control, and adherence to privacy regulations (e.g., GDPR, HIPAA).
- Clinical integration: Sequencing must be seamlessly embedded into existing health infrastructures. This includes interoperability with Electronic Health Records (EHRs), integration into clinical workflows, and compatibility with Clinical Decision Support System (CDSS) interfaces.
- Workforce readiness: Pharmacists and other healthcare providers must be equipped with genomic literacy. This necessitates curriculum reforms in pharmacy and medical education to include genomic pharmacotherapy, bioinformatics, and ethical considerations.

### A Transformative Role for Sequencing in Pharmacy

The convergence of high-speed sequencing, AI, and personalized medicine is reshaping the pharmacist's role within the healthcare ecosystem [69]. Sequencing technologies will no longer be confined to specialized laboratories but will become routine instruments in everyday clinical decision-making. Soon, pharmacists may routinely conduct or interpret genomic tests to:

- Screen for drug–gene interactions
- Adjust dosage regimens based on metabolism profiles
- Prevent adverse drug reactions
- Monitor treatment response and resistance

As sequencing technologies mature and their integration into health systems becomes more seamless, they will enable pharmacists to offer precise, safe, and cost-effective care tailored to the genetic makeup of each individual.

## 4.4 Mass Spectrometry Devices

Mass spectrometry (MS) is a highly sensitive and versatile analytical technique used for both qualitative identification and quantitative measurement of a wide array of analytes with clinical relevance. When integrated with gas chromatography (GC) or liquid chromatography (LC), MS extends its utility to a broad spectrum of clinical, pharmaceutical, and biomedical applications. Among its most transformative roles, MS serves as a cornerstone in proteomics, enabling precise detection, quantification, and structural analysis of proteins and peptides [70].

At the core of MS is the measurement of the mass-to-charge ratio (m/z) of ions, where m refers to the molecular mass (typically in Daltons) and z represents the number of charges carried by the ion. For small molecules (<1000 Da), single-charged ions are typically observed, meaning the m/z value is numerically equivalent to the molecular mass. In contrast, larger biomolecules, such as peptides or intact proteins, often acquire multiple charges, resulting in m/z values that are fractional representations of their actual molecular masses.

The success of MS-based analysis is highly dependent on adequate sample preparation, especially in complex biological matrices commonly encountered in clinical settings. Sample preparation strategies may involve protein precipitation, centrifugation, filtration, solid-phase extraction, liquid-liquid extraction, affinity enrichment, or chemical derivatization [71]. Derivatization refers to the chemical modification of analytes to enhance their analytical properties, such as volatility, thermal stability, chromatographic retention, ionization efficiency, or fragmentation behavior, depending on the analytical objective [72].

Mass spectrometry functions by converting neutral molecules into charged ions, which are then manipulated using electric and magnetic fields for analysis. This process occurs across three key functional components:

- Ion Source: Where the analytes are ionized upon entry into the instrument.
- Mass Analyzer: Where ions are separated based on their m/z values.
- Detector: Where separated ions are measured and the resulting mass spectrum is recorded.

Ionization is the initial step in mass spectrometry (MS), in which molecules are given a positive charge by either removing an electron or adding a proton, depending on the ionization technique employed. These charged species often undergo fragmentation, and the resulting cationic fragments are guided into the mass analyzer, while neutral species are discarded or remain undetected within the system [73].

The mass spectrum produced is typically plotted with m/z values on the x-axis and relative ion abundance on the y-axis. The most abundant ion in a sample is termed the base peak, assigned a relative intensity of 100%. Other ion peaks are expressed relative to this standard. The molecular ion peak, also known as the parent peak, corresponds to the intact ionized molecule and directly reflects the sample's molecular mass [74]. For instance, hexane has a molecular weight of 86 g/mol; thus, an ion peak at m/z = 86 would represent its molecular ion. Isotopic variants, such as a $^{13}C$ isotope, produce an m + 1 peak observed at m/z = 87.

Before ionization, samples must be converted into an appropriate gaseous or liquid phase, typically using chromatographic separation, to enable efficient entry and processing within the mass spectrometer.

Gas Chromatography (GC) separates components of a gas mixture based on physical and chemical properties such as molecular weight, volatility, and boiling point. In GC, the sample is vaporized and passed through a chromatographic column, where molecules are separated as they interact differently with the stationary phase. Only compounds that can be volatilized without decomposition are suitable for GC-MS analysis. Once separated, the analytes are introduced into the mass spectrometer for further identification.

Liquid Chromatography (LC), in contrast, separates molecules based on their polarity and interaction with both the mobile and stationary phases. Components that differ significantly in polarity from the mobile phase will elute faster, forming distinct bands as they pass through the liquid chromatography (LC) column. These bands can then be analyzed by mass spectrometry [75]. Additional sample preparation and ionization techniques include:

- Fast Atom Bombardment (FAB): Generates ions from solid-phase samples using a high-energy neutral atom beam.
- Electrospray Ionization (ESI): Uses high voltage to produce charged droplets from liquid samples for mass spectrometric analysis.

Mass spectrometry can accommodate a diverse range of biomolecules, including proteins, lipids, fatty acids, and nucleic acids.

**Ionization**

Ionization is the process by which atoms or molecules gain a positive charge, forming cations suitable for mass spectrometric detection. Even molecules that are naturally uncharged or negatively charged (e.g., neon or fluoride) can be ionized in this way. Ionization typically involves an electric field that removes electrons or adds protons, generating ions that can then be analyzed [76, 77].

- Electron Ionization (EI) is widely used in GC/MS. A heated filament emits high-energy electrons (~70 eV), which bombard sample molecules, fragmenting them into predictable ion patterns that reflect molecular structure.
- LC/MS, in contrast, relies on soft ionization techniques such as:
  - Electrospray Ionization (ESI): High voltage is applied to a liquid stream exiting the chromatography column, producing charged microdroplets. As the solvent evaporates, ions transfer to the gas phase and enter the mass analyzer.
  - Atmospheric Pressure Chemical Ionization (APCI): Combines heat and corona discharge to ionize molecules in the gas phase via interactions with ionized solvent molecules.

Unlike the highly reproducible fragmentation patterns observed with EI, LC/MS ionization methods yield spectra with greater variability between instruments due to softer fragmentation and different ionization mechanisms.

**Ion Acceleration and Deflection**
After ionization, all cations must be accelerated to standard kinetic energy before entering the mass analyzer. Once accelerated, ions pass through slits that align them into a narrow beam directed into the analyzer. In the deflection stage, ions are bent by a magnetic or electric field based on their mass-to-charge ratio (m/z). Heavier ions or those with lower charge are deflected less, while lighter or more highly charged ions are deflected more. This separation enables precise calculation of m/z values [78, 79]. For example, a molecule with a mass of 120 Da and a charge of +3 would have an m/z value of 40. In most practical cases, ions bear a single positive charge (1+), meaning m/z is numerically equivalent to the molecular mass.

**Detection**
The detector in a mass spectrometer counts the number of ions at each m/z and produces a signal proportional to their abundance. Neutral species are excluded, either being evacuated by vacuum or ignored by the detection system. The electron multiplier is the most common detection mechanism. It consists of a cascade of dynodes with increasing electrical potential. Ions strike the first dynode, releasing secondary electrons that are accelerated to subsequent dynodes, creating an amplified signal [80]. This cascade enhances the signal by factors of up to $10^6$ or more.

**Vacuum Environment**
Mass spectrometry requires a high vacuum environment to minimize collisions between ions and neutral gas molecules. Operating at low pressure ensures that ions travel unimpeded through the analyzer and into the detector, thereby improving resolution and sensitivity.

However, interference can occur at multiple stages:

- Poor sample preparation.
- Cross-contamination.
- Improper chromatographic separation.
- Contaminants and isobaric ions in the sample matrix.

Such interferences can distort the mass spectrum, leading to inaccurate identification or quantification of target analytes. Rigorous quality control, calibration, and sample handling procedures are crucial for minimizing these effects.

### *4.4.1 History*

The origins of mass spectrometry trace back to the late nineteenth century, when scientists began exploring the behavior of charged particles. In 1898, German physicist Wilhelm Wien designed an apparatus that deflected ions using electric and magnetic fields, effectively creating a "velocity filter." This foundational concept—separating ions based on their mass-to-charge ratio (m/z)—became central to the future of mass spectrometric analysis.

In 1912, British physicist J.J. Thomson, renowned for discovering the electron, constructed the first true mass spectrograph. His device enabled the analysis of ionized atoms by simultaneously applying magnetic and electric forces, thereby revealing their mass-to-charge ratios. One of Thomson's most pivotal contributions was the discovery of neon isotopes, providing the first evidence that elements could exist in multiple atomic weight forms. This insight fundamentally changed atomic theory. Building upon this foundation, Francis W. Aston developed the first high-resolution mass spectrograph in the early 1920s. Aston's innovations enabled the precise measurement of atomic masses, leading to the discovery of numerous isotopes. His work earned him the Nobel Prize in Chemistry in 1922, solidifying mass spectrometry as a critical tool in both physics and chemistry. It is important to note that Aston's instrument remained a spectrograph, producing photographic records of ion separation, unlike the spectrometer, which converts ion signals into electronic data.

Advancements accelerated in the 1930s and 1940s. Arthur Jeffrey Dempster (1918) and Kenneth Bainbridge (1930s) developed more refined mass spectrometers capable of highly accurate mass determinations. These instruments played crucial roles in nuclear physics and isotope separation, particularly during World War II, when the Manhattan Project utilized mass spectrometry to separate uranium isotopes. The postwar era witnessed a surge in technological progress, driven by both military and industrial demands. The development of quadrupole mass filters in the 1950s introduced a compact and durable method for ion filtering based on oscillating electric fields. These remain a staple in many modern analytical platforms [81].

In the 1960s, Time-of-Flight (TOF) analyzers emerged, measuring the time it takes ions to reach a detector—an approach where lighter ions arrive at the detector faster than heavier ones. The following decades saw breakthroughs such as:

- Ion Trap technologies and
- Fourier Transform Ion Cyclotron Resonance (FT-ICR) in the 1970s and 1980s, which dramatically enhanced mass resolution and detection sensitivity.

Simultaneously, progress in computational analysis allowed faster data interpretation and expanded the utility of mass spectrometry in environmental science, organic chemistry, and natural products research.

One of the most transformative milestones was the invention of soft ionization techniques, which enabled the analysis of large and fragile biomolecules without extensive fragmentation:

- Electrospray Ionization (ESI), pioneered by John Fenn, facilitated the gentle ionization of proteins and macromolecules.
- Matrix-Assisted Laser Desorption/Ionization (MALDI), developed by Koichi Tanaka and colleagues, further expanded this capability to include polymers and peptides. Both Fenn and Tanaka were recognized with a share of the 2002 Nobel Prize in Chemistry for their contributions.

These breakthroughs established mass spectrometry as a cornerstone of proteomics, genomics, and drug discovery. Today, the technique is integral to a wide range of fields, including:

- Forensic science
- Environmental monitoring
- Clinical diagnostics
- Biomedical research

Modern mass spectrometers are highly specialized, ranging from benchtop instruments to portable field devices, and from high-throughput screening systems to ultra-high resolution analyzers. This diversity continues to grow, reflecting the ever-expanding role of mass spectrometry in contemporary science and medicine (Fig. 4.5).

### 4.4.2 *Technical Characteristics*

This section focuses on the technical components of the MALDI (Matrix-Assisted Laser Desorption/Ionization) mass spectrometer, a widely used platform for analyzing large macromolecules, particularly in biomedical research and clinical diagnostics.

#### Hardware

In MALDI mass spectrometry, the analyte is mixed with an excess of a suitable organic matrix and spotted onto a metal target plate. The mixture dries at room temperature to form a crystalline solid solution. Upon exposure to nanosecond laser pulses—commonly from UV nitrogen lasers (337 nm)—the matrix absorbs the energy, facilitating the desorption and ionization of the analyte.

The matrix absorbs the laser energy, leading to rapid heating and sublimation. This causes the co-crystallized analyte molecules to ionize. Ion formation occurs either via protonation (M+H)+ in positive ion mode or deprotonation (M−H)− in negative ion mode. Additionally, small ions such as $Na^+$, $K^+$, or ammonium present

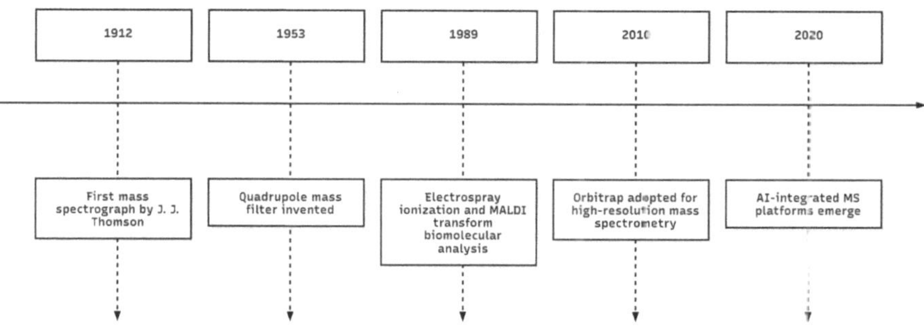


**Fig. 4.5** Timeline of the historical development of mass spectrometry

in the solution may contribute to analyte ionization. For optimal performance, the MALDI matrix must:

- Be a non-volatile solid with an aromatic structure to absorb laser energy efficiently
- Promote efficient energy transfer with minimal analyte degradation
- Be chemically inert and stable under vacuum conditions

Typical matrix-to-analyte ratios range between 100:1 and 1000:1. Common sample preparation techniques include dried droplet, fast evaporation, and repeated stacking. To improve ion yield and analytical sensitivity, methods such as air-pressure matrix-assisted laser desorption/ionization (AP-MALDI) and liquid AP-MALDI have been developed. For instance, AP-MALDI has been successfully used to distinguish goat and sheep milk samples with high accuracy. Once ionized, analyte molecules are transferred electrostatically into the mass analyzer [82]. Several types of analyzers can be used in conjunction with MALDI, each offering distinct advantages. Among them:

- Time-of-Flight (ToF) analyzers: Measure the ion travel time to determine the m/z ratio. Reflectron and orthogonal acceleration modes enhance resolution, often achieving resolutions of 10,000 or higher.
- Quadrupole Ion Traps and Orbitraps: Offer high resolution and are helpful for complex biological analyses.
- FT-ICR (Fourier Transform Ion Cyclotron Resonance): Provides ultra-high mass accuracy.
- Hybrid Systems: Instruments such as Time-of-Flight (ToF)/ToF and quadrupole-Orbitrap combine multiple analyzers for accurate precursor and product ion measurements.

These analyzers have enabled MALDI to achieve sensitivity ranging from picomoles to femtomoles, which is critical for proteomics, metabolomics, and clinical applications.

## Software

Two primary MALDI-TOF MS identification systems are widely used for microbial diagnostics:

- MALDI Biotyper (Bruker Daltonics)
- VITEK® MS (bioMérieux)

While both platforms operate on similar mass spectrometric principles, they differ in database structures and algorithm design. The MALDI Biotyper reports scores from 0 to 3.0:

- 2.0: Species-level identification
- 1.7–2.0: Genus-level identification
- <1.7: Unreliable match

Conversely, the VITEK® MS system outputs a confidence percentage. Scores close to 99% represent high-confidence identifications, whereas values below 60% indicate unidentified organisms. MALDI-TOF has been especially successful in identifying yeast species. However, its application to filamentous fungi and dermatophytes remains limited due to insufficient database entries and challenges in sample preparation. Many misidentifications stem from incomplete or low-quality reference spectra. To improve fungal species identification, enhancements in sample preparation protocols and database enrichment are essential [83, 84]. When MALDI-TOF and biochemical methods fail to yield conclusive results, full-length 16S rRNA gene sequencing is often used as a confirmatory approach. These hardware and software integrations make MALDI-TOF MS a robust, rapid, and accurate platform for identifying a wide range of microorganisms and biomolecules, reinforcing its value in both clinical and research laboratories [85].

### *4.4.3 Types of Devices*

Mass spectrometry devices exist in a wide array of configurations, each optimized for specific analytical tasks involving diverse molecular types—from proteins and amino acids to small organic and inorganic compounds. Although the underlying principle of ion generation, separation, and detection remains consistent across platforms, the choice of instrument depends heavily on the nature of the sample, analytical goals, budget, and operational requirements. Some instruments are optimized for the analysis of organic molecules, such as peptides and metabolites, while others are suited for the elemental analysis of inorganic substances [86–88]. Factors such as instrument sensitivity, resolution, speed, and maintenance requirements also significantly influence the selection process.

#### Time-of-Flight (TOF) Analyzers

TOF analyzers measure the time it takes for ions to travel from the ionization source to the detector. Since lighter ions travel faster than heavier ones, the arrival times correspond to specific mass-to-charge (m/z) ratios. TOF systems are widely used in microbiology and clinical diagnostics, particularly when combined with MALDI (Matrix-Assisted Laser Desorption/Ionization). TOF analyzers are valued for their high speed, broad mass range, and compatibility with soft ionization techniques.

#### MALDI-TOF Systems

These systems couple MALDI with TOF detection, enabling rapid and high-throughput analysis of biomolecules. MALDI selectively ionizes analytes using a laser-absorbing matrix, and TOF subsequently measures ion flight time. These systems are broadly adopted in clinical microbiology, proteomics, and pharmaceutical research due to their speed, reliability, and ease of operation.

#### Quadrupole Mass Analyzers

Quadrupole devices utilize oscillating electric fields generated by four parallel rods to filter ions of a specific m/z ratio selectively. They are widely used in routine pharmaceutical and biochemical applications due to their low cost, robustness, and ease of integration with liquid or gas chromatography systems.

#### Ion Trap Mass Spectrometers

Ion traps create electric fields that confine ions in a small space, allowing them to be selectively ejected and detected. These instruments are beneficial for analyzing peptides and small biomolecules. They are user-friendly and offer capabilities for tandem mass spectrometry (MS/MS), which enables the structural elucidation of compounds.

#### Orbitrap Mass Analyzers

Orbitrap instruments utilize a central electrode around which ions orbit. The frequency of ion oscillation depends on their m/z ratio, allowing for highly accurate mass determination. These systems are renowned for their exceptional resolution and mass accuracy, making them ideal for proteomics and the analysis of complex mixtures.

#### Fourier Transform Ion Cyclotron Resonance (FT-ICR)

FT-ICR instruments trap ions in a magnetic field and excite them using radiofrequency pulses. The ions' cyclotron frequencies are detected and translated into mass spectra using Fourier transform techniques. FT-ICR provides unparalleled resolving power and accuracy, though it is among the most expensive and technically demanding platforms.

#### Triple Quadrupole Mass Spectrometers

This system comprises three quadrupole units: the first filters the precursor ions, the second serves as a collision cell to generate fragments, and the third analyzes the product ions. Triple quadrupoles are extensively used in clinical research, pharmacokinetics, toxicology, and food safety due to their speed, specificity, and quantitative precision.

#### Magnetic Sector Instruments

These devices generate a magnetic field to deflect ions based on their m/z ratio. The extent of deflection depends on both mass and charge, enabling precise mass analysis. While older in design, magnetic sector instruments are still valued for their accuracy and are used in specialized applications such as isotope ratio analysis. Each type of mass spectrometer brings specific strengths to clinical diagnostics, pharmaceutical research, proteomics, metabolomics, and forensic science. Matching the device's capabilities to the analytical question is crucial to obtaining reliable, actionable data.

### 4.4.4 Clinical Applications

Mass spectrometry (MS) has evolved into a cornerstone analytical technique across numerous scientific and clinical domains, including metabolomics, proteomics, pharmacology, forensic science, environmental monitoring, and biopharmaceutical research. Its versatility stems from the ability to provide both qualitative and quantitative insights into a wide range of analytes, from small metabolites to complex macromolecules [89].

#### Disease Diagnosis Through Biomarker Detection

One of the most impactful uses of MS in clinical medicine is the detection and quantification of biomarkers—molecular indicators of physiological and pathological states. Mass spectrometry enables the high-precision measurement of biomarkers across various biological matrices, including blood, urine, saliva, sweat, and skin secretions.

For example, elevated serum amylase is a diagnostic marker for pancreatitis, while B-type natriuretic peptides (BNPs) are used to monitor heart failure and predict patient prognosis. In pharmacology, MS is used to assess drug metabolism profiles, providing feedback on therapeutic efficacy and dosing optimization. When coupled with liquid chromatography (LC-MS) or gas chromatography (GC-MS), mass spectrometry (MS) enhances both specificity and sensitivity, enabling the analysis of complex biological samples with high resolution [90, 91]. These technologies facilitate comparative proteomics, where changes in the proteome between healthy and diseased states can be systematically quantified using isotope-labeled spectral tags. In lipidomics, MS supports the profiling of lipid species, shedding light on metabolic disorders and endocrine dysregulation by mapping lipid oxidation products and signaling molecules.

#### COVID-19 Diagnostics

During the COVID-19 pandemic, mass spectrometry emerged as a valuable tool for virus detection, particularly in the face of global supply shortages of diagnostic kits. Clinical laboratories have developed protocols to analyze nasal swab samples using MS, with the resulting spectral patterns used to distinguish between patients with SARS-CoV-2-positive and negative results [48]. This approach provided a rapid, accurate, and scalable alternative during periods of testing scarcity.

#### Pharmaceutical and Drug Monitoring

In pharmaceutical sciences, MS is indispensable for drug discovery, quality control, and therapeutic monitoring. The ionization capabilities of MS enable precise molecular identification, facilitating pharmacokinetic studies, impurity profiling, and the real-time assessment of drug levels in patient samples. This improves drug safety and efficacy, especially for medications with narrow therapeutic indices [47, 92]. Triple quadrupole and high-resolution mass analyzers are commonly used for these applications, supporting high-throughput drug screening, metabolite identification, and compliance with regulatory standards.

#### Glycomics: Analysis of Glycans

Mass spectrometry plays a pivotal role in characterizing glycans, complex oligosaccharides formed through glycosidic linkages. Unlike proteins and nucleic acids, glycans exhibit extensive structural diversity, with variations in monosaccharide sequence, branching, and stereochemistry. MS enables the determination of glycan composition, isomer position, linkage orientation, and branching architecture. These insights are critical in fields such as vaccine development, cancer diagnostics, and therapeutic antibody design, where glycosylation patterns influence biological activity.

#### Oligonucleotide Characterization

Oligonucleotides, including DNA and RNA, often undergo natural and synthetic modifications that affect their structure and function. MS offers high-resolution detection of these modifications, allowing researchers to determine sequence integrity, molecular weight, and structural variants. This is particularly valuable in epigenetics, RNA therapeutics, and gene editing technologies, where modified nucleotides play crucial roles in gene expression and cellular function.

#### Environmental and Forensic Applications

Mass spectrometry extends beyond healthcare into environmental science and forensic analysis. In environmental testing, MS is used for:

- Detection of pesticide and herbicide residues
- Trace-level analysis of heavy metals and soil contaminants
- Monitoring of air and water pollution
- Evaluation of carbon emissions and isotope ratios

In forensic science, MS is integral for:

- Identifying narcotics, explosives, and accelerants in criminal investigations
- Analyzing trace materials like paint chips, textile fibers, or biological fluids
- Confirming substance abuse and toxicological profiles in postmortem samples

### 4.4.5 Regulatory Considerations

Mass spectrometry-based laboratory-developed tests (LDTs), particularly those utilizing liquid chromatography–tandem mass spectrometry (LC-MS/MS), are subject to evolving regulatory frameworks aimed at ensuring analytical accuracy, clinical validity, and patient safety.

#### U.S. Regulatory Landscape

In the United States, the Food and Drug Administration (FDA) defines an LDT as "an in vitro diagnostic (IVD) test that is designed, manufactured, and used within a single laboratory". While most IVDs are regulated as medical devices under the Federal Food, Drug, and Cosmetic Act (FFDCA) and the 1976 Medical Device Amendments (MDA), laboratory-developed tests (LDTs) have historically been subject to a regulatory gray area. In 1992, the FDA adopted a policy of enforcement discretion, choosing not to regulate LDTs despite their classification under the MDA actively. This approach remained in place until 2014, when the FDA issued draft guidance proposing more rigorous oversight, including premarket review and the eventual phase-out of enforcement discretion. However, regulatory authority over laboratory practices is primarily exercised through the Clinical Laboratory Improvement Amendments of 1988 (CLIA'88), which are administered by the Centers for Medicare & Medicaid Services (CMS).

Under CLIA, LDTs do not require FDA approval; however, they must meet specific quality standards, particularly in areas such as personnel qualifications, test validation, and quality assurance. For LC-MS/MS LDTs, accreditation organizations with deemed status under CLIA, such as the College of American Pathologists (CAP), may impose additional validation requirements. One such example is CAP's matrix effect validation for LC-MS/MS assays, ensuring test performance in real patient samples rather than simplified reference matrices.

### Clinical Necessity and Superiority of LC-MS/MS

The clinical justification for LC-MS/MS-based LDTs is often tied to their superior analytical specificity and accuracy compared to immunoassays (IAs), especially in the detection of low-concentration analytes [93]. For instance:

- Low-level testosterone is frequently over- or under-estimated by IA, while LC-MS/MS provides reliable quantification.
- Aldosterone levels in chronic kidney disease patients may be significantly overestimated by IA but remain accurate using LC-MS/MS.
- Thyroglobulin (Tg) measurement in the presence of autoantibodies—a key marker for thyroid cancer monitoring—is compromised by IA but not by LC-MS/MS.

Commercial FDA-cleared tests are often unavailable for niche targets, new compounds, or low-volume assays, particularly in therapeutic drug monitoring or oncology. LC-MS/MS enables laboratories to rapidly develop and validate such assays in-house, ensuring timely and clinically relevant results.

### Industry Limitations and Justification for Local Validation

Despite its advantages, LC-MS/MS assays are rarely offered as FDA-approved kits. Vendors may supply LC systems, mass spectrometers, and general protocols, but typically do not provide complete, validated methods. Moreover, these vendor-developed methods are often optimized using artificial or simplified matrices and do not account for endogenous interferences found in actual clinical samples. This underscores the need for site-specific validation—a process ensuring each laboratory independently verifies accuracy, precision, and reliability using native patient matrices. CAP has provided clear guidance on matrix effect testing, which should be considered a minimum requirement for all quantitative LC-MS/MS LDTs used in clinical care.

### Toward Standardized High-Quality Validation

To ensure consistency across clinical laboratories—including academic centers, hospital laboratories, outpatient clinics, and reference laboratories—a more uniform set of validation criteria is necessary. At a minimum, this should include:

- Matrix effect evaluation using real patient samples
- Defined minimums for precision, accuracy, and method comparison studies
- Multiple-day reproducibility testing
- Justification for acceptance criteria when deviating from established norms

As emphasized by experts in clinical mass spectrometry, such as Dr. Russell Grant, inadequate validation increases the likelihood of false or misleading results, potentially leading to treatment errors, method redevelopments, or regulatory non-compliance.

### 4.4.6 Future Perspectives

The growing recognition of mass spectrometry imaging (MSI) as a powerful tool for spatially resolved molecular analysis has led to rapid advancements and increased adoption across diverse scientific and clinical disciplines. Unlike conventional imaging methods, MSI enables the simultaneous detection of thousands of biomolecules—such as metabolites, lipids, and proteins—directly from tissue surfaces without the need for molecular tags or labeling. This makes MSI an increasingly attractive complement or alternative to existing histological and molecular imaging techniques. Despite its potential, several challenges remain. A critical issue is the lack of standardized protocols for sample preparation, which can significantly affect data quality and reproducibility. Although recent studies have attempted to address inter-laboratory variability, consistent and universally accepted guidelines for sample handling, matrix application, and acquisition parameters are still lacking. Establishing robust quality control frameworks is essential for translating MSI into routine diagnostic and biomedical research workflows.

A parallel trend in MSI development is the drive toward enhanced spatial resolution, which is crucial for subcellular and single-cell-level investigations. Submicrometer spatial resolution is now being approached with advanced instrumentation and beam-focusing technologies. Additionally, the emergence of 3D MSI, which involves serial sectioning and volumetric reconstruction, has exponentially increased the amount of data generated per experiment. This shift demands sophisticated data analysis infrastructures capable of handling terabyte-scale datasets while preserving spectral fidelity and spatial coherence [94]. To meet these demands, there is an urgent need for more scalable, interoperable, and user-friendly computational tools. Open-source platforms have made substantial contributions in this area, yet many still require expert knowledge for practical use. Ideally, future software solutions should support modular integration of diverse analytical tools into cohesive pipelines, allowing researchers to customize workflows for specific MSI modalities or research questions. Simplifying quantitative analysis and visualization will be crucial to enabling widespread adoption by non-specialist users in clinical environments.

The integration of artificial intelligence (AI) and machine learning (ML) in MSI analysis is another area of rapid development. However, variability in experimental conditions—such as ionization methods, detector sensitivity, and instrument configurations—poses significant barriers to developing generalized AI models. Adopting standardized data formats, including comprehensive metadata annotations (e.g., mass analyzer type, resolution settings), is a foundational step toward building interoperable AI frameworks [95]. There is growing recognition of the need for benchmark datasets and standardized evaluation protocols to allow meaningful comparisons between AI models across different MSI platforms. Transparent models that offer interpretability—such as confidence scoring, feature importance mapping, and uncertainty quantification—will improve user trust and regulatory acceptance. Techniques such as transfer learning and active learning offer promising solutions to the challenge of limited annotated datasets, enabling AI models to generalize from smaller or more heterogeneous training data. Advanced neural architectures such as convolutional neural networks (CNNs) and recurrent neural networks (RNNs) are increasingly applied to MSI data for segmentation, classification, and molecular feature extraction. These models have demonstrated the potential to support automated biomarker discovery, spatially resolved disease classification, and tissue phenotype prediction at molecular resolution. Looking forward, the routine clinical integration of MSI will depend on parallel progress in the following domains:

- Optimization of sample preparation and matrix application for reproducibility
- Enhancement of instrumental throughput and spatial resolution
- Development of cloud-compatible, AI-integrated software pipelines
- Establishment of interoperable standards for data structure, metadata, and validation

## References

1. Cao H, Oghenemaro EF, Latypova A, Abosaoda MK, Zaman GS, Devi A. Advancing clinical biochemistry: addressing gaps and driving future innovations. Front Med. 2025;12:1521126.
2. Park J, Han DH, Park JK. Towards practical sample preparation in point-of-care testing: user-friendly microfluidic devices. Lab Chip. 2020;20(7):1191–203.
3. Naphade M, Ankur PS, Rajendra SR. Quality control in clinical biochemistry laboratory – a glance. J Clin Diagn Res. 2023;17(2).
4. Berger D. A brief history of medical diagnosis and the birth of the clinical laboratory. Part 1—ancient times through the 19th century. MLO Med Lab Obs. 1999;31(7):28–30.
5. Song XD, Li SX, Qin ZM, Chen DL, Guo LL, Liu CR, Dai EH. Ensure the accuracy and consistency of biochemical analyzer test results: chemometrics for instrument and inter-instrument item comparison in Chinese hospital laboratory. Heliyon. 2024;10(1).
6. Nazir S, Farooq M, Khan R, Khan AU, Husnain A, Hassan MA, Neubauer H. Comparative evaluation of diagnostic tests for brucellosis in humans and animals: a meta-analytical approach. Vet Sci. 2025;12(7):638.
7. Plebani M. Errors in clinical laboratories or errors in laboratory medicine? Clin Chem Lab Med. 2006;44(6):750–9.

8. World Health Organization. Report on laboratory automation. WHO; 2011.
9. Lippi G, Jackson B, Plebani M. Improving diagnosis in health care: laboratory medicine. Diagnosis. 2025;12(4):570–7.
10. Nam Y, Park HD. Revolutionizing laboratory practices: pioneering trends in total laboratory automation. Ann Lab Med. 2025;45(5):472–83.
11. Al Naam YA, Elsafi S, Al Jahdali MH, Al Shaman RS, Al-Qurouni BH, Al Zahrani EM. The impact of total automation on the clinical laboratory workforce: a case study. J Healthc Leadersh. 2022;55–62.
12. Sachdeva S, Davis RW, Saha AK. Microfluidic point-of-care testing: commercial landscape and future directions. Front Bioeng Biotechnol. 2021;8:602659.
13. Sackmann EK, Fulton AL, Beebe DJ. The present and future role of microfluidics in biomedical research. Nature. 2014;507(7491):181–9.
14. Plebani M, Nichols JH, Luppa PB, Greene D, Sciacovelli L, Shaw J, Lippi G. Point-of-care testing: state-of-the-art and perspectives. Clin Chem Lab Med. 2025;63(1):35–51.
15. De Olazarra AS, Wang SX. Advances in point-of-care genetic testing for personalized medicine applications. Biomicrofluidics. 2023;17(3).
16. Wang XY, Zhang F, Zhang C, Zheng LR, Yang J. The biomarkers for acute myocardial infarction and heart failure. Biomed Res Int. 2020;2020(1):2018035.
17. Raja Aljehani M, Mohammed Terkustani W, Oqla Alahmadi N, Hamad Abdulrahim Alamri M, Abdulfttah Abulula N, Ahmed Alqarni K, Mansour Basaid B. Clinical applications of laboratory chemistry in early detection of metabolic and endocrine disorders. Egypt J Chem. 2025;68(12):35–40.
18. Chume FC, Schiavenin LG, Freitas PAC, Pimentel AL, Camargo JL. The usefulness of glycated albumin in patients with diabetes and renal disease: a scoping review. J Lab Precis Med. 2022;7:12.
19. Zhang H, Xu B, Lai NS. Recent progress on the application of biosensors in biomechanics for the early detection of infectious diseases. Mol Cell Biomech. 2025;22(3).
20. Mejia-Salazar JR, Rodrigues Cruz K, Materon Vasques EM, Novais de Oliveira Jr O. Microfluidic point-of-care devices: new trends and future prospects for e-health diagnostics. Sensors. 2020;20(7):1951.
21. U.S. Food and Drug Administration (FDA). Clinical Chemistry and Clinical Toxicology Devices Panel: Regulatory guidance and review considerations. FDA; 2023.
22. European Union. Regulation (EU) 2017/746 on in vitro diagnostic medical devices (IVDR). Off J Eur Union. 2017.
23. International Organization for Standardization (ISO). ISO 13485:2016 – Medical devices — Quality management systems — Requirements for regulatory purposes. ISO; 2016.
24. Martelli E, Capoccia L, Di Francesco M, Cavallo E, Pezzulla MG, Giudice G, Panagrosso M. Current applications and future perspectives of artificial and biomimetic intelligence in vascular surgery and peripheral artery disease. Biomimetics. 2024;9(8):465.
25. Li G, Wen D. Wearable biochemical sensors for human health monitoring: sensing materials and manufacturing technologies. J Mater Chem B. 2020;8(16):3423–36.
26. Sengupta J, Hussain CM. Graphene and its derivatives for analytical lab on chip platforms. TrAC Trends Anal Chem. 2019;114:326–37.
27. Bartlett JM, Stirling D, editors. PCR protocols. Humana Press; 2003;226:3–525.
28. Mullis KB, Faloona FA. Specific synthesis of DNA in vitro via a polymerase-catalyzed chain reaction. Methods Enzymol. 1987;155:335–50.
29. Mullis K. The unusual origin of the polymerase chain reaction. Sci Am. 1990;262:56–65.
30. Saiki RK, et al. Primer-directed enzymatic amplification of DNA with a thermostable DNA polymerase. Science. 1988;239:487–91.
31. Green MR, Sambrook J. Molecular cloning: a laboratory manual. 4th ed. Cold Spring Harbor Laboratory Press; 2012;4.
32. Brown TA. Gene cloning and DNA analysis: an introduction. 2016;65–80.

33. Huggett JF, Garson JA, Whale AS. Digital PCR and its potential application to microbiology. Molecular Microbiology: Diagnostic Principles and Practice. ASM Press; 2016;49–57.
34. Bustin SA, Nolan T. Pitfalls of quantitative real-time reverse-transcription polymerase chain reaction. J Biomol Tech. 2004;15(3):155.
35. Mackay IM, Arden KE, Nitsche A. Real-time PCR in virology. Nucleic Acids Res. 2002;30:1292.
36. Deumić S, Lavić A, Crnčević N, Pramenković E, Deumić A. Biosensor for rapid methods for the detection of viruses. Mediterranean Conference on Medical and Biological Engineering and Computing. 2023;423–9.
37. Lay MJ, Wittwer CT. Real-time fluorescence genotyping of factor V Leiden during rapid-cycle PCR. Clin Chem. 1997;43(12):2262–7.
38. Kubista M, Andrade JM, Bengtsson M, Forootan A, Jonák J, Lind K, Zoric N. The real-time polymerase chain reaction. Mol Aspects Med. 2006;27(2–3):95–125.
39. Higuchi R, Fockler C, Dollinger G, Watson R. Kinetic PCR analysis: real-time monitoring of DNA amplification reactions. Bio/technology. 1993;11(9):1026–30.
40. Bio-Rad Laboratories. PCR technology guide. PCR Applications and Workflow Reference Manual. Bio-Rad; 2023.
41. Shen HH, Fan SK, Kim CJ, Yao DJ. EWOD microfluidic systems for biomedical applications. Microfluid Nanofluid. 2014;16(5):965–87.
42. World Health Organization. Molecular assays for COVID-19 diagnostics: policy brief. WHO; 2020.
43. U.S. Food and Drug Administration (FDA). Guidance for industry and FDA staff: In vitro diagnostic (IVD) device studies—design, documentation, and reporting. FDA; 2017.
44. Badnjević A, Pokvić LG, Hasičić M, Bandić L, Mašetić Z, Kovačević Ž, Pecchia L. Evidence-based clinical engineering: machine learning algorithms for prediction of defibrillator performance. Biomed Signal Process Control. 2019;54:101629.
45. Badnjević A, Pokvić LG, Deumić A. Post-market surveillance of medical devices: a review. Technol Health Care. 2022;30:1315–29.
46. Kovačević Ž, Gurbeta Pokvić L, Spahić L, Badnjević A. Prediction of medical device performance using machine learning techniques: infant incubator case study. Health Technol. 2020;10(1):151–5.
47. Peruničić Ž, Lalatović I, Spahić L, Ašić A, Pokvić LG, Badnjević A. Enhancing mechanical ventilator reliability through machine learning based predictive maintenance. Technol Health Care. 2025;33(3):1288–97.
48. Badnjević A, Pokvić LG, Smajlhodžić-Deljo M, Spahić L, Bego T, Meseldžić N, Bedak O. Application of artificial intelligence for the classification of the clinical outcome and therapy in patients with viral infections: the case of COVID-19. Technol Health Care. 2024;32(3):1859–70.
49. Zeeshan F, Razzak S. Next generation sequencing and its role in clinical microbiology and molecular epidemiology. Ann Jinnah Sindh Med Univ. 2020;6(1):31–2.
50. Bhat AI, Rao GP. Next-generation sequencing for diagnosis of viruses. Characterization of Plant Viruses: Methods and Protocols. 2020;389–95.
51. Zhong Y, Xu F, Wu J, Schubert J, Li MM. Application of next generation sequencing in laboratory medicine. Ann Lab Med. 2021;41(1):25–43.
52. Kathiresan N, Ramachandran S, Kulanthaivel L. Next-generation sequencing to study the DNA interaction. Reverse Engineering of Regulatory Networks. 2023;249–64.
53. Hess JF, Kotrová M, Calabrese S, Darzentas N, Hutzenlaub T, Zengerle R, Paust N. Automation of amplicon-based library preparation for next-generation sequencing by centrifugal microfluidics. Anal Chem. 2020;92(19):12833–41.
54. Satam H, Joshi K, Mangrolia U, Waghoo S, Zaidi G, Rawool S, Malonia SK. Next-generation sequencing technology: current trends and advancements. Biology. 2023;12(7):997.
55. Bhaskaran S, Saikumar C. A review of next generation sequencing methods and its applications in laboratory diagnosis. J Pure Appl Microbiol. 2022;16(2).

56. Ferros AE, Ray A, Raj A. Next-generation sequencing and its data analysis. Information Technology & Bioinformatics: International Conference on Advance IT, Engineering and Management (SACAIM). 2022;1:196.
57. Hrvat F, Spahić L, Pokvić LG, Badnjević A. Artificial neural networks for prediction of medical device performance based on conformity assessment data: infusion and perfusor pumps case study. 2020 9th Mediterranean Conference on Embedded Computing (MECO). 2020;1–4. IEEE.
58. Mittal S, Jena MK, Pathak B. Machine learning empowered next generation DNA sequencing: perspective and prospectus. Chem Sci. 2024;15:12169–88.
59. Spahić L, Sredović U, Kurpejović Z, Mrdanović E, Pokvić G, Badnjević A. Machine learning for improved medical device management: a focus on infant incubators. Technol Health Care. 2025;33:2034–40.
60. Badnjevic A, Spahic L, Jordamovic NB, Pokvic LG. A novel method for conformity assessment testing of infant incubators for post-market surveillance purposes. Technol Health Care. 2023;31(1):389–9.
61. Hilt EE, Ferrieri P. Next generation and other sequencing technologies in diagnostic microbiology and infectious diseases. Genes. 2022;13(9):1566.
62. Zhou Y, Lauschke VM. Challenges related to the use of next-generation sequencing for the optimization of drug therapy. Precision Medicine. 2022;237–60.
63. Nair SV, Madhulaxmi T, Thomas G, Ankathil R. Next-generation sequencing in cancer. J Maxillofac Oral Surg. 2021;20(3):340–4.
64. Khan S, ul Hasnain MJ, Pervez MT, Hussain T, Maqsood K. Next-generation sequencing in clinical virology: a review of its applications. Pure Appl Biol. 2020;9(4):2356–60.
65. Badnjević A, Pokvić LG, Džemić Z, Bečić F. Risks of emergency use authorizations for medical products during outbreak situations: a COVID-19 case study. BioMed Eng OnLine. 2020;19:75.
66. Edward P, Handel AS. Metagenomic next-generation sequencing for infectious disease diagnosis: a review of the literature with a focus on pediatrics. J Pediatric Infect Dis Soc. 2021;10(Suppl 4):S71–S77.
67. Pokvić LG, Deumić A, Lutovac B, Badnjević A. Possibility of managing medical device post-market surveillance using artificial intelligence and standardized methodology. 2021 10th Mediterranean Conference on Embedded Computing (MECO). 2021;1–4. IEEE.
68. Spahić L, Softić A, Durak-Nalbantić A, Begić E, Stanetić B, Vranić H. Integrating machine learning in clinical decision support for heart failure diagnosis: case study. Mediterranean Conference on Medical and Biological Engineering and Computing. 2023;696–705. Springer Nature Switzerland.
69. Liu Y, Ma Y. Clinical applications of metagenomics next-generation sequencing in infectious diseases. J Zhejiang Univ Sci B. 2024;25:471–84.
70. Matthiesen R, Bunkenborg J. Introduction to mass spectrometry-based proteomics. Mass Spectrometry Data Analysis in Proteomics. 2013;1–45.
71. Urban PL. Quantitative mass spectrometry: an overview. Philos Trans R Soc A Math Phys Eng Sci. 2016;374(2079):20150382.
72. Domon B, Aebersold R. Mass spectrometry and protein analysis. Science. 2006;312:212–7.
73. Wilschefski SC, Baxter MR. Inductively coupled plasma mass spectrometry: introduction to analytical aspects. Clin Biochem Rev. 2019;40:115–33.
74. Olshina MA, Sharon M. Mass spectrometry: a technique of many faces. Q Rev Biophys. 2016;49:e18.
75. Finoulst I, Pinkse M, Van Dongen W, Verhaert P. Sample preparation techniques for the untargeted LC-MS-based discovery of peptides in complex biological matrices. Biomed Res Int. 2011;2011(1):245291.
76. Huang MZ, Yuan CH, Cheng SC, Cho YT, Shiea J. Ambient ionization mass spectrometry. Annu Rev Anal Chem. 2010;3(1):43–65.

77. Maciel EVS, Pereira dos Santos NG, Vargas Medina DA, Lanças FM. Electron ionization mass spectrometry: quo vadis? Electrophoresis. 2022;43(15):1587–600.
78. Morato NM, Cooks RG. Desorption electrospray ionization mass spectrometry: 20 years. Acc Chem Res. 2023;56(18):2526–36.
79. Wilm M. Principles of electrospray ionization. Mol Cell Proteomics. 2011;10(7).
80. Lee JK, Banerjee S, Nam HG, Zare RN. Acceleration of reaction in charged microdroplets. Q Rev Biophys. 2015;48(4):437–44.
81. Karas M, Hillenkamp F. Laser desorption ionization of proteins with molecular masses exceeding 10,000 daltons. Anal Chem. 1988;60(20):2299–301.
82. Pitman CN, LaCourse WR. Desorption atmospheric pressure chemical ionization: a review. Anal Chim Acta. 2020;1130:146–54.
83. Vertes A. Soft laser desorption ionization—MALDI, DIOS and nanostructures. Laser Ablation and Its Applications. 2007;505–28.
84. Leopold J, Popkova Y, Engel KM, Schiller J. Recent developments of useful MALDI matrices for the mass spectrometric characterization of lipids. Biomolecules. 2018;8(4):173.
85. Badnjevic A, Gurbeta L, Jimenez ER, Iadanza E. Testing of mechanical ventilators and infant incubators in healthcare institutions. Technol Health Care. 2017;25(2):237–50.
86. Clark AE, Kaleta EJ, Arora A, Wolk DM. Matrix-assisted laser desorption ionization–time of flight mass spectrometry: a fundamental shift in the routine practice of clinical microbiology. Clin Microbiol Rev. 2013;26(3):547–603.
87. Haag AM. Mass analyzers and mass spectrometers. Adv Exp Med Biol. 2016;919:157–69.
88. Cadene M, Chait BT. A robust, detergent-friendly method for mass spectrometric analysis of integral membrane proteins. Anal Chem. 2000;72(22):5655–8.
89. Rappold BA. Review of the use of liquid chromatography-tandem mass spectrometry in clinical laboratories: part I–development. Ann Lab Med. 2022;42(2):121–40.
90. Shan L, Gao H, Zhang J, Li W, Su Y, Guo Y. Plasma and serum exosome markers analyzed by matrix-assisted laser desorption/ionization time-of-flight mass spectrometry coupled with electron multiplier. Talanta. 2022;247:123560.
91. Badnjević A, Gurbeta L, Custovic E. An expert diagnostic system to automatically identify asthma and chronic obstructive pulmonary disease in clinical settings. Sci Rep. 2018;8:11645.
92. Züllig T, Köfeler HC. High-resolution mass spectrometry in lipidomics. Mass Spectrom Rev. 2021;40:162–76.
93. Zubarev RA, Makarov A. Orbitrap mass spectrometry. Anal Chem. 2013;85(11):5288–5296.
94. Buchberger AR, DeLaney K, Johnson J, Li L. Mass spectrometry imaging: a review of emerging advancements and future insights. Anal Chem. 2017;90(1):240–65.
95. Alexandrov T, Chernyavsky I, Becker M, von Eggeling F, Nikolenko S. Analysis and interpretation of imaging mass spectrometry data by clustering mass-to-charge images according to their spatial similarity. Anal Chem. 2013;85(23):11189–95.

# Chapter 5
# Review, Practice Problems, and Future Directions

This section consolidates the key concepts of biomedical engineering, revisiting foundational principles, core disciplines, medical devices, clinical engineering, laboratory technologies, and ethical, legal, and societal considerations. The section presents curated practice problems and exercises, enabling readers to apply theoretical knowledge, analyze case studies, and develop critical thinking and problem-solving skills relevant to both academic and professional contexts (Sect. 5.1). This forward-looking perspective emphasizes ongoing innovation and the evolving impact of biomedical engineering on healthcare delivery and patient outcomes.

## 5.1 Practice Problems and Exercises

### *5.1.1 Definition and Scope of Biomedical Engineering*

1.1. Biomedical engineering is best described as the bridge between:

(a) Physics and Chemistry
(b) Engineering and Medicine
(c) Computer Science and Law
(d) Mathematics and Astronomy

1.2. Which principle in biomedical engineering involves viewing biological systems as interconnected networks?

(a) Mechanical design
(b) Systems thinking
(c) Independent analysis
(d) Random experimentation



A. Badnjević et al., *Biomedical Instrumentation*, Series in BioEngineering,
https://doi.org/10.1007/978-3-032-10978-1_5

1.3. What regulatory body in the United States ensures the safety and efficacy of medical devices?

(a) WHO
(b) CDC
(c) FDA
(d) NIH

1.4. What field uses engineered substances designed to interact with biological systems?

(a) Biomechanics
(b) Biomaterials
(c) Bioinformatics
(d) Rehabilitation Engineering

1.5. Which imaging method allows the visualization of brain activity in real time?

(a) CT scan
(b) Ultrasound
(c) Functional MRI
(d) PET scan

1.6. The creation of prosthetic limbs that use myoelectric signals is a part of:

(a) Biomedical Imaging
(b) Tissue Engineering
(c) Rehabilitation Engineering
(d) Bioinformatics

1.7. Which area focuses on creating 3D scaffolds for tissue regeneration?

(a) Robotics
(b) Tissue Engineering
(c) Imaging Systems
(d) Electrical Engineering

1.8. Bioinformatics mainly deals with the analysis of:

(a) Engineering designs
(b) Physical therapy routines
(c) Large biological datasets
(d) Surgical techniques

1.9. Which development has allowed non-invasive visualization of the body?

(a) Prosthetics
(b) Rehabilitation devices
(c) Biomedical imaging
(d) Robotic surgeries

1.10. What type of engineering is primarily concerned with helping individuals with physical disabilities regain independence?

(a) Mechanical Engineering
(b) Rehabilitation Engineering
(c) Electrical Engineering
(d) Genetic Engineering

1.11. Biomedical engineering combines __________ principles with biology and medical sciences.
1.12. The study of the mechanical properties of biological systems is called __________.
1.13. __________ imaging provides non-invasive visualization of internal body structures.
1.14. A __________ heart is an example of an engineered device that mimics organ function.
1.15. In rehabilitation engineering, __________ prosthetics use muscle signals to control movement.
1.16. The regulatory body __________ ensures the safety and effectiveness of medical devices in the USA.
1.17. __________ are engineered materials designed to interact safely with biological systems.
1.18. __________ medicine uses scaffolds, stem cells, and growth factors to repair tissues.
1.19. An important ethical principle in biomedical engineering is ensuring patient __________ and safety.
1.20. __________ allows analysis of genetic data to personalize medical treatments.

## *5.1.2 History and Evolution of Biomedical Engineering*

2.1. Which of the following best defines BME?

(a) A field combining medicine and architecture
(b) A branch of engineering focused on automobile design
(c) A discipline integrating engineering principles with biological and medical sciences
(d) A study of ancient medical texts

2.2. Which civilization is known to have used prosthetics made from wood and leather?

(a) Greeks
(b) Romans
(c) Egyptians
(d) Chinese

2.3. Who is often called the "Father of Medicine"?

(a) Galen
(b) Hippocrates
(c) Sushruta
(d) Leonardo da Vinci

2.4. What significant contribution did Galen of Pergamon make to medicine?

(a) Development of artificial limbs
(b) Detailed anatomical studies based on human dissections
(c) Advancements in robotic surgery
(d) Research on regenerative medicine

2.5. Which medical imaging technology was discovered first?

(a) X-ray
(b) MRI
(c) CT scan
(d) Ultrasound

2.6. Which medical device was invented by René Laennec in 1816?

(a) X-ray machine
(b) Stethoscope
(c) MRI scanner
(d) CT scanner

2.7. Which event was crucial in formally recognizing biomedical engineering as a professional field?

(a) The Renaissance
(b) The Industrial Revolution
(c) World War II
(d) The discovery of DNA

2.8. Which of the following is NOT a specialization within Biomedical Engineering?

(a) Medical device design
(b) Bioinformatics
(c) Neural engineering
(d) Aerospace engineering

2.9. What modern innovation allows paralyzed individuals to control prosthetic limbs using their thoughts?

(a) Electrocardiograms
(b) Brain-Computer Interfaces
(c) AI-assisted radiology
(d) Nanotechnology

2.10. Which scientist conducted early anatomical studies and produced detailed human body sketches?

(a) Sushruta
(b) Andreas Vesalius
(c) Leonardo da Vinci
(d) Al-Zahrawi

2.11. What is the purpose of AI in biomedical engineering?

(a) Enhancing diagnostic tools and patient monitoring
(b) Replacing doctors in surgical procedures
(c) Creating mechanical prosthetics only
(d) Manufacturing vaccines

2.12. Which ancient text details early surgical techniques and medical procedures in India?

(a) Ebers Papyrus
(b) De Humani Corporis Fabrica
(c) Sushruta Samhita
(d) Hippocratic Corpus

2.13. Which imaging technique allows visualization of soft tissues using magnetic fields?

(a) X-ray
(b) MRI
(c) CT scan
(d) Ultrasound

2.14. Which advancement in biomedical engineering has significantly improved personalized medicine?

(a) 3D printing of organs
(b) AI-driven drug discovery
(c) Wearable health monitors
(d) All of the above

2.15. The ancient ______ civilization developed the Ebers Papyrus, which contained medical treatments and surgical techniques.
2.16. The first X-ray image was taken in the year ______ by Wilhelm Röntgen.
2.17. Biomedical engineering became a formalized academic and professional field during the mid-______ century.
2.18. The AI-driven system used to assist in complex surgeries is the ______ Surgical System.
2.19. The interdisciplinary nature of biomedical engineering combines principles from ______, ______, and _____.

### 5.1.3 Key Disciplines and Applications

3.1. BME is an interdisciplinary field that integrates:

(a) Physics, chemistry, and literature
(b) Engineering, biology, and medicine
(c) Architecture, chemistry, and music
(d) Computer science, mathematics, and economics

3.2. Which of the following is NOT a core discipline of Biomedical Engineering?

(a) Biomechanics
(b) Biomaterials
(c) Medical Imaging
(d) Astrophysics

3.3. Which discipline of BME focuses on studying the mechanical properties of biological systems?

(a) Bioinformatics
(b) Biomechanics
(c) Medical Imaging
(d) Regenerative Medicine

3.4. What is a significant application of biomechanics in healthcare?

(a) Studying genetic sequences
(b) Developing prosthetic limbs and orthopedic implants
(c) Designing MRI machines
(d) Manufacturing vaccines

3.5. Biomaterials are used in the development of:

(a) Stents and prosthetic limbs
(b) Antibiotics
(c) Vaccines
(d) Genetic sequencing

3.6. Which properties are essential for biomaterials used in medical implants?

(a) High electrical conductivity
(b) Biocompatibility
(c) Radioactivity
(d) Magnetic properties

3.7. Which imaging technique is best suited for visualizing soft tissues?

(a) X-ray
(b) MRI
(c) Ultrasound
(d) PET scan

3.8. Which field of BME uses computational and statistical techniques to analyze biological data?

(a) Biomechanics
(b) Bioinformatics
(c) Biomaterials
(d) Rehabilitation Engineering

3.9. Which of the following is NOT a commonly used medical imaging technique?

(a) X-ray
(b) MRI
(c) Computed tomography
(d) Electrocardiogram

3.10. What is one of the primary goals of computational modeling in biomedical engineering?

(a) Predict biological system behaviors
(b) Replace all medical doctors
(c) Manufacture surgical instruments
(d) Develop music therapy techniques

3.11. Which of the following is an example of a biodegradable biomaterial?

(a) Titanium implants
(b) Cobalt-chromium alloys
(c) Biodegradable polymers
(d) Lead-based alloys

3.12. Which medical imaging technique uses sound waves to create images?

(a) X-ray
(b) MRI
(c) Ultrasound
(d) CT scan

3.13. How does AI contribute to medical imaging?

(a) By eliminating the need for medical professionals
(b) By enhancing image interpretation and abnormality detection
(c) By increasing radiation exposure to improve clarity
(d) By making medical imaging obsolete

3.14. ______ is the study of the mechanical behavior of biological systems, particularly focusing on the forces exerted by muscles and bones.

3.15. Materials designed to interact with biological systems for medical purposes are known as ______.

3.16. Medical imaging technologies, such as ______ and ______, allow healthcare professionals to visualize internal body structures without invasive procedures.

3.17. ______ is a computational field in BME that analyzes biological data, including genetic sequences.
3.18. One of the significant applications of biomaterials is the development of ______, which are used to replace or support damaged bones or joints.

### *5.1.4 Ethical, Legal, and Social Considerations*

4.1. Which three domains must biomedical engineers consider when developing new technologies?

(a) Physics, chemistry, and biology
(b) Ethical, legal, and social
(c) Engineering, marketing, and finance
(d) Scientific, cultural, and artistic

4.2. The ethical principle of "not harm" is known as:

(a) Beneficence
(b) Autonomy
(c) Non-maleficence
(d) Justice

4.3. Which of the following is a legal consideration in biomedical engineering?

(a) Patient autonomy
(b) Cultural acceptance of medical devices
(c) Compliance with regulatory standards
(d) Ethical implications of gene editing

4.4. Which field of biomedical engineering raises ethical concerns about data privacy and algorithmic bias?

(a) Biomechanics
(b) AI in diagnostics
(c) Tissue engineering
(d) Medical device design

4.5. Which international regulatory body oversees medical devices in the European Union?

(a) FDA
(b) EMA
(c) WHO
(d) CDC

4.6. What is a significant concern regarding the social implications of biomedical advancements?

(a) Increased revenue for medical companies
(b) The creation of social inequalities in healthcare access
(c) The ability to patent more technologies
(d) The elimination of all genetic diseases

4.7. Which of the following is a concern with CRISPR gene editing technology?

(a) Reduced medical costs
(b) Ethical issues regarding human genetic modifications
(c) Its inability to alter DNA
(d) Lack of medical applications

4.8. Which regulatory framework classifies medical devices based on risk level?

(a) Genetic Modification Act
(b) The Medical Device Regulation (MDR)
(c) The Artificial Intelligence Ethics Act
(d) International Bioengineering Treaty

4.9. How can AI in healthcare potentially contribute to social inequalities?

(a) By making healthcare decisions for doctors
(b) By reducing the need for trained medical professionals
(c) By favoring patients from specific socioeconomic backgrounds due to algorithmic bias
(d) By making medical treatments more affordable

4.10. Which ethical principle ensures that patients have the right to make informed decisions about their healthcare?

(a) Non-maleficence
(b) Autonomy
(c) Confidentiality
(d) Fairness

4.11. How do one-way biomedical engineers ensure fairness in healthcare innovation?

(a) Focus only on profitable technologies
(b) Design technologies that are inclusive and accessible to all populations
(c) Patent their discoveries to prevent public access
(d) Ignore ethical concerns in favor of innovation

4.12. Which of the following is a significant legal issue in biomedical engineering?

(a) AI outperforms human doctors
(b) Protection of intellectual property rights
(c) Limited use of medical implants
(d) The popularity of robotic-assisted surgery

4.13. What is a significant challenge in ensuring the responsible use of biomedical technologies?

(a) Ethical dilemmas related to patient consent and safety
(b) Lack of technological advancements
(c) The disappearance of traditional medical practices
(d) The elimination of healthcare regulations

4.14. The principle of ______ ensures that biomedical engineers strive to create technologies that benefit patients and improve their health.

4.15. Legal frameworks in biomedical engineering help regulate technologies to ensure ______ and ______.

4.16. Biomedical engineers must consider the societal impact of new technologies and ensure that they do not worsen ______ in healthcare access.

4.17. The ______ plays a central role in regulating medical devices in the United States.

4.18. A significant concern with AI in healthcare is the potential for ______ bias, which can result in unequal access to accurate medical diagnoses.

### *5.1.5 Overview of Medical Devices*

5.1. Which of the following is NOT considered a medical device?

(a) MRI scanner
(b) Cardiac pacemaker
(c) Antibiotic medication
(d) Wearable health monitor

5.2. Which emerging technology is revolutionizing the production of patient-specific implants and prosthetics?

(a) Blockchain
(b) 3D Printing
(c) Nanotechnology
(d) Virtual Reality

5.3. What is a primary challenge in ensuring the cybersecurity of medical devices?

(a) Battery life
(b) Unauthorized access and cyberattacks
(c) Cost of manufacturing
(d) Patient compliance

5.4. Which category of medical devices includes AI-powered diagnostic platforms?

(a) Life support devices

(b) Therapeutic devices
(c) Diagnostic devices
(d) Assistive devices

5.5. What is the primary role of the European Medicines Agency (EMA) in medical device regulation?

(a) Approving only pharmaceuticals
(b) Regulating artificial intelligence in healthcare
(c) Categorizing and approving medical devices for patient safety
(d) Overseeing medical education programs

5.6. Which of the following is an example of a life support device?

(a) Pacemaker
(b) MRI scanner
(c) Mechanical ventilator
(d) Cochlear implant

5.7. Why is post-market surveillance essential for medical devices?

(a) To collect user feedback for marketing purposes
(b) To track long-term safety and device malfunctions
(c) To reduce the cost of device manufacturing
(d) To eliminate the need for regulatory approval

5.8. Which of the following standards helps ensure interoperability between medical devices and healthcare systems?

(a) HTTP
(b) FHIR
(c) HTML
(d) CSS

5.9. What role does AI play in modern medical diagnostics?

(a) Reduces the need for doctors
(b) Enhances disease detection accuracy and predictive analytics
(c) Replaces traditional medical devices
(d) Eliminates the need for laboratory testing

5.10. Which of the following is an example of an implantable medical device?

(a) Stethoscope
(b) X-ray machine
(c) Insulin pump
(d) Blood pressure cuff

5.11. Which of these medical imaging techniques is best suited for detecting metabolic activity in tissues?

(a) X-ray

(b) Ultrasound
(c) PET scan
(d) MRI

5.12. Which material advancement has significantly improved the longevity and biocompatibility of orthopedic implants?

(a) Copper wiring
(b) Biocompatible polymers and titanium alloys
(c) Carbon fiber plastics
(d) Aluminum sheets

5.13. Which class of medical devices in the FDA system requires the most rigorous approval process?

(a) Class I
(b) Class II
(c) Class III
(d) Class IV

5.14. Which key feature of nanotechnology makes it promising for future medical device applications?

(a) Large size and weight
(b) Ability to target specific cells and tissues
(c) High power consumption
(d) Low cost of manufacturing

5.15. The ________________________ is responsible for regulating medical devices in the United States.
5.16. One major challenge in medical device cybersecurity is preventing __________________ unauthorized access to patient data.
5.17. The use of ___________________ technology allows for the on-demand creation of patient-specific implants, reducing costs and improving compatibility.
5.18. One key advantage of AI-driven diagnostics is its ability to provide more _______________ and faster detection of diseases.
5.19. Wearable medical devices, such as smartwatches with ECG capabilities, allow for ________________ patient monitoring and enable early detection of health issues.

### 5.1.6 Basic Components and Functions

6.1. What is the primary function of a resistor in a biomedical circuit?

(a) Amplify voltage
(b) Store electrical charge

(c) Resist current flow
(d) Generate magnetic fields

6.2. Which component is responsible for temporarily storing electrical charge?

(a) Inductor
(b) Capacitor
(c) Diode
(d) Transistor

6.3. What does a high Common Mode Rejection Ratio (CMRR) indicate in amplifiers?

(a) Better ability to amplify noise
(b) Better rejection of standard noise signals
(c) Higher current consumption
(d) Higher voltage gain

6.4. Which of the following is *not* a commonly monitored biosignal?

(a) ECG
(b) EEG
(c) LCD
(d) EMG

6.5. Which technology is most power-hungry in wearable medical devices?

(a) Sensors
(b) Amplifiers
(c) Wireless communication modules
(d) Microcontrollers

6.6. What type of filter is typically used to remove 50/60 Hz interference?

(a) High-pass filter
(b) Low-pass filter
(c) Notch filter
(d) Band-pass filter

6.7. Which property does an inductor mainly oppose?

(a) Voltage
(b) Resistance
(c) Change in current
(d) Signal frequency

6.8. Which material is typically used for the base of integrated circuits?

(a) Carbon
(b) Aluminum
(c) Copper
(d) Silicon

6.9. What is the function of biosensors in health monitoring systems?

(a) Generate power
(b) Process analog signals
(c) Convert physiological signals into electrical signals
(d) Encrypt data for wireless transmission

6.10. Which parameter is critical in amplifier design for biosignals?

(a) Bandwidth above 10 MHz
(b) Low input impedance
(c) High CMRR
(d) Low power gain

6.11. A ________________ is a device used to resist the flow of electric current.
6.12. The unit of capacitance is the ________________.
6.13. A diode conducts current in only ______________ direction.
6.14. The basic building blocks of all electronics are resistors, capacitors, inductors, diodes, and ______________.
6.15. Electrodes are used to acquire ______________ biosignals like ECG and EEG.
6.16. Notch filters are used to remove ________________ Hz interference from power lines.
6.17. The energy in an inductor is stored in the form of a ______________ field.
6.18. The formula for resistance in series is $R_{total} = R_1 +$ ______ $+ R_n$.
6.19. A wearable system should prioritize ergonomics, low power consumption, and ____________.
6.20. Kirchhoff's Voltage Law is based on the principle of ______________ of energy.
6.21. Calculate the equivalent resistance of a circuit with resistors of 10, 20, and 30 Ω connected in series.
6.22. Determine the total capacitance of three capacitors (5, 10, and 20 μF) connected in parallel.
6.23. Use Ohm's law to calculate the current flowing through a 100 Ω resistor connected to a 5 V source.
6.24. Draw a basic ECG acquisition system schematic using resistors, op-amps, and electrodes.
6.25. Identify the component that resists changes in current flow and calculate the voltage across a 2H inductor if the current changes at 3 A/s.
6.26. Explain the importance of CMRR in biomedical amplifiers using an example.
6.27. Calculate power consumption using the formula $P = V \times I$ for a sensor drawing 10 mA at 3.3 V.
6.28. List and label all components in a block diagram of a wireless health monitoring system.

### 5.1.7 *Imaging Devices*

7.1. Which imaging modality uses strong magnetic fields and radio waves to produce detailed images of soft tissues?

(a) X-ray
(b) CT
(c) MRI
(d) Ultrasound

7.2. What principle guides the safe use of X-ray imaging in medicine?

(a) As High As Technically Possible
(b) Only When Necessary
(c) As Low As Reasonably Achievable
(d) Always Use Radiation

7.3. Which imaging device is most commonly used for real-time visualization during pregnancy?

(a) MRI
(b) Ultrasound
(c) CT
(d) X-ray

7.4. What technological advancement has improved image interpretation in modern diagnostic imaging?

(a) Manual drawing
(b) Analog signals
(c) Artificial intelligence
(d) Darkroom processing

7.5. What component in an X-ray tube emits electrons?

(a) Anode
(b) Cathode
(c) Filament
(d) Coil

7.6. Which imaging modality is most sensitive for detecting neurological disorders?

(a) Ultrasound
(b) CT
(c) MRI
(d) X-ray

7.7. Which of the following uses ionizing radiation?

(a) MRI

(b) Ultrasound
(c) CT
(d) None of the above

7.8. Which technique in ultrasound is used to visualize blood flow?

(a) 2D Ultrasound
(b) Elastography
(c) Doppler Ultrasound
(d) 3D Ultrasound

7.9. Portable imaging devices have significantly improved access to imaging. In which setting have they been improved?

(a) Urban hospitals
(b) Medical universities
(c) Remote and underserved areas
(d) Laboratories

7.10. What does the integration of AI in imaging help reduce?

(a) Radiation dose
(b) Scan time
(c) Human error
(d) Power consumption

7.11. ______________ imaging uses high-frequency sound waves to create real-time images of internal structures.
7.12. The first X-ray image was taken by ______________ in 1895.
7.13. MRI imaging is beneficial for examining __________ tissues.
7.14. CT scanning provides ____________________ images of the body.
7.15. In Doppler ultrasound, the change in frequency of sound waves is used to assess ________ flow.
7.16. The cathode in an X-ray tube emits ________________.
7.17. The principle used to minimize X-ray exposure is called ________________ ____________________.
7.18. Artificial intelligence helps in ________________________ and ________________________.
7.19. MRI scanners align ____________________ nuclei in the body using strong magnetic fields.
7.20. __________________ imaging allows clinicians to view moving structures in real-time.

## Case Studies

Case Study 1: Portable Ultrasound for Rural Clinics

**Scenario**: A medical startup introduces a low-cost, portable ultrasound device for rural clinics.
**Challenge**:

- Image resolution vs. portability
- Minimal training for healthcare workers
- Durability

**Student Question**: *How would you design a portable ultrasound device that balances image quality, battery life, and ease of use for healthcare workers in remote areas?*

Case Study 2: AI-Enhanced MRI Scans for Faster Diagnosis

**Scenario**: A hospital uses AI to reconstruct MRI images faster.
**Challenge**:

- Diagnostic accuracy
- AI integration
- Legal responsibility

**Student Question**: *Should hospitals rely on AI to speed up imaging scans, and how would you ensure the results remain accurate and trustworthy for patient care?*

Case Study 3: Real-Time Imaging During Robotic Surgery

**Scenario**: Real-time 3D imaging is used during robotic surgeries.
**Challenge**:

- Data processing speed
- Surgeon usability
- High cost

**Student Question**: *How can real-time imaging systems be improved to help surgeons during operations without overwhelming them with too much data?*

Case Study 4: Low-Dose CT Imaging for Pediatric Patients

**Scenario**: A hospital adopts low-dose CT scans for children.
**Challenge**:

- Image quality vs. radiation risk
- Equipment calibration
- Communication with families

**Student Question**: *What strategies would you use to ensure low-dose CT scans provide accurate diagnoses while minimizing radiation risks for pediatric patients?*

Case Study 5: Handheld Thermal Imaging for Emergency Medicine

**Scenario**: Emergency teams use thermal cameras in the field.
**Challenge**:

- Environmental variability
- Device durability
- Battery management

**Student Question**: *How could thermal imaging devices be optimized to improve emergency care in outdoor or unpredictable environments?*

Case Study 6: Wearable Imaging for Brain Monitoring

**Scenario**: Wearable NIRS devices monitor brain activity in real-world settings.
**Challenge**:

- Motion artifacts
- Wireless transmission
- Comfort

**Student Question**: *How would you design a wearable brain imaging system that remains reliable during daily activities like sports or work?*

Case Study 7: Development of Low-Cost Retinal Imaging Devices

**Scenario**: Smartphone-based retinal imaging devices for low-resource areas.
**Challenge**:

- Smartphone optics adaptation
- Diagnostic resolution
- Data management

**Student Question**: *What are the major engineering and ethical considerations when designing a low-cost retinal imaging device for developing countries?*

Case Study 8: Advanced PET-CT for Early Cancer Detection

**Scenario**: Hospitals adopt high-resolution PET-CT for early cancer detection.
**Challenge**:

- Managing hypersensitive diagnostics
- Personalized treatment integration
- Costs

**Student Question**: *Should hospitals invest in expensive high-resolution PET-CT machines for early cancer detection, and how should their use be prioritized ethically and economically?*

### *5.1.8 Electrocardiographs*

8.1. What does the P wave represent in the ECG?

(a) Ventricular depolarization
(b) Atrial depolarization
(c) Ventricular repolarization
(d) Atrial repolarization

8.2. The PR interval typically lasts:

(a) 80–120 ms
(b) 200–300 ms
(c) 120–200 ms
(d) 300–400 ms

8.3. Which of the following electrodes acts as a ground/reference in a 12-lead ECG?

(a) RA
(b) LA
(c) LL
(d) RL

8.4. Which lead is calculated as LA − RA?

(a) Lead I
(b) Lead II
(c) Lead III
(d) aVF

8.5. The QRS complex represents:

(a) Atrial repolarization
(b) Ventricular repolarization
(c) Atrial depolarization

(d) Ventricular depolarization

8.6. The frequency range of a typical ECG signal is:

(a) 0.1–20 Hz
(b) 0.05–150 Hz
(c) 1–500 Hz
(d) 10–200 Hz

8.7. The purpose of a notch filter in ECG is to:

(a) Amplify QRS
(b) Remove baseline wander
(c) Remove 50/60 Hz powerline noise
(d) Detect P waves

8.8. What is Einthoven's triangle?

(a) A triangle of precordial leads
(b) The shape of the heart
(c) Configuration of limb leads RA, LA, LL
(d) Shape of the QRS

8.9. Which component digitizes the ECG signal?

(a) Differential amplifier
(b) Filter
(c) ADC
(d) DAC

8.10. A heart rate of less than 60 bpm is called:

(a) Tachycardia
(b) Ischemia
(c) Bradycardia
(d) Ventricular fibrillation

8.11. The P wave represents ____________________.
8.12. The QRS complex indicates ________________________.
8.13. The isoelectric line shows _____________________________.
8.14. The reference electrode in ECG is the _________________.
8.15. Lead II measures voltage between _________ and __________.
8.16. The standard ECG paper speed is ____________.
8.17. The T wave represents ___________________________.
8.18. The frequency range for ECG signals is typically ____________________.
8.19. In ECG devices, small signals are boosted using ______________________.
8.20. A 12-lead ECG uses ________ electrodes.
8.21. Calculate the Nyquist rate for ECG signals with a maximum frequency of 100 Hz.
8.22. Determine how many samples are recorded in 3 min at 340 Hz sampling rate.

8.23. Calculate memory size for a 2-channel ECG at 360 Hz and 2 bytes per sample for 1 min.
8.24. Label a 12-lead ECG electrode placement diagram.
8.25. Draw and identify components in a block diagram of an ECG system.

## Case Studies

Case Study 1: Home-Based Continuous ECG Monitoring

**Scenario**: A 75-year-old patient is provided with a wireless ECG monitor for 48-h continuous monitoring at home.
**Challenge**:

- Long battery life
- Reducing motion artifacts
- Reliable wireless data transmission

**Student Question**: *How would you design a home-based ECG monitoring device to ensure continuous, high-quality signal recording with minimal user intervention?*

Case Study 2: Smart Textile ECG Integration for Athletes

**Scenario**: A bright T-shirt integrates ECG sensors to monitor athletes during intense physical activities.
**Challenge**:

- Wearability and comfort
- Reliable signal acquisition during movement
- Seamless data transfer to a mobile app

**Student Question**: *What materials and signal processing strategies would you use to create an ECG-embedded smart garment for real-time athletic monitoring?*

Case Study 3: ECG Remote Monitoring Via ZigBee Networks in Rural Clinics

**Scenario**: Wearable ECG devices use ZigBee communication to remotely monitor patients' heart health in rural clinics.
**Challenge**:

- Low power usage
- Stable communication in remote areas
- Simple design for elderly patients

**Student Question**: *How would you optimize a ZigBee-based ECG monitoring system for reliability and user-friendliness in low-resource rural settings?*

Case Study 4: Early Detection of Arrhythmias Using AI-Processed ECG

**Scenario**: A hospital introduces AI software that automatically detects arrhythmias from ECG signals.
**Challenge**:

- Accuracy of automatic diagnosis
- Trust between human doctors and AI systems
- Reducing false positives and negatives

**Student Question**: *Would you recommend using AI to assist ECG interpretation for arrhythmia detection, and how would you balance automation with human oversight?*

Case Study 5: ECG Monitoring in Wearable Smartwatches

**Scenario**: A new smartwatch includes a feature for on-demand ECG readings and continuous heart rate monitoring.
**Challenge**:

- Ensuring medical-grade accuracy
- Power and battery constraints
- Managing noise from daily activities

**Student Question**: *What technical and regulatory hurdles must be overcome to ensure smartwatch-based ECG monitoring is both medically reliable and consumer-friendly?*

Case Study 6: High-Resolution ECG for Cardiac Research

**Scenario**: A research institute develops a high-resolution ECG system to detect micro-variations in cardiac electrophysiology.
**Challenge**:

- Handling high data volumes
- Minimizing environmental noise
- Balancing invasiveness vs. resolution

**Student Question**: *How would you design a high-resolution ECG system that captures micro-events in cardiac activity without compromising patient safety or comfort?*

Case Study 7: Low-Cost ECG Devices for Developing Countries

**Scenario**: An NGO plans to distribute ultra-low-cost ECG machines to rural clinics in low-income countries.
**Challenge**:

- Affordability
- Simple setup and maintenance
- Minimal training requirements

**Student Question**: *What are the essential features you prioritize when designing a low-cost, reliable ECG device for under-resourced healthcare systems?*

Case Study 8: Implantable ECG Sensors for Long-Term Monitoring

**Scenario**: A biotech company develops an implantable miniaturized ECG sensor to monitor high-risk patients for sudden cardiac arrest.
**Challenge**:

- Biocompatibility and safety
- Data transmission and storage
- Power supply for long-term function

**Student Question**: *What considerations must be addressed in the design of an implantable ECG sensor for continuous, long-term cardiac monitoring?*

Case Study 9: Pediatric ECG Monitoring Systems

**Scenario**: A children's hospital needs specialized ECG monitors designed for pediatric patients, including neonates.
**Challenge**:

- Smaller electrodes and lower signal amplitudes
- Minimizing discomfort
- Avoiding false alarms

**Student Question**: *How would you adapt ECG monitoring technology to meet pediatric patients' unique physiological and comfort needs?*

Case Study 10: Tele-ECG for Emergency Medical Services

**Scenario**: Paramedics transmit real-time ECG data from ambulances to hospital emergency rooms before arrival.
**Challenge**:

- Real-time wireless transmission reliability
- Signal clarity during ambulance movement
- Fast integration into ER systems

**Student Question**: *What technical solutions would you propose to ensure robust, real-time ECG transmission from ambulances to hospitals for faster emergency response?*

### 5.1.9 Blood Pressure Monitors

9.1. What is the main determinant of arterial blood pressure?

(a) Body temperature
(b) Blood viscosity
(c) Cardiac output and peripheral resistance
(d) Pulse pressure

9.2. Which value represents the average blood pressure during a cardiac cycle?

(a) Systolic pressure
(b) Diastolic pressure
(c) Pulse pressure
(d) Mean arterial pressure

9.3. Korotkoff sounds are used to measure blood pressure in which method?

(a) Oscillometric
(b) Invasive
(c) Auscultatory
(d) Doppler

9.4. What is considered hypertension in terms of systolic and diastolic values?

(a) >140/90 mmHg
(b) >120/80 mmHg
(c) >100/60 mmHg
(d) <90/60 mmHg

9.5. Which device requires no calibration due to its construction?

(a) Aneroid sphygmomanometer
(b) Mercury manometer
(c) Digital monitor
(d) Hybrid sphygmomanometer

9.6. What does MAP stand for?

(a) Manual Arterial Pulse
(b) Maximum Arterial Pressure

(c) Mean Arterial Pressure
(d) Minimum Arterial Pressure

9.7. In an oscillometric method, MAP corresponds to:

(a) Onset of oscillations
(b) Maximum oscillation
(c) Disappearance of sound
(d) First Korotkoff sound

9.8. Which of the following is a non-invasive BP measurement?

(a) Direct catheter insertion
(b) Oscillometry
(c) Central venous line
(d) Pulmonary wedge

9.9. A hybrid sphygmomanometer combines features of:

(a) Mercury and invasive monitors
(b) Digital and Doppler monitors
(c) Mercury and digital monitors
(d) Analog and thermistor monitors

9.10. Which pressure value is calculated using the DP + (PP/3) formula?

(a) Pulse pressure
(b) Systolic pressure
(c) Diastolic pressure
(d) Mean arterial pressure

9.11. The maximum pressure during heart contraction is called the ____________ pressure.
9.12. The Korotkoff sounds were introduced by ______________.
9.13. Blood pressure is usually measured in units of ____________.
9.14. The difference between systolic and diastolic pressure is called __________ pressure.
9.15. The most common artery used for non-invasive BP measurement is the ____________ artery.
9.16. In an auscultatory method, the disappearance of sound indicates ____________ pressure.
9.17. A cuff that is too narrow can result in a falsely __________ BP reading.
9.18. Oscillometric monitors detect blood flow via __________ pressure changes.
9.19. MAP stands for ________________________.
9.20. A mercury manometer uses a __________ column to display pressure.
9.21. Calculate MAP: If SP = 130 mmHg and DP = 70 mmHg, use MAP = DP + (PP/3).
9.22. Determine MAP using Method #2: SP = 120 mmHg, DP = 80 mmHg
9.23. Interpret Korotkoff sounds phases I and V.

9.24. Compare invasive and non-invasive methods.
9.25. Calculate pulse pressure: SP = 140 mmHg, DP = 90 mmHg.

**Case Studies**

Case Study 1: Home Blood Pressure Monitoring for Hypertensive Patients

**Scenario**: A healthcare provider recommends home-use blood pressure monitors for patients with hypertension.
**Challenge**:

- Device calibration and accuracy
- Ease of use for elderly patients
- Data sharing with doctors

**Student Question**: *How would you design a user-friendly home blood pressure monitor that maintains clinical accuracy and allows easy data sharing with healthcare providers?*

Case Study 2: Wearable Blood Pressure Monitoring in Athletes

**Scenario**: A company develops a wrist-worn blood pressure monitor for continuous tracking during athletic performance.
**Challenge**:

- Accuracy during physical movement
- Battery life and size constraints
- Comfort and waterproofing

**Student Question**: *What engineering solutions would you implement to ensure continuous, accurate blood pressure monitoring in wearable devices used during sports activities?*

Case Study 3: Cuffless Blood Pressure Monitoring Via Smartphone

**Scenario**: Researchers are developing an app that estimates blood pressure using sensors and algorithms through a smartphone camera and finger placement.
**Challenge**:

- Validation against clinical standards
- User consistency in measurements
- Handling environmental factors (e.g., lighting)

**Student Question**: *Is relying on smartphone-based, cuffless blood pressure monitoring feasible? What steps would you take to improve its reliability and clinical acceptance?*

Case Study 4: Blood Pressure Monitoring in ICU Settings

**Scenario**: An ICU upgrades to automated, real-time blood pressure monitoring systems for critically ill patients.
**Challenge**:

- Continuous monitoring without signal artifacts
- Integration with electronic health records
- Alarms for critical readings

**Student Question**: *How would you design a blood pressure monitoring system suitable for intensive care, ensuring both reliability and rapid response to critical changes?*

Case Study 5: Blood Pressure Monitoring for Pregnant Women (Preeclampsia Detection)

**Scenario**: A health initiative introduces remote blood pressure monitoring for pregnant women to detect early signs of preeclampsia.
**Challenge**:

- Frequent, accurate readings
- Ensuring compliance in remote areas
- Simple and safe home operation

**Student Question**: *What key features would you incorporate in a blood pressure monitor aimed at early detection of preeclampsia in expectant mothers?*

Case Study 6: Blood Pressure Monitoring in Remote Villages with No Internet

**Scenario**: A non-profit organization aims to supply blood pressure monitors to rural communities without stable electricity or internet access.
**Challenge**:

- Power-independent operation (solar, hand-crank?)
- Manual recording and safe data storage
- Durable, low-maintenance design

**Student Question**: *How would you design a blood pressure monitoring solution for remote areas lacking reliable power and internet connectivity?*

Case Study 7: Continuous Blood Pressure Monitoring for Sleep Studies

**Scenario**: Researchers want to monitor blood pressure continuously during sleep to study sleep apnea and nocturnal hypertension.
**Challenge**:

- Non-intrusive and comfortable overnight monitoring
- Accurate readings without waking the patient
- Long battery life

**Student Question**: *What design features are essential for a noninvasive, continuous blood pressure monitor that patients can comfortably wear during sleep studies?*

Case Study 8: Smartwatch with Blood Pressure and ECG Integration

**Scenario**: A tech company is launching a smartwatch to monitor blood pressure and ECG.
**Challenge**:

- Accuracy across a variety of wrist sizes and skin tones
- Balancing multiple sensor types without overwhelming users
- FDA approval for medical-grade claims

**Student Question**: *What engineering and regulatory challenges must be addressed when combining blood pressure and ECG monitoring into a wearable device?*

Case Study 9: Pediatric Blood Pressure Monitoring

**Scenario**: A hospital needs blood pressure monitors designed for children of various ages and sizes.
**Challenge**:

- Different cuff sizes for different ages
- Ensuring minimal discomfort and quick readings
- Pediatric-specific calibration

**Student Question**: *How would you adapt blood pressure monitoring technology to accommodate the unique physiological needs of pediatric patients?*

Case Study 10: Blood Pressure Data Management with AI Prediction

**Scenario**: An insurance company proposes using AI to predict hypertension risks based on trends from wearable BP monitors.
**Challenge**:

- Large-scale data collection and privacy concerns
- Ensuring predictive algorithms are unbiased
- Avoiding over-reliance on predictions over clinical judgment

**Student Question**: *What ethical, technical, and clinical factors should be considered when using AI-driven predictions based on continuous blood pressure monitoring data?*

### *5.1.10 Patient Monitors*

10.1. Which of the following is NOT a standard parameter a patient monitor measures?

(a) Blood pressure
(b) Oxygen saturation
(c) Blood sugar
(d) Heart rate

10.2. Which component converts biological signals into electrical signals in a patient monitor?

(a) Microprocessor
(b) Filter
(c) Transducer
(d) Actuator

10.3. Telemetry monitors are primarily used for:

(a) Invasive blood pressure monitoring
(b) Short-term surgical use
(c) Wireless patient monitoring
(d) Transport of patients

10.4. What is the primary function of the Analog-to-Digital Converter (ADC) in a patient monitor?

(a) Amplify signals
(b) Filter signals
(c) Convert digital to analog
(d) Convert analog to digital

10.5. The process of patient monitoring is mainly used in:

(a) Laboratories
(b) Waiting rooms
(c) Intensive care units
(d) Cafeterias

10.6. What is the typical sampling rate for ECG signals to avoid distortion?

(a) 25 Hz
(b) 50 Hz
(c) 100 Hz
(d) 500 Hz

10.7. Which parameter is typically measured using a light-emitting diode and a light sensor?

(a) Blood pressure
(b) $SpO_2$
(c) Respiration
(d) ECG

10.8. Which part of the system triggers alarms in a patient monitor?

(a) Display module
(b) Battery system
(c) Microprocessor
(d) AC power supply

10.9. What is the primary purpose of the information monitor at the bedside?

(a) Power backup
(b) Alarm control
(c) Access and display patient data
(d) Ventilator control

10.10. Which type of monitoring system allows seamless transition during patient transport?

(a) Telemetry monitor
(b) Stand-alone monitor
(c) Integrated acute medical system
(d) Compact monitor

10.11. The term ________________ describes continuous measurement of vital signs and organ functions.

10.12. The device that converts biological signals to electrical signals is called a ________________.

10.13. In the ICU, bedside monitors are used to collect and display ________________ signals.

10.14. The ECG measures electrical activity from the ____________.

10.15. $SpO_2$ is a measure of blood _______________ saturation.

10.16. A 10-bit ADC can detect ________ discrete analog levels.

10.17. The component responsible for processing data in the monitor is the ____________________.

10.18. ________________ monitors allow mobility and wireless data transmission.

10.19. The display unit shows physiological parameters in the form of _______________ and values.
10.20. Sampling ECG at 25 Hz can result in _____________ distortion.
10.21. Identify the number of measurement modules in a patient monitor display and list their measured values.
10.22. Given an 8-bit ADC with a 0–5 V range, calculate the analog voltage for a digital output of 11001011.
10.23. Draw a block diagram of a modern patient monitor, including key signal flow components.
10.24. Mark the P wave, QRS complex, and T wave in a patient monitor's ECG waveform.
10.25. Determine the number of discrete levels for a 12-bit ADC.
10.26. Calculate the ADC output value for a 3.3 V input signal using a 10-bit ADC with 0–10 V range.
10.27. Write down a use case where the patient monitor's battery backup system is critical.
10.28. Design a simple user interface mock-up for a patient monitor that displays ECG, $SpO_2$, heart rate, and NIBP readings. Label key features such as alarm indicators, waveform display areas, and numerical readouts.

**Case Studies**

Case Study 1: Portable Multi-Parameter Patient Monitors for Ambulances

**Scenario**: Emergency medical services adopt portable monitors to track ECG, blood pressure, $SpO_2$, and respiration in ambulances.
**Challenge**:

- Reliability during transport and vibrations
- Long battery life
- Fast and simple user interface

**Student Question**: *How would you design a rugged, reliable multi-parameter patient monitor suitable for use during ambulance transport?*

Case Study 2: Wireless ICU Patient Monitoring

**Scenario**: An ICU upgrades to a wireless patient monitoring system to reduce cable clutter and improve mobility.
**Challenge**:

- Ensuring secure, stable wireless data transmission
- Preventing interference from other hospital equipment
- Maintaining real-time vital sign updates

**Student Question**: *What technical and safety considerations would you prioritize when developing a wireless patient monitoring system for an ICU?*

Case Study 3: Wearable Monitors for Post-Surgery Recovery

**Scenario**: Hospitals begin using wearable patches that continuously monitor heart rate, oxygen levels, and body temperature after surgery.
**Challenge**:

- Ensuring accuracy despite patient movement
- Comfort for long-term wear
- Managing wireless data and alerts

**Student Question**: *How would you design a wearable patient monitoring patch that maintains comfort and accuracy during recovery?*

Case Study 4: Remote Patient Monitoring at Home

**Scenario**: Clinics deploy remote monitoring kits for chronic patients to measure vital signs (heart rate, blood pressure, temperature) at home.
**Challenge**:

- Device usability for non-technical users
- Secure remote data transmission
- Alerting doctors only for meaningful events

**Student Question**: *How would you optimize a remote patient monitoring system to ensure reliability, data security, and patient adherence at home?*

Case Study 5: Continuous Neonatal Monitoring in NICU

**Scenario**: A neonatal ICU (NICU) installs advanced monitors to continuously track preemies' heart rate, $SpO_2$, temperature, and respiratory rates.
**Challenge**:

- Non-invasive, gentle sensors for fragile newborns
- Reducing false alarms
- Continuous, highly sensitive monitoring

**Student Question**: *What special considerations are needed when designing continuous monitoring systems for fragile neonatal patients?*

Case Study 6: Patient Monitoring in Disaster Zones

**Scenario**: Relief organizations deploy lightweight, battery-powered patient monitors in natural disaster zones.
**Challenge**:

- Durability under extreme conditions
- Offline functionality (no internet)
- Fast deployment and easy training

**Student Question**: *What features would you prioritize for a patient monitor designed for emergency use in disaster zones?*

Case Study 7: AI-Based Early Warning Systems for Patient Deterioration

**Scenario**: A hospital implements AI software that analyzes vital signs to predict and alert for early signs of patient deterioration.
**Challenge**:

- Ensuring the AI model's accuracy across different patient populations
- Avoiding alarm fatigue among staff
- Integrating predictions into the workflow

**Student Question**: *How would you design an AI-supported patient monitoring system that helps detect patient deterioration without overwhelming clinical staff?*

Case Study 8: Low-Cost Vital Signs Monitor for Rural Clinics

**Scenario**: An NGO develops an ultra-low-cost vital signs monitor (heart rate, blood pressure, oxygen) for rural healthcare workers.
**Challenge**:

- Keeping costs low while maintaining accuracy
- Training minimally skilled users
- Durability in harsh environments

**Student Question**: *What compromises and innovations would you propose to create a low-cost vital signs monitor for resource-limited settings?*

Case Study 9: Integration of Monitoring Data into Electronic Health Records (EHRs)

**Scenario**: Hospitals want to automatically integrate real-time patient monitoring data into EHR systems.
**Challenge**:

- Standardizing data formats
- Ensuring data privacy and security
- Avoiding system overload

**Student Question**: *What are the technical and privacy challenges when integrating real-time patient monitoring data into electronic health records?*

Case Study 10: Patient Monitoring for Space Missions

**Scenario**: NASA develops a remote patient monitoring system for astronauts on long space missions.
**Challenge**:

- Ultra-reliability in harsh conditions
- Compact, multi-parameter monitoring
- Minimal maintenance and calibration

**Student Question**: *How would you design a patient monitoring system suitable for extreme environments like space missions?*

### *5.1.11 Mechanical Ventilators*

11.1. What is the primary function of a mechanical ventilator?

(a) Humidify the air
(b) Perform dialysis
(c) Assist or replace spontaneous breathing
(d) Monitor brain activity

11.2. Which of the following gases is commonly used in mechanical ventilation?

(a) Helium
(b) Nitrous Oxide
(c) Oxygen
(d) Methane

11.3. What is PEEP used for in ventilators?

(a) Increase heart rate
(b) Prevent alveolar collapse
(c) Remove $CO_2$
(d) Humidify gas

11.4. Where is the expiratory valve typically located in a dual-hose system?

(a) Near the ventilator
(b) Near the humidifier

(c) Near the patient
(d) In the oxygen tank

11.5. Which component heats and humidifies the breathing gas?

(a) Gas mixer
(b) Pressure generator
(c) Breathing circuit
(d) Gas humidifier

11.6. Which mode allows both mandatory and spontaneous breaths?

(a) Volume-controlled ventilation
(b) Pressure-controlled ventilation
(c) SIMV
(d) CPAP

11.7. What is the typical expiratory time in PC-APRV?

(a) 2 seconds
(b) 0.5 seconds
(c) 5 seconds
(d) 3 seconds

11.8. What does the AutoFlow function optimize?

(a) Oxygen purity
(b) Gas scavenging
(c) Tidal volume at the lowest pressure
(d) Alarm sensitivity

11.9. What kind of ventilator is ideal for neonates due to constant gas flow?

(a) Demand flow
(b) Continuous flow
(c) Hybrid flow
(d) Jet ventilation

11.10. What happens in pressure-cycled ventilation?

(a) Volume remains constant
(b) Expiration is patient-triggered
(c) Inspiration ends at target pressure
(d) Flow is irrelevant

11.11. __________ is the pressure remaining in the lungs at the end of expiration.
11.12. A ____________________ is used to warm and moisten inhaled gases.
11.13. Volume-controlled ventilation maintains constant ______________ delivery.
11.14. ____________ is the pressure set in pressure-controlled modes.

11.15. ________________________ support changes pressure based on the patient's effort.
11.16. PC-APRV is known for its brief ______________________________ ____ phase.
11.17. The ______________________ valve controls gas exit during exhalation.
11.18. In CPAP, the patient must have an intact _______________________ drive.
11.19. ______________________ ventilators do not rely on compressed air but use turbines.
11.20. The breathing circuit used in emergency care often has a ________________ configuration.

**Case Studies**

Case Study 1: Portable Ventilators for Ambulances

**Scenario**: Emergency teams need lightweight, portable ventilators that can be quickly deployed in ambulances during trauma cases.
**Challenge**:

- Compact size and rugged design
- Reliable battery life
- Simple and fast setup in emergencies

**Student Question**: *How would you design a portable ventilator that balances lightweight mobility, robustness, and reliable emergency performance in ambulances?*

Case Study 2: Ventilator Sharing During Resource Shortages

**Scenario**: Hospitals consider ventilator sharing (using one ventilator for two patients) during critical shortages, like pandemics.
**Challenge**:

- Individualized control for each patient
- Preventing cross-contamination
- Managing different lung compliances

**Student Question**: *Should ventilators be adapted for multiple-patient use during crises, and what technical and ethical issues must be addressed?*

Case Study 3: Home Use Ventilators for Chronic Respiratory Diseases

**Scenario**: Patients with chronic respiratory diseases (like ALS or COPD) require ventilators that they can safely operate at home.
**Challenge**:

- User-friendly interface for patients and caregivers
- Remote monitoring capability
- Compact, quiet design

**Student Question**: *What features are most critical when designing ventilators for long-term home use by patients with chronic illnesses?*

Case Study 4: Ventilators for Neonatal ICU (NICU) Use

**Scenario**: NICUs require highly sensitive ventilators that deliver precise, gentle breaths to premature infants.
**Challenge**:

- Extremely low tidal volumes without causing lung damage
- Accurate synchronization with infant breathing efforts
- Minimal noise and invasiveness

**Student Question**: *What design adaptations are necessary to create ventilators suitable for fragile newborns in neonatal intensive care units?*

Case Study 5: Ventilator Design for Low-Resource Settings

**Scenario**: A non-profit designs simple, cost-effective ventilators for rural hospitals with unstable power supplies.
**Challenge**:

- Manual backup (hand-pumpable) options
- Simple mechanical designs (e.g., no need for compressed air)
- Easy maintenance

**Student Question**: *How would you design a low-cost, power-independent ventilator that is easy to maintain and use in remote and low-resource hospitals?*

Case Study 6: AI-Driven Smart Ventilator Systems

**Scenario**: A hospital installs ventilators with AI that auto-adjust settings based on real-time patient data (lung compliance, blood gases).
**Challenge**:

- AI reliability and explainability
- Avoiding over-reliance on automation
- Clinician override features

**Student Question**: *How can AI be safely integrated into ventilators to optimize respiratory care while maintaining human clinician control and patient safety?*

Case Study 7: Emergency DIY Ventilators During a Pandemic

**Scenario**: Engineers and universities collaborate to build DIY ventilators quickly during a sudden pandemic ventilator shortage.
**Challenge**:

- Basic life-support capability vs. sophisticated features
- Meeting emergency-use regulatory standards
- Safe, rapid deployment

**Student Question**: *In a crisis, how should emergency ventilators be designed to balance production speed, safety, and essential functionality?*

Case Study 8: Long-Term Ventilation in Rehabilitation Centers

**Scenario**: Rehabilitation centers use ventilators for patients recovering from severe lung injury or neurological damage.
**Challenge**:

- Supporting partial or gradually improving lung function
- Patient-ventilator weaning protocols
- Ensuring mobility and comfort

**Student Question**: *What features would you prioritize in ventilators for long-term recovery and rehabilitation use?*

Case Study 9: Noise Reduction in Ventilators for ICU Settings

**Scenario**: ICUs aim to reduce ventilator noise levels to improve patient comfort and sleep quality.
**Challenge**:

- Noise from airflow and compressors
- Maintaining performance while reducing sound
- Impact of noise on staff and patients

**Student Question**: *How could you redesign ventilators to operate more quietly in ICUs while maintaining optimal ventilation performance?*

Case Study 10: Ventilator Integration with Hospital Information Systems

**Scenario**: Modern hospitals seek to integrate ventilator data (flow rates, pressures, alarms) directly into patient electronic health records (EHRs).
**Challenge**:

- Standardized data formats and communication protocols
- Real-time secure transmission
- Avoiding information overload for clinicians

**Student Question**: *What technical and security considerations must be considered when integrating ventilator monitoring data into hospital EHR systems?*

### *5.1.12 Anesthesia Machines*

12.1. What is the primary function of a vaporizer in an anesthesia machine?

(a) Regulate pressure
(b) Remove $CO_2$
(c) Deliver volatile anesthetics
(d) Filter oxygen

12.2. What prevents hypoxia in case of oxygen failure?

(a) Vaporizer
(b) Hypoxic guard
(c) Capnograph
(d) Gas scavenger

12.3. Which gas is **not** commonly used in anesthesia machines?

(a) Oxygen
(b) Nitrous Oxide
(c) Helium
(d) Air

12.4. What kind of ventilator uses compressed gases to function?

(a) Pneumatic
(b) Electric
(c) Manual
(d) Dual-mode

12.5. Which circuit allows for rebreathing of gases after $CO_2$ removal?

(a) Mapleson
(b) Circle system
(c) Open system
(d) Semi-open system

12.6. What system is used to remove excess anesthetic gases?

(a) Vaporizer
(b) Breathing circuit
(c) Scavenging system

(d) $O_2$ flush valve

12.7. What monitors end-tidal $CO_2$?

(a) Pulse oximeter
(b) Capnograph
(c) Flowmeter
(d) Vaporizer

12.8. What is the typical unit for oxygen supply pressure in anesthesia machines?

(a) 50 mmHg
(b) 345 kPa
(c) 2 atm
(d) 100 psi

12.9. What does the oxygen fail-safe system do?

(a) Increase nitrous oxide delivery
(b) Shut off $N_2O$ if oxygen pressure is low
(c) Ventilate the patient automatically

12.10. What is a component of the scavenging system?

(a) Reservoir bag
(b) Check valve
(c) Expiratory limb
(d) Vacuum line

12.11. The ____________ system delivers gases to the anesthesia machine.
12.12. The gas flow is controlled using ______________.
12.13. __________________ convert liquid anesthetics to vapor.
12.14. ____________________ ventilation is when the machine delivers a fixed pressure.
12.15. The __________________ circuit allows rebreathing with $CO_2$ absorption.
12.16. Capnographs measure _______ in exhaled air.
12.17. _______________ alarms alert for low oxygen or pressure changes.
12.18. Hypoxic guard maintains a minimum ____________ concentration.
12.19. __________________ safety valves stop gas flow in case of failure.
12.20. A __________________ system removes anesthetic waste gases from the OR.

## Case Studies

Case Study 1: Portable Anesthesia Machines for Field Hospitals

**Scenario**: A humanitarian organization needs portable anesthesia machines for emergency surgeries in field hospitals.
**Challenge**:

- Compact, lightweight design
- Operation with limited oxygen supply
- Durability in harsh environments

**Student Question**: *How would you design a portable anesthesia machine that ensures safe anesthesia delivery in low-resource, emergency settings?*

Case Study 2: Low-Flow Anesthesia for Environmental Sustainability

**Scenario**: A hospital aims to implement low-flow anesthesia techniques to reduce environmental impact and gas waste.
**Challenge**:

- Precise control of anesthetic agent concentration
- Monitoring inspired and expired gas volumes
- Training staff in low-flow techniques

**Student Question**: *What technical features should be prioritized when designing anesthesia machines for safe and efficient low-flow anesthesia practices?*

Case Study 3: Integration of Anesthesia Machine Data into EHRs

**Scenario**: A hospital upgrades anesthesia machines to directly feed real-time anesthesia and vital data into the electronic health record (EHR) system.
**Challenge**:

- Real-time secure data transmission
- Standardization across devices
- Avoiding clinician information overload

**Student Question**: *How would you design a system to securely and efficiently integrate anesthesia machine data into a hospital's EHR?*

Case Study 4: Closed-Loop Anesthesia Systems with AI

**Scenario**: Using AI algorithms, researchers develop anesthesia machines that automatically adjust anesthetic delivery based on patient monitoring data.
**Challenge**:

- Maintaining patient safety with automation
- Transparency and override capability for anesthetists
- Managing unexpected patient reactions

**Student Question**: *Should anesthesia delivery be automated with AI systems, and how would you ensure that safety, transparency, and clinician control are maintained?*

Case Study 5: Anesthesia Machines for Pediatric Patients

**Scenario**: Hospitals require specialized anesthesia machines tailored for newborns and young children.
**Challenge**:

- Precise delivery of tiny gas volumes
- Sensitive monitoring of pediatric physiology
- Minimizing risks of overdose

**Student Question**: *What special features are necessary in anesthesia machines to safely manage anesthesia for neonates and pediatric patients?*

Case Study 6: Emergency Manual Mode in Anesthesia Machines

**Scenario**: Anesthesia machines must be able to operate manually if there is an electronic system failure during surgery.
**Challenge**:

- Quick switch to manual mode
- Mechanical reliability without digital controls
- Easy usability under stressful conditions

**Student Question**: *How would you design an emergency manual mode for anesthesia machines to ensure uninterrupted anesthesia delivery during system failures?*

Case Study 7: Low-Cost Anesthesia Machines for Rural Clinics

**Scenario**: A non-profit designs simple anesthesia machines for rural clinics that cannot afford advanced machines.
**Challenge**:

- Minimize complexity and cost
- Ensure safe delivery without relying on compressed gases
- Easy cleaning and maintenance

**Student Question**: *How would you design a low-cost, safe, and maintainable anesthesia machine for clinics in rural or low-income settings?*

Case Study 8: Anesthesia Machines with Integrated Ventilators

**Scenario**: Newer anesthesia machines integrate advanced ventilators for patient support during surgery.
**Challenge**:

- Coordinating anesthesia delivery with ventilation modes
- Ensuring synchronized control between anesthesia and ventilation
- Managing alarms for multiple systems simultaneously

**Student Question**: *What challenges arise when integrating ventilation systems into anesthesia machines, and how would you ensure safe and synchronized operation during surgeries?*

Case Study 9: Minimizing Human Error in Anesthesia Machine Use

**Scenario**: Human factors engineers are asked to redesign anesthesia machine interfaces to reduce the likelihood of user errors.
**Challenge**:

- Simplifying controls and displays
- Prioritizing critical information
- Designing intuitive alarm systems

**Student Question**: *What design improvements would you suggest to anesthesia machines to minimize the risk of human error during surgeries?*

Case Study 10: Anesthesia Monitoring for Outpatient Surgery Centers

**Scenario**: Outpatient surgery centers require anesthesia machines optimized for short procedures and fast recovery.
**Challenge**:

- Rapid induction and emergence capabilities
- Efficient scavenging of anesthetic gases
- Compact designs for smaller operating rooms

**Student Question**: *What design elements would be most important for anesthesia machines explicitly used in outpatient surgery centers where speed and efficiency are critical?*

### *5.1.13 Pacemakers and Defibrillators*

13.1. What is the primary purpose of a defibrillator?

(a) Monitor ECG
(b) Stimulate muscle contractions
(c) Deliver an electrical shock to restore normal heart rhythm
(d) Measure oxygen levels

13.2. Which rhythm requires immediate defibrillation?

(a) Atrial flutter
(b) Bradycardia
(c) Ventricular fibrillation
(d) Sinus arrhythmia

13.3. Which waveform is commonly used in modern AEDs?

(a) Monophasic
(b) Trapezoidal
(c) Biphasic
(d) Sinusoidal

13.4. What does AED stand for?

(a) Automated Electric Defibrillator
(b) Adult Emergency Device
(c) Automated External Defibrillator
(d) Automatic Extrinsic Defibrillator

13.5. What do biphasic defibrillators deliver the typical energy range?

(a) 20–100 J
(b) 150–200 J
(c) 300–400 J
(d) 500–600 J

13.6. What component stores energy in a defibrillator?

(a) Resistor
(b) Diode
(c) Capacitor
(d) Inductor

13.7. Which of the following factors increases thoracic impedance?

(a) Larger electrode area
(b) Wet skin
(c) Small electrode surface
(d) Using gel pads

13.8. What is the synchronization feature used for?

(a) Charging the capacitor faster
(b) Reducing patient movement
(c) Ensuring the shock is applied during the QRS complex

(d) Displaying the ECG

13.9. Which type of defibrillator is implanted inside the body?

(a) AED
(b) Manual defibrillator
(c) ICD
(d) CRT

13.10. What is the main risk of applying a shock during the T wave?

(a) Syncope
(b) Bradycardia
(c) Ventricular fibrillation
(d) Hypertension

13.11. The capacitor stores energy in a defibrillator and releases it during a __________.
13.12. The waveform commonly used in modern defibrillators is __________.
13.13. Thoracic impedance typically ranges from __________ to __________ ohms.
13.14. The electrical shock delivered by a defibrillator is measured in __________.
13.15. Defibrillation is most effective when applied within __________ minutes of cardiac arrest.
13.16. AEDs are designed to be used by individuals with minimal ____________.
13.17. The ________________ electrode method is preferred for arrhythmia therapy in emergencies.
13.18. A pacemaker that coordinates signals between ventricles is called a __________ device.
13.19. Implantable defibrillators provide therapy via antitachycardia pacing, cardioversion, and _______________.
13.20. A ______________ shock is applied without synchronization to the ECG.
13.21. Draw and label the circuit of an RCL defibrillator with patient resistance.
13.22. Derive the differential equations for capacitor charging and discharging in a defibrillator.
13.23. Calculate the capacitor value required for a 4 ms discharge time with 50 Ω patient resistance.
13.24. Compute the resistor value that receives $2 \times 10^5$ J from a 0.9 V battery over 4 h.
13.25. A defibrillator passes 16 A for 1.6 ms—calculate the charge and the number of electrons transferred
13.26. A 20 μF capacitor charged to 4 kV—compute stored charge, energy, and average current/power for 2 ms discharge.
13.27. Sketch the strength–duration curve; mark rheobase and chronaxy.
13.28. For a 15 V and 80 μF AED capacitor, calculate the charge and the resistor for a 3 s charge time.
13.29. Draw and identify defibrillator waveforms—trapezoidal, biphasic, damped sine.

13.30. Simulate the discharge curve of a capacitor into a 50 Ω patient and annotate major features.

## Case Studies

Case Study 1: Leadless Pacemaker Design

**Scenario**: A company develops a leadless pacemaker that sits entirely inside the heart, eliminating traditional lead wires.
**Challenge**:

- Miniaturization without losing battery life
- Secure fixation inside the heart tissue
- Safe retrieval or replacement if needed

**Student Question**: *What design strategies would you propose to ensure long-term reliability and safety for leadless pacemakers?*

Case Study 2: MRI-Compatible Pacemakers

**Scenario**: A hospital mandates that all new pacemaker implants must be safe for patients undergoing MRI scans.
**Challenge**:

- Preventing device heating during MRI
- Avoiding interference with MRI signals
- Maintaining pacing functionality during imaging

**Student Question**: *How would you modify pacemaker designs to ensure complete safety and compatibility with MRI procedures?*

Case Study 3: Wearable External Defibrillators for High-Risk Patients

**Scenario**: Patients at high risk for sudden cardiac arrest are given wearable defibrillator vests before receiving an implantable device.
**Challenge**:

- Ensuring comfort for long-term daily wear
- Reliable detection of dangerous arrhythmias
- Automatic but safe shock delivery

**Student Question**: *What technical and human-centered features would you prioritize when designing a wearable external defibrillator?*

Case Study 4: Battery Life Management in Implantable Devices

**Scenario**: Patients often require surgical replacement of pacemakers and defibrillators when batteries deplete.
**Challenge**:

- Extending battery life without increasing size
- Wireless energy harvesting possibilities
- Early low-battery detection alerts

**Student Question**: *What strategies would you implement to maximize battery longevity and minimize surgical interventions in pacemakers and defibrillators?*

Case Study 5: Pediatric Pacemaker Challenges

**Scenario**: Children with congenital heart defects require pacemakers that can adapt as they grow.
**Challenge**:

- Adjusting pacing thresholds over time
- Minimizing device size for smaller bodies
- Enabling minimally invasive upgrades

**Student Question**: *How would you adapt pacemaker technology to meet pediatric patients' unique physiological and developmental needs?*

Case Study 6: Remote Monitoring of Pacemakers and ICDs

**Scenario**: Hospitals implement remote monitoring systems for patients with implanted cardiac devices.
**Challenge**:

- Secure and reliable wireless data transmission
- Real-time detection of device malfunctions
- Patient-friendly monitoring equipment

**Student Question**: *What technical and privacy challenges must be addressed to implement remote monitoring for pacemakers and defibrillators successfully?*

Case Study 7: Dual-Chamber Pacemakers for Complex Arrhythmias

**Scenario**: Patients with atrial and ventricular rhythm disorders require dual-chamber pacing devices.
**Challenge**:

- Coordinating the timing between chambers accurately
- Avoiding unnecessary pacing to conserve battery
- Managing device settings remotely

**Student Question**: *What innovations could improve synchronization and efficiency in dual-chamber pacemaker systems?*

Case Study 8: Public Access Defibrillators (AEDs) in Smart Cities

**Scenario**: Cities deploy smart AEDs (automated external defibrillators) that alert emergency services automatically upon use.
**Challenge**:

- Ensuring AEDs are accessible, functional, and easy to use
- Enabling real-time geolocation tracking
- Regular maintenance and status monitoring

**Student Question**: *How would you design a smart public AED system to maximize survival rates and integrate with emergency services?*

Case Study 9: Minimizing Post-Implantation Infections

**Scenario**: Patients undergoing pacemaker or ICD implantation sometimes develop site infections.
**Challenge**:

- Antimicrobial device coatings
- Minimally invasive implantation techniques
- Monitoring for early signs of infection

**Student Question**: *What measures can be taken during design and implantation to reduce infection risk for pacemakers and defibrillators?*

Case Study 10: Ethical Issues in Implantable Defibrillator Deactivation

**Scenario**: Terminally ill patients sometimes wish to deactivate their implantable cardioverter-defibrillators (ICDs) to avoid unnecessary shocks.
**Challenge**:

- Clear patient consent processes
- Programming safe deactivation protocols
- Supporting ethical and legal frameworks

**Student Question**: *How should medical teams approach the technical and ethical challenges of deactivating ICDs at a patient's request?*

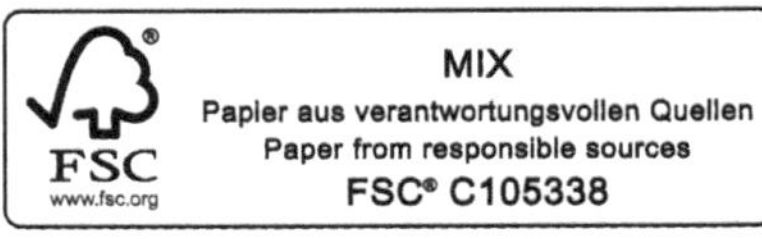


If you have any concerns about our products,
you can contact us on
**ProductSafety@springernature.com**

In case Publisher is established outside the EU,
the EU authorized representative is:
**Springer Nature Customer Service Center GmbH**
**Europaplatz 3, 69115 Heidelberg, Germany**

Printed by Libri Plureos GmbH
in Hamburg, Germany